Essential Revision Notes for the FRCS (Urol)

2nd edition

Jack Donati-Bourne

Volume 1

Foreword by
Keith Yeates Gold Medal Winners
Rachel Barratt and Sotonye Tolofari

First published in 2025 by Libri Publishing

ISBN 978-1-911451-36-5

Cover and Design by Carnegie Publishing

Libri Publishing
Brunel House
Volunteer Way
Faringdon
Oxfordshire
SN7 7YR

Tel: +44 (0)845 873 3837

www.libripublishing.co.uk

CONTENTS

DEDICATION

This book is dedicated to Zakariya, my beautiful precious boy.

ABOUT THE AUTHOR AND CONTRIBUTOR

Jack Donati-Bourne works as a Consultant Urological Surgeon in Sandwell and West Birmingham Hospitals NHS Trust. He qualified in medicine (2010) and then obtained a Master's degree in anatomy (2013), both at the University of Birmingham, proceeding subsequently to complete Membership (2013) and Fellowship (2019) of the Royal College of Surgeons of England.

He has published 20 articles in peer-reviewed journals and his work has been presented in eight different countries. The first edition of the *Essential Revision Notes for the FRCS (Urol)* textbook was sold across the world.

Jack has a passion for the NHS and teaching, aiming to support and inspire trainees along the way, which was the driving force behind the production of the textbooks.

Fiona McCaig is a Consultant Urological and Renal Transplant Surgeon at the Royal Free Hospital in London. She graduated from Edinburgh University in 2001 and was subsequently awarded a Doctorate of Medicine before completing her surgical training. Fiona completed fellowships in London and Paris in renal transplantation and has a passion for everything related to transplant urology.

FOREWORD

I had sat through three years of high-class urology teaching and yet, as I approached my exam year, I realised I had no clue where or how to start my revision for the FRCS (Urol) exam. I started making notes – scraping information from any source I could find – followed by a mad month of cramming at the end. Sadly, I sat my FRCS (Urol) at the same time as Jack Donati-Bourne and didn't have the fortune to have a textbook that gave me such a solid foundation from which to start my revision. So, congratulations – if you are reading this then you are already a step ahead. Whilst I also advise writing additional notes yourself, this book will allow you to really focus your time on assimilating and understanding the information.

Revision for Part 1 is, to put it mildly, dull, lonely and life consuming. Everyone has their own way of revising for written exams. I spent three months writing notes (a job this book makes easier for you!) with a revision timetable roughly split to give more time to larger topics and less to shorter topics or those with which I was already more familiar. I am a planner by nature but, for this exam, I would recommend some sort of timetable, no matter how approximate. And as everyone will tell you, Part 1 is a marathon not a sprint. Allow plenty of time. I planned to start revision in July (for a Part 1 exam in January) and, after a few false starts, finally got going in mid-September.

Everyone revises differently but here are my top three tips:

1. Delete social media – you will find there are plenty enough (more worthwhile – see point 3) things to do with any free moments. It's just not worth wasting that time checking Instagram.

2. Mix up the type of revision – I am primarily someone who learns by reading but I realised that I would need variety in order to maintain the revision momentum. I made notes (they are also useful to use for Part 2 later) and in between times practised questions. There are lots of question banks available but it's worth noting that none are specific to the FRCS (Urol). However, they can be useful in small measure for practising the art of answering an MCQ.

3. Take breaks – if you haven't quite left yourself enough time to cover everything then this might just be a short walk with a podcast, a quick gym session or a good TV show (but don't pick anything too addictive!). If you have planned well then make sure to make time for date night with your partner, a trip to the park with the kids or coffee with a friend and, if possible, have days with no or minimal revision.

Once you've sat in your (typically driving) test centre and passed your Part 1 there is often little time to turn around and prepare for Part 2 (unless you are planning a break or we hit another global pandemic that delays exams). Part 2 can be approached as more of a middle-distance race – eight weeks should be plenty of time (if you are attending the BAUS FRCS course then this is normally a reasonable time to start the big last push to the revision finish line). Take a decent break from the books and, if you can, go on holiday before starting revision again for Part 2.

The viva is about using the information you have from Part 1 and making sensible day-one urology consultant decisions. That's not to say that these are straightforward decisions – and the scenarios sometimes seem so improbable and uncommon that it's almost laughable. You wonder when you might actually need to know about emphysematous pyelonephritis or transuretero-ureterostomy, but trust me – I managed to encounter all 16 tables' worth of bizarre FRCS (Urol) scenarios during my first consultant on-call and have never been more grateful that I had sat the exam.

Revision for Part 2 is simple: practise, practise, practise (with a little bit of note revision and guideline reading – assuming you haven't immediately forgotten all of your Part 1 knowledge). Get a viva group together – aim for no more than three or four people at a time, but these can be drawn from a wider group. Aim to practise as often as you can – you can learn both from your own vivas as well as from vivaing others and observing others being viva'd, so make sure you make the most of every opportunity. Of course, work is like a perpetual FRCS exam: treat it as such, and make the most of the consultants and more senior trainees – say yes to any offer to be viva'd (no matter how embarrassing) and don't be afraid to ask for viva practice either. Courses are good but expensive in the main – if you can attend one this will help but don't feel like you must attend all of them.

Top three tips for the viva:

1. Listen to the question – if the question asks "how would you *manage* this patient" do not start talking about history/examination – the examiner wants to start straight with the first rung of the management ladder.

2. Try to learn history/exam/initial-investigation patter for key conditions of each table – this doesn't work all the time (for example, some scenarios start halfway through and technology is often just rapid-fire questions) but for most vivas it will give you a minute at the beginning of the station to recall the relevant information you need for the onward scenario, making the next nine minutes a bit easier.

3. Papers – there is no need to quote these ad nauseam. They need to be relevant and ideally only used to validate your decision making on more complex questions. Finally, only quote it if you really know it – examiners will rightly quiz you on it if you mention a paper. Save for a few key papers (mainly BPH and Oncology), knowledge of papers is not necessary to pass the FRCS.

People say you should enjoy the FRCS (Urol) viva, and if you do then congratulations – I didn't particularly. But preparing for this exam gives you the final pieces of the toolkit you will need for the rest of your consultant career – in a slightly perverse way, we should all be grateful for it. I wish you all good luck. Remember, "by failing to prepare, you prepare to fail" – so stop reading this and get reading the book!

Rachel Barratt

Keath Yeates Gold Medal Winner 2019
Consultant Urologist
UCLH

FOREWORD

I remember it like it was yesterday, that nauseating feeling of impending doom when I walked into the FRCS (Urol) examination hall to see what felt like an endless sea of examiners sat at tables, all eagerly awaiting to question me with varying degrees of intensity and ferocity. However, in hindsight, I've come to realise that in that brief moment of my career, I knew more about urology than I ever had done before or ever have done since. Arguably, the candidates sitting the FRCS (Urol) have a much wider depth of knowledge than many of the examiners, which is really quite an empowering feeling.

Now that you've opened this book, you have embarked on a journey that takes you to the end of your training career and the start of your consultant career. Inevitably, there are a mixture of feelings. For myself, there was nervous excitement at the thought of completing the final hurdle to commencing my consultant career. However, of course there was an overarching feeling of anxiety and fear: *"what if I fail?"*, *"who will employ me?"*, *"what are my next steps?"*. To reassure you, all of these thoughts and feelings are entirely normal for any candidate sitting any FRCS examination.

The FRCS (Urol) is an examination of two parts. The first is MCQ based, which requires the use of multiple resources. You can improve your pattern recognition by reviewing as many online or paper MCQs as you can find. Additionally, it's important to read well-known urology handbooks to ensure you have sufficient knowledge in common question themes, which include basic science, physiology, pharmacology, anatomy and urological nomenclature.

As I often say at the BAUS FRCS (Urol) viva course, my advice to all candidates for the second part of the FRCS (Urol) would be firstly to set up a viva group early with colleagues – ideally six-to-eight weeks before the exam. The magic number for your viva group is three, with one person to examine, one person to be the examinee and one person to give feedback. Secondly, get used to talking through scenarios, and practise, practise, practise. Unsurprisingly, the more you get used to talking through scenarios, the slicker and more polished you become. Never be too embarrassed to practise with people, no matter how good they say they are. Any experience is good experience. During the viva, always remember to take occasional pauses between your responses to allow time to gather your thoughts and invite the next question from the examiner. This way you can control the scenario and the pace of the examiner, which ultimately gives an impression of a confident and organised candidate. You will not know everything. If you don't know the answer on the day, don't be afraid to say "I'm afraid I can't recall" or "can I come back to that?". Again, this gives you control of the narrative and makes you appear relaxed and in control of the scenario (even though we know you'll be quaking in your boots under the table). Finally, never catastrophise; I can tell you now, you will more than likely have one "car crash" station where you feel you didn't represent yourself well. Compartmentalise this and move on. Each table is a new examiner who has no idea how your last station went, so you have a new opportunity to perform well.

Whilst the FRCS (Urol) is certainly a challenging and daunting experience, it is certainly a necessary rite of passage. You will find that you have developed more knowledge about the field of urology than you ever have done before. As a result, you will feel empowered and deserving of the coveted urology consultant appointment for which you have strived so hard for all these years.

Ultimately, this exam will be a nerve-racking experience. Try to remain calm, don't catastrophise and always ensure you are structured and safe in your responses. For what it's worth, try to enjoy the experience as much as you can, you will never know this much about urology ever again. One important thing to remember is that once you've completed the FRCS (Urol) the real challenge starts, which is actually convincing someone to give you a consultant job! Good luck and Godspeed.

Sotonye K. Tolofari BSc (Hons), MBChB, FRCS (Urol)

Keith Yeates Gold Medallist 2019
Consultant Urological Surgeon
Northern Care Alliance, Manchester

ACKNOWLEDGEMENTS

Compiling a more-than-600-page textbook is a rather time-consuming exercise, I have to say, and not straightforward to slot in between childcare and working as a full-time NHS consultant. Most of this textbook was written during night-time sessions between the hours of 10pm and 1am (or later). I therefore wish to apologise to everyone for having been more tired, strained and unsociable for the last six months.

I am indebted to Roger Amos and his team from Libri Publishing – without you this project would not have been possible, and you should be proud that you have had a key role in training future urologists around the world. Roger you are an absolute pleasure to work with and I hope we will collaborate on more projects together in the future.

I wish to thank Fiona McCaig for writing the renal transplantation chapter. I appreciate you trying to sketch a dialysis machine the day after recovering from a late-night operation on a bleeding transplant kidney! Your contribution is invaluable and a great addition to the textbook.

I am very grateful to Rachel Barratt and Sot Tolofari for their forewords – it was very kind of you to share your advice and memories of the exam, and I am honoured that you both agreed to contribute to the textbook.

Thank you to my friends and colleagues for supporting me during a difficult time.

Thank you Shamah for all your love, care and attention for our son.

Thank you Mum for literally everything I can think of.

Thank you Dad. Unfortunately you never got to see the textbooks – but if indeed I do have any writing skills I am pretty sure they came from you.

And finally, thank you to my son, Zakariya – my love for you has changed the whole way I live and view life since you came along. You are a beautiful shining star and I am proud of you every day.

INTRODUCTION

Dear colleague, thank you so much for choosing the second edition of *Essential Revision Notes for the FRCS (Urol)*. I sincerely hope it serves you as a valuable, helpful and trustworthy companion throughout the long odyssey that is the FRCS (Urol), and that ultimately the book supports you in passing the exam.

I wish to briefly share with you the story behind the first and second editions of my book, for some light-heartedness prior to hundreds of pages of facts and figures.

As I began to prepare and write my personal revision notes for the FRCS (Urol), within no more than a week the idea came to me that as (all being well) I would likely be sat at the same desk revising for the best part of seven months, I might as well construct and format my notes as I studied along the way such that by the end of the process I would have a manuscript ready for publication. By the end I even had it neatly printed, bound and laminated ready to present to a publishing company.

As it happened, the euphoria of passing the exam, then moving house and general life busyness resulted in the manuscript being put in a box (but fortunately not being lost in the house move) and in my heart I gave up on the idea of publishing it. Ultimately I was simply grateful that I had passed the exam.

When the COVID-19 pandemic struck, however, between self-isolation, lockdowns, support bubbles and erratic work rotas I found myself unexpectedly having extended periods of time at home. I found the box with the manuscript. I recall literally blowing dust off the top of it. I went about organising interviews with various publishers until Roger Amos and John Sivak from Libri Publishing saved the day – and the rest is history.

The tentative first-edition project proved to be more successful than we would have ever imagined and above all the feedback I got from colleagues was that they found my book handy for their revision and were grateful. (However, from a financial point of view I do not recommend becoming a writer of medical textbooks – stick to being a doctor!)

The fact that I knew I had helped people made the production of a second edition imperative.

The atmosphere in my mind when writing the second edition was different – this is because whilst producing the first edition we were expecting our son, Zakariya. I thus felt I had a race against time to complete as I presumed that, once he was born, I would barely have time to eat – and I was right. This time round therefore, as he was now more grown up, I thought I would have more free time and spare energy – but I was wrong. Parenting does not get any easier!

In order to ensure I would be providing as accurate, tidy, relevant and up-to-date information as possible to my colleagues, I committed to painstakingly reviewing every single word, line and punctuation mark you will find in the book. This took a *lot* longer than I had anticipated.

Not that I think I have quite reached a stage where I can compare myself to Leonardo da Vinci just yet; but the best comparison I can make of the contrast between the production of the two editions is with his painting of the Last Supper – about three years to paint it (first edition) and more than 21 years for its restoration (second edition).

So here I present to you, only eight months contractually late (sorry Roger), the completed second edition of *Essential Revision Notes for the FRCS (Urol)*.

There are many new features in this edition that I really hope you will find helpful:

- All information robustly fact-checked, with relevant NICE and EAU guidance up-to-date as of 2024
- More than 170 new sample MCQs
- Bonus chapter "Viva Tips & Tricks", where I share my advice having been faculty member on multiple different FRCS (Urol) revision courses over the years
- Bonus chapter "Renal Transplantation", which I wish to thank Fiona McCaig for writing, as I felt it more appropriate for an expert in the field to be entrusted to guide you with what you need to know on this topic
- Important scientific papers for you to be aware of and read up about are now highlighted with the symbol **KEY PAPER**, with 17 additional papers featuring in the book as well as those present in the first edition
- I share practical advice for the FRCS (Urol) viva section, which can be identified with the symbol **VIVA**, with 48 of these now featuring
- Errata corrige (thank you to those who contacted me highlighting any mistakes in the first edition)
- More consistent, succinct and fluent reading style.

As ever I recommend that you use this book as the roadmap/skeleton for your revision. You cannot pass the FRCS (Urol) using a single resource, however: you must complement this with other textbooks, courses and online material.

I am very grateful to Rachel Barratt and Sot Tolofari for their invaluable contributions to the book with their advice on how to master the FRCS (Urol) – as Gold Medal winners you really ought to follow their recommendations on that rather than mine.

I would, however, wish to briefly share with you my thoughts, memories and advice on the FRCS (Urol) journey.

It is a long expedition. Clear the mental deck if you can – by which I mean avoid taking the exam at the same time as major life events like getting married or moving house. Start revising early (I began three months before Section 1). Talk to as many colleagues as you can who have recently passed the exam to find common themes in how they did it and what resources they used. Do not cram – if someone tells you they successfully did that, it probably isn't true. Vary your revision to keep you engaged – you can read notes, watch videos, practise MCQs, use flash cards. For the viva section, it is all about practice – form a small revision group and commit to practising every evening if possible, from the moment after attending the BAUS FRCS (Urol) revision course.

Above all, try to enjoy it. This should be your last hurdle after having completed innumerable exams to reach the end of your surgical training, and arguably all the information you will learn and absorb during the FRCS (Urol) journey will be relevant to your future practice as a urologist. You will hopefully be interested to discover the evidence behind a lot of the practice you currently do (many trainees, like me before, mostly know what they should do but not *why* they do it) and you will hopefully enjoy the feeling of really finally *knowing your stuff*.

Having expertise to be able to help a sick patient in their time of need is truly a gift. This consideration galvanised me to master the FRCS (Urol) exam and continues to motivate me to keep improving my practice as a doctor every day, to learn more, do more, serve more and teach more. I hope this will inspire you.

I do wish you all the very best.

Jack Donati-Bourne

GLOSSARY OF ABBREVIATIONS

AAST – American Association for the Surgery of Trauma
ABU – anastomotic bulbar urethroplasty
ACEi – angiotensin converting enzyme inhibitor
ACR – albumin creatinine ratio
ACT – α1 anti-chymotrypsin
ACTH – adreno-corticotropic hormone
ADC – apparent diffusion coefficient
ADH – anti-diuretic hormone
ADT – androgen deprivation therapy
AFP – alpha feto-protein
AKI – acute kidney injury
ALP – alkaline phosphatase
ALPP – abdominal leak-point pressure
AMG – α2 macro globulin
AML – angiomyolipoma
AP – antero-posterior
APC – adenomatous polyposis coli
APD – antero-posterior diameter
APLS – Advanced Paediatric Life Support
ARR – absolute risk reduction
AS – active surveillance
ASAP – atypical small acinar proliferation
ATLS – Advanced Trauma Life Support
ATN – acute tubular necrosis
ATP – adenosine triphosphate
AUA – American Urology Association
AUR – acute urinary retention
AUS – artificial urethral sphincter
AVF – arterio-venous fistula
BAPU – British Association of Paediatric Urologists
BAUS – British Association of Urological Surgeons
BCG – Bacillus Calmette–Guerin
BCI – bladder contractility index
BHD – Birt–Hogg–Dubé
BMD – bone mineral density
BNF – British National Formulary
BNI – bladder neck incision
BOO – bladder outlet obstruction

BOOI – bladder outlet obstruction index
BPE – benign prostatic enlargement
BPH – benign prostatic hyperplasia
BPS – bladder pain syndrome
BTB – blood–testis barrier
BTx – brachytherapy
BXO – balanitis xerotica obliterans
CAH – congenital adrenal hyperplasia
CAIS – complete androgen insensitivity syndrome
CAP – continuous antibiotic prophylaxis
CAPD – continuous ambulatory peritoneal dialysis
CBAVD – congenital bilateral absence of vas deferens
CBP – chronic bacterial prostatitis
CCG – clinical commissioning group
CCI – Charlson Comorbidity Index
CCrISP – Care of the Critically Ill Surgical Patient
CF – cystic fibrosis
CFU – colony forming units
cGMP – cyclic guanosine monophosphate
CI – confidence interval
CIS – carcinoma in situ
CKD – chronic kidney disease
CMV – cytomegalovirus
CN – cytoreductive nephrectomy
CNS – central nervous system
COPD – chronic obstructive pulmonary disease
CPEX – cardio-pulmonary exercise testing
CPG – Cambridge prognostic group
CPPS – chronic pelvic pain syndrome
CRP – C-reactive protein
CRPC – castrate resistant prostate cancer
CSF – cerebrospinal fluid
CSS – cancer specific survival
CT – computed tomography
CT TAP – computed tomography of thorax abdomen and pelvis
CTU – computed tomography urogram
CVA – cerebrovascular accident
CVVH – continuous veno-venous haemofiltration
CXR – chest x-ray
DCE – dynamic contrast enhanced
DEXA – dual energy absorptiometry scan

DFS – disease-free survival
DHT – dihydrotestosterone
DLPP – detrusor leak-point pressure
DMSA – dimercaptosuccinic acid
DNA – deoxyribonucleic acid
DO – detrusor overactivity
DRE – digital rectal examination
DetSD – detrusor sphincter dyssynergia
DSD – differences in sex development
DSNB – dynamic sentinel node biopsy
DTPA – diethylene-triamine-pentaacetate
DVC – dorsal venous complex
DVT – deep-vein thrombosis
DWI-MRI – diffusion-weighted magnetic resonance imaging
EAU – European Association Urology
EBL – estimated blood loss
EBRT – external beam radiotherapy
ECG – electro-cardiogram
ECOG – Eastern Cooperative Oncology Group
ED – erectile dysfunction
EDTA – ethylenediaminetetraacetic acid
EMA – European Medicines Agency
EMRT – emergency medical response team
EORTC – European Organisation for Research and Treatment of Cancer
EPE – extra-prostatic extension
EPLND – extended pelvic lymph-node dissection
EPN – emphysematous pyelonephritis
EPO – erythropoietin
EPR – extra-peritoneal
ERSPC – European Randomised Study of Screening for Prostate Cancer
ESRF – end-stage renal failure
ESWL – extra-corporeal shockwave lithotripsy
ETS – E26 transformation specific
EUA – examination under anaesthesia
FBC – full blood count
FDA – Food and Drug Administration
FDG – fluorodeoxyglucose
FFP – fresh frozen plasma
FNA – fine-needle aspiration
FSGS – focal segmental glomerulosclerosis
FSH – follicle stimulating hormone

FUD – female urethral diverticulum
FURS – flexible ureteroscopy
FVC – frequency–volume chart
f/t PSA – free to total prostate-specific antigen
GA – general anaesthesia
GAG – glycosaminoglycans
GCNIS – germ cell neoplasia in situ
GCS – Glasgow coma scale
GCT – germ cell tumour
GFR – glomerular filtration rate
GnRH – gonadotropin-releasing hormone
GS – Gram stain
GTN – glyceryl trinitrate
GUCG – Genito-Urinary Cancer Group
HDL – high-density lipoprotein
HDP – hydroxydiphosphonate
HEPA – high-efficiency particulate air
HFEA – Human Fertilisation and Embryology Authority
HG – high grade
HGPIN – high-grade prostatic intra-epithelial neoplasia
HIF – hypoxia-inducible factor
HIFU – high-intensity focused ultrasound
HIV – human immunodeficiency virus
HK – human kallikrein
HLA – human leucocyte antigen
HLRCC – hereditary leiomyomatosis and renal cell carcinoma
HoLEP – holmium laser enucleation of the prostate
HPCRU – high-pressure chronic retention of urine
HPF – high-powered field
HPG – hypothalamo–pituitary–gonadal
HPRC – hereditary papillary renal carcinoma
HPV – human papilloma virus
HU – Hounsfield unit
IBD – inflammatory bowel disease
ICCS – International Children's Continence Society
ICD – implanted cardiac defibrillator
ICIQ-UI – International Consultation on Incontinence Questionnaire
ICS – International Continence Society
ICSI – intra-cytoplasmic sperm injection
IDO – idiopathic detrusor overactivity
IGCCCG – International Germ Cell Cancer Collaborative Group

IGF – insulin growth factor
IHD – ischaemic heart disease
IHT – intermittent hormone therapy
IIEF – International Index of Erectile Function
IM – intra-muscular
IMRT – intensity-modulated radiation therapy
INR – international normalised ratio
IPR – intra-peritoneal
IPSS – International Prostate Symptom Score
IR – interventional radiology
ISC – intermittent self-catheterisation
ISD – intermittent self-dilatation
ISUP – International Society of Urological Pathology
ITGCN – intra-tubular germ cell neoplasia
ITU – intensive therapy unit
IUI – intra-uterine insemination
IV – intra-venous
IVC – inferior vena cava
IVF – in-vitro fertilisation
IVU – intra-venous urogram
kD – kilo Dalton
KSS – kidney-sparing surgery
KUB – kidneys ureter bladder
LASER – light amplification by stimulated emission of radiation
LDL – low-density lipoprotein
LFT – liver function tests
LG – low grade
LH – luteinising hormone
LHRH – luteinising hormone releasing hormone
LN – lymph node
LND – lymph-node dissection
LOH – late onset hypogonadism
LOS – length of stay
LTC – long-term catheter
LUT – lower urinary tract
LUTD – lower urinary tract dysfunction
LUTS – lower urinary tract symptoms
LVI – lympho-vascular invasion
MAB – maximum androgen blockade
MAG3 – mercapto acetyltriglycine
MAP – mean arterial pressure

MCDK – multi-cystic dysplastic kidney
mCRPC – metastatic castrate resistant prostate cancer
MCUG – micturating cysto-urethrogram
MDP – methylene diphosphonate
MDRD – Modification of Diet in Renal Disease
MDT – multi-disciplinary team
MET – medical expulsive therapy
mg – milligram
MHRA – Medicines and Healthcare products Regulatory Agency
MHz – megahertz
MI – myocardial infarction
MIBC – muscle-invasive bladder cancer
MIBG – metaiodobenzylguanidine
MIS – Mullerian inhibiting substance
mL – millilitre
MMC – mitomycin-C
MNE – monosymptomatic nocturnal enuresis
mPCa – metastatic prostate cancer
mpMRI – multi-parametric magnetic resonance imaging
mRCC – metastatic renal cell carcinoma
MRI – magnetic resonance imaging
MRU – magnetic resonance urogram
MS – multiple sclerosis
MSU – midstream urine
MUI – mixed urinary incontinence
MV – megavoltage
NA – noradrenaline
NAAT – nucleic acid amplification test
NAC – neo-adjuvant chemotherapy
NBI – narrow-band imaging
NCCT – non-contrast computed tomography
Nd – neodymium
NDO – neurogenic detrusor overactivity
NEWS2 – National Early Warning Score 2
ng – nanogram
NGT – nasogastric tube
NHS – National Health Service
NICE – National Institute of Clinical Excellence
NICU – neonatal intensive care unit
NIDDK – National Institute of Diabetes, Digestive and Kidney Diseases
NMIBC – non-muscle-invasive bladder cancer

NNS – number needed to screen
NNT – number needed to treat
NO – nitric oxide
NPV – negative predictive value
NS – nerve sparing
NSAID – non-steroidal anti-inflammatory drug
NSGCT – non-seminomatous germ cell tumour
NVB – neurovascular bundle
NVH – non-visible haematuria
OAB – overactive bladder
OD – once daily
OS – overall survival
PAE – prostate artery embolisation
PCa – prostate cancer
PCN – percutaneous nephrostomy
PCNL – percutaneous nephrolithotomy
PDD – photo dynamic diagnosis
PDE5i – phosphodiesterase-5 inhibitor
PDGF – platelet-derived growth factor
PE – pulmonary embolism
PeIN – penile intraepithelial neoplasia
PET – positron emission tomography
PID – pelvic inflammatory disease
PI-RADS – Prostate Imaging Reporting and Data System
PFE – pelvic-floor exercises
PFMT – pelvic-floor muscle training
PFS – progression free survival
PFUDD – pelvic fracture urethral distraction defects
PGE1 – prostaglandin E1
PGF2 – prostaglandin F2
PN – partial nephrectomy
PO – per oral
POP – pelvic organ prolapse
PPI – proton pump inhibitor
PPS – prostate pain syndrome
PPV – patent processus vaginalis
PR – per rectum
PRN – pro re nata
PSA – prostate-specific antigen
PSAD – prostate-specific antigen density
PSADT – prostate-specific antigen doubling time

PSATZD – prostate-specific antigen transitional zone density
PSAV – prostate-specific antigen velocity
PSMA – prostate-specific membrane antigen
PTFE – polytetrafluoroethane
PTH – parathyroid hormone
PTLD – post-transplant lympho-proliferative disease
PTNS – posterior tibial nerve stimulation
PUJ – pelviureteric junction
PUJO – pelviureteric junction obstruction
PUNLMP – papillary urothelial neoplasm of low malignant potential
PUV – posterior urethral valves
PVD – peripheral vascular disease
PVR – post-void residual
QDS – quarter die sumendum (four times daily)
QOL – quality of life
qSOFA – quick sepsis-related organ failure assessment
RBC – red blood cell
RCC – renal cell carcinoma
RCT – randomised controlled trial
RFA – radio-frequency ablation
RN – radical nephrectomy
RNA – ribonucleic acid
RNU – radical nephroureterectomy
RP – radical prostatectomy
RR – relative risk
RRT – renal replacement therapy
RTA – renal tubular acidosis
RTB – renal tumour biopsy
RTx – radiotherapy
RU – retrograde urethrography
rUTI – recurrent urinary tract infection
SCC – spinal cord compression
SCCa – squamous cell carcinoma
SCI – spinal cord injury
SD – standard deviation
SFR – stone-free rate
SHBG – sex hormone binding globulin
SIADH – syndrome of inappropriate secretion of anti-diuretic hormone
SIRS – systemic inflammatory response syndrome
SNM – sacral neuromodulation
SOFA – sequential organ failure assessment

SPC – suprapubic catheter
SPECT – single-photon emission computed tomography
sPSA – super-sensitive prostate-specific antigen
SRM – small renal mass
SSRI – selective serotonin reuptake inhibitor
STI – sexually transmitted infection
SUI – stress urinary incontinence
Sv – sievert
TB – tuberculosis
Tc – technetium
TC – testicular cancer
TCC – transitional cell carcinoma
TDS – ter die sumendum (three times daily)
TENS – trans-cutaneous electrical nerve stimulation
TESE – testicular sperm extraction
TIN – testicular intra-epithelial neoplasia
TKI – tyrosine kinase inhibitor
TLR – toll-like receptor
TMPRSS2 – trans-membrane protease serine 2
TOT – trans-obturator tape
TPN – total parenteral nutrition
TRT – testosterone replacement therapy
TRUS – trans-rectal ultrasound
TSG – tumour suppressor gene
TUIP – trans-urethral incision of prostate
TURBT – trans-urethral resection of bladder tumour
TURED – trans-urethral resection of ejaculatory ducts
TURP – trans-urethral resection of prostate
TVT – tension-free vaginal tape
UDS – urodynamics
UDT – undescended testis
UE – urea and electrolytes
ULD – ultra low-dose
URS – ureteroscopy
US – ultrasound
USA – United States of America
USANZ – Urological Society of Australia and New Zealand
UTI – urinary tract infection
UTUC – upper-tract urothelial cancer
UUI – urge urinary incontinence
VEGF – vascular endothelial growth factor

VH – visible haematuria
VHL – Von Hippel–Lindau syndrome
VIP – vaso-active intestinal peptide
VI-RADS – Vesical Imaging-Reporting and Data System
VLPP – Valsalva leak-point pressure
VTE – venous thrombo-embolism
VUDS – video urodynamics
VUJ – vesico-ureteric junction
VUR – vesico-ureteric reflux
VVF – vesicovaginal fistula
WCC – white cell count
WHO – World Health Organization
WLE – wide local excision
WW – watchful waiting
XGP – xanthogranulomatous pyelonephritis
XR – x-ray
YAG – yttrium aluminium garnet
ZA – zoledronic acid
5-ALA – 5-aminolaevulinic acid
5AR – 5-alpha reductase
5ARIs – 5-alpha reductase inhibitors
5-FU – 5-fluorouracil

STATION 1
UROLOGICAL ONCOLOGY 1

HAEMATURIA

DEFINITIONS

VH was formerly known as "gross" or "macroscopic haematuria":

- It is the most common presenting symptom of bladder cancer.
- VH with associated storage LUTS is potentially concerning for CIS of the bladder.

NVH can be categorised as:

- Symptomatic NVH (s-NVH), i.e. in the presence of LUTS
- Asymptomatic NVH (a-NVH).

Table 1 – Definition of NVH according to differing guidelines [1]

AUA	≥ 3 RBC per high-powered field
USANZ	> 10 RBC per high-powered field

NON-VISIBLE HAEMATURIA

Trace dipstick haematuria finding is considered negative.

Prevalence of NVH noted in 2.5% of men and 10% of women; transient urine sample contamination may arise from vigorous exercise, sexual intercourse or menstruation.

Overall ≤ 10% of patients with NVH will have urological malignancy.

Table 2 – Degree of NVH on urine dipstick in relation to number of RBCs per high-powered field [1]

Dipstick Result	RBCs per High-powered Field
+	1–10
++	10–40
+++	40–100

Mechanism of Action

Urine dipstick for NVH relies on oxidation of a chromogen by the peroxidase activity of haemoglobin, resulting in colour change on strip which is compared to known standards.

False negative – community/GP samples have a high false-negative rate due to red-cell lysis in transit.

False positive – occurs in presence of myoglobinuria, bacterial peroxides, povidone.

CAUSES

Table 3 – Summary of causes of VH

Stones	Anywhere in urinary tract
Infection	Bacterial, mycobacterial (TB), parasitic (schistosomiasis)
Oncological	Renal, ureteric, bladder, prostate, urethral cancers
Benign	BPH
Nephrological	(further listed below)

Haematuria in BPH

Aetiological causes include:

- Increased prostatic vascularity due to higher microvessel density in hyperplastic prostatic tissue
- Elevated expression of VEGF.

BPH-related haematuria can usually be successfully treated with 5AR inhibitors as first-line option – alternatives in refractory cases include ADT, emergency TURP or prostatic artery embolisation.

Finasteride decreases VEGF expression, microvessel density and prostatic blood flow. [2]

Screening for Bladder Cancer

Studies by Britton et al. (1992) [3] and Messing et al. (2006) [4] screened thousands of patients via dipstick test, finding 15–20% had NVH.

False-positive rates were ≤ 90%, which would yield prohibitively high patient numbers for investigation.

Khadra et al. (2000) reviewed almost 2,000 haematuria clinic patients, finding urinary tract malignancy in 13% (9.4% of NVH referrals and 24.2% in VH referrals). [5]

NICE GUIDELINES HAEMATURIA

NICE released guidance (last updated 2023) for "Suspected cancer: recognition and referral" for haematuria under the bladder-cancer category (Table 4).

| VIVA | It is imperative you know confidently the contents of Table 4 below and can relay this rapidly and without doubt to the FRCS (Urol) viva examiners. |

Table 4 – NICE 2023 Guidelines for referral of haematuria [6]

Aged > 45 years	Unexplained VH without UTI or VH that persists or recurs after UTI treatment
Aged > 60 years	Unexplained NVH + (raised WCC or dysuria)
Non-urgent bladder-cancer referral	Aged > 60 years with new unexplained recurrent UTI

| KEY PAPER | Price et al. (2014) – haematuria study in primary care [7] |

The criteria used to devise the NICE guideline for NVH were drawn from this primary-care study.

Almost 5,000 patients with known bladder cancer were compared with > 20,000 matched controls, to estimate the positive predictive value for bladder cancer of certain clinical findings.

Positive predictive value was highest for raised WCC (PPV = 3.9) and dysuria (4.5).

INVESTIGATIONS

Ideally, eligible patients should be referred to a one-stop haematuria clinic.

History:

- Onset of haematuria, duration, associated symptoms
- Past medical history, drug history
- Smoking status and occupational exposure to carcinogens

Examination:

- Abdominal examination, external genitalia, pelvic examination in women, DRE in men

MSU and Urine Cytology

Blood tests:

- FBC/UE/clotting screen
- PSA to be considered if VH, LUTS or ED (NICE)

Flexible cystoscopy

Imaging:

- US and/or CTU

URINE CYTOLOGY

Urine examination for exfoliated cancer cells has very high sensitivity in HG/G3 tumours (≤ 84%) and CIS (≤ 100%) bur far less so in LG tumours (≤ 16%).

Positive cytology can indicate urothelial carcinoma anywhere in the urinary tract.

Positive cytology is highly specific (95%), high positive predictive value due to very low false positives.

To maximise accuracy of sampling:

- Mid-morning sample (not early morning as these provide degenerate specimens)
- Whole stream analysis is preferable, as mid-stream is the most acellular fraction
- Catheter specimens can be analysed but may be unreliable
- Analysis must be fast; if prolonged delay expected, refrigerate samples or fix with 50% alcohol.

A standardised reporting system known as the "Paris System" (2022) is recommended by EAU 2024 to be used for urine cytology reporting:

- Negative for urothelial carcinoma
- Atypical for urothelial carcinoma (atypia)
- Suspicious for HG urothelial carcinoma (suspicious)
- HG/G3 urothelial carcinoma (malignant).

> **VIVA** The use of urine cytology in one-stop haematuria clinics is not mandatory. However, in your FRCS (Urol) viva you may be expected to discuss the pros and cons of employing cytology to assess for urothelial cancer, so I recommend learning the sensitivity and specificity percentages.

The scenario of positive urine cytology but negative haematuria investigations (CTU and flexible cystoscopy) is challenging and the clinician must meticulously search for urothelial carcinoma.

The patient should be consented and proceed to:

- Rigid cystoscopy and bladder biopsies of trigone, right and left lateral walls, posterior wall and dome and consider bilateral retrograde studies and ureteroscopy.

Alternative Urinary Molecular Markers

The low sensitivity of urine cytology in detecting LG bladder tumours prompted exploration of various alternative urinary tests, but none are currently accepted in routine practice.

Examples include *Nuclear-matrix protein 22 (NMP 22)* and *UroVysion test (FISH)*.

NEW METHODS OF TUMOUR VISUALISATION

NICE 2015 recommends offering white-light guided TURBT plus one of PDD, NBI, urine cytology or urinary biomarker test (e.g. FISH, UroVysion) to patients with suspected bladder cancer.

White light alone may miss cancers that are not visible, prompting development of new technologies.

Photodynamic Diagnostic Cystoscopy

Relies on the molecular handling of 5-ALA (a light-sensitising drug) by tumour cells.

PDD is more sensitive than white light for detection of malignant tumours and particularly CIS.

How to perform PDD cystoscopy:

- Instil 5-ALA into bladder 2–4 hours prior to cystoscopy (taken up by urothelium)

- 5-ALA is converted to protoporphyrin which is preferentially taken up by malignant cells
- As blue light (380–450 nm wavelength) illuminates bladder, areas of red fluorescence from abnormal mucosa will light up surrounding normal bladder mucosa
- Any resection of abnormal blue-light area should be undertaken with white light, then at final check under blue light, the affected area should no longer be visible.

False positives may arise from recent inflammation, BCG or TURBT treatments.

EAU 2024 supports the use of PDD cystoscopy in cases of negative cystoscopy but positive cytology.

KEY PAPER   PHOTO Trial [8]

Randomised, open-label, parallel-group trial undertaken in 22 UK NHS hospitals.

500+ patients recruited with suspected first diagnosis of NMIBC with intermediate or high risk of recurrence based on visual inspection.

Randomised (1:1) to: standard white-light guided TURBT vs. PDD-guided TURBT.

Primary outcome was time to recurrence at three-years follow-up.

Key finding was that PDD-guided TURBT did not reduce recurrence rates and was not cost-effective.

Narrow-band Imaging

Optical filter technology that enhances the contrast between hyper-vascular cancer-tissue vessels and normal urothelium beyond what white-light imaging achieves.

NBI is not yet in routine use in many centres across the UK.

NEPHROLOGY REFERRAL

Joint Consensus Statement on the Initial Assessment of Haematuria prepared on behalf of the Renal Association and BAUS 2008 outlined guidelines for referral to nephrology.

Patients with negative urological investigations need nephrology referral if other factors present:

- Declining eGFR by > 10mL/min within last 5 years or > 5mL/min within last 1 year
- Stage 4 or 5 CKD
- Significant proteinuria (albumin to creatinine ratio [ACR] > 30mg/mmol).

Consider primary nephrology referral in patients under 40 years of age with NVH if there is:

- Significant proteinuria (albumin to creatinine ratio [ACR] > 30mg/mmol)
- Hypertension (BP > 140/90)
- eGFR < 60mL/min.

NEPHROLOGICAL CAUSES OF HAEMATURIA

Glomerular Causes:

- *IgA nephropathy* (Berger's disease) – deposition of IgA after an upper respiratory tract infection
- *Alport's syndrome* – involves X-linked collagen mutation resulting in nephritis
- *Goodpasture's syndrome* – auto-immune disease where antibodies attack basement membrane of kidneys resulting in NVH
- *Nephrotic syndrome* – results from non-inflammatory injury to the glomerulus, associated with proteinuria, hypoalbuminaemia, hypercholesterolaemia and hyperlipidaemia
- *Henoch–Schonlein purpura* – a systemic vasculitis characterised by deposition of IgA

Non-glomerular Causes:

- *Renal artery stenosis* (when stenosis > 70%)
- *Papillary necrosis* due to pyelonephritis, obstructive uropathy, sickle cell, TB, trauma, cirrhosis, analgesic nephropathy, renal vein thrombosis, diabetes (POSTCARD acronym)
- *Interstitial nephritis* involves inflammatory infiltrate affecting nephron function

NON-MUSCLE-INVASIVE BLADDER CANCER

EPIDEMIOLOGY

Eighth most common cancer in men in UK.

Majority (75%) of new bladder-cancer patients present with non-muscle-invasive disease (Ta/T1, CIS).

The most common presenting symptom is painless VH, and the concomitant presence of irritative LUTS may suggest presence of CIS.

5% of patients will have metachronous upper-tract TCC.

RISK FACTORS

Smoking	Most important risk factor, accounting for 50% of cases (aromatic amines are renally excreted) with 2–5x increased risk (electronic cigarette risk not yet known)
Age	Most commonly diagnosed > 80 years
Occupational	10% of all cases, from exposure to aromatic amines (paint, dye, petroleum, rubber) and chlorination of drinking water
Inflammation	Chronic inflammatory conditions such as schistosomiasis
Drugs	Cyclophosphamide (chemotherapy agent to treat haematological cancers)
Radiotherapy	Pelvic RTx to treat cancer can increase risk 2–4x
Genetic	Family history not known influence, no clear genetic causes found, although karyotypic changes of chromosomes 9, 17 (p53) & 13 (retinoblastoma loci)

PATHOLOGY

95% of patients with bladder cancer have TCC, the remaining have SCCa (4%) or rarer variants such as adenocarcinoma, small cell, sarcomatoid and nested variants.

The most common bladder sarcoma is leiomyosarcoma, which is not associated with smoking.

The most common NMIBC histology found in new diagnoses is pTa LG (50–70%).

Bladder cancer may metastasise via the following routes:

- *Haematogenous*, to liver, lung, adrenal gland and bone
- *Lymphatic*, iliac and para-aortic lymph nodes
- *Implantation*, via direct seeding (e.g. SPC insertion)
- *Direct invasion*, to prostate, adnexa, bowel.

CARCINOMA IN SITU (CIS)

CIS is a flat, high-grade, non-invasive urothelial carcinoma, may be mistaken for an inflammatory lesion if not biopsied, is often multi-focal and may occur in upper tracts.

Urine cytology is very sensitive and specific for detecting CIS ($\leq$ 100%).

Aggressive and high-risk: > 50% progress if untreated, $\leq$ 80% progression in G3 + CIS.

CIS may be classified as:

- *Primary*, isolated CIS with no concurrent or previous history of bladder cancer
- *Secondary*, CIS detected during patient follow-up with no previous bladder cancer or CIS
- *Concurrent*, CIS detected in the presence of any urothelial tumour in the bladder.

SQUAMOUS CELL CARCINOMA

Rare in UK (4%), associated with chronic bladder irritation (e.g. LTC, bladder stones, schistosomiasis).

In areas where schistosomiasis is endemic, 75% of bladder cancers are SCCa in origin.

Cystoscopy reveals ulcerated lesion on trigone or lateral walls.

ADENOCARCINOMA

Can be *primary* (associated with urachal remnant) or *secondary* (distant metastasis).

A urachal remnant may present with VH and mucous discharge, histological analysis shows mucous secreting cells.

PRE-MALIGNANT LESIONS

The majority of bladder tumours are malignant; however, there are pre-malignant lesions:

Keratinising squamous metaplasia (leukoplakia)

- Thick raised white plaques of squamous metaplasia on bladder surface
- Seen in bladder exstrophy, schistosomiasis, chronic bladder inflammation, rUTI
- Associated with bladder-cancer development; annual cystoscopic surveillance advised

Urothelial dysplasia

- Flat non-invasive lesion typified by nuclear clustering, considered precursor to bladder cancer

Cystitis cystica and non-keratinising squamous metaplasia are <u>not</u> considered pre-malignant lesions.

INVESTIGATIONS

As per "Haematuria" section (history, examination, investigations, cystoscopy, proceed to TURBT).

TRANS-URETHRAL RESECTION OF BLADDER TUMOUR

| VIVA | You may be asked how to perform a TURBT in your FRCS (Urol) viva. As this is considered to be a bread-and-butter operation in urological practice, you would be expected to answer the question rapidly, efficiently and highlighting the key steps only:

- In a suitably consented patient, prepped and draped in lithotomy position with all facets of the WHO Checklist complete and cystoscopy/ CTU report on the operating room monitor
- I would perform bi-manual EUA (palpable tumour suggests MIBC)
- Proceeding to full diagnostic cystoscopy with a continuous flow 26F resectoscope
- Tumour resection with mono- or bipolar diathermy loop, rollerball for haemostasis and fulguration of tumour edge to destroy any residual malignant tissue

- Biopsy any other abnormal areas searching for CIS, biopsy healthy mucosa in context of high-grade cytology and/or solid tumour, prostatic biopsies considered
- Repeat bi-manual EUA at the end (presence of mass strongly suggests T3 disease)
- Placement of a three-way catheter and initiation of irrigation +/- MMC if applicable
- Write a detailed operation note with clear documented time of when the MMC should be drained.

Mono- or bipolar diathermy are currently both considered acceptable for TURBT (EAU 2024).

En-bloc Resection

En-bloc resection during TURBT is an alternative to the standard fractionated/piecemeal technique.

It implies removal of whole bladder tumour as single piece (exophytic tumour + base).

The increasing interest in en-bloc TURBT stems from the perceived advantages of:

- Providing intact specimens, thus improving histological analysis
- Avoiding fragmentation and thus minimising floating tumour cells and distant seeding.

Currently, superiority of en-bloc technique over conventional TURBT is debatable (EAU 2024 suggests either technique is acceptable).

Obturator Kick

Tumours on the postero-lateral aspect of the bladder lie close to the obturator nerve which can be stimulated by the electric current and cause obturator kick/spasm.

The risk of this can be reduced by:

- Keeping bladder under-filled during resection
- Neuromuscular blockade (paralysis) under GA or direct obturator nerve block by lignocaine infiltration 2cm infero-lateral to pubic tubercle
- Reducing the voltage on the diathermy
- Short and small controlled swipes using the loop.

SECOND RESECTION

Key aims of a second TURBT are to clear any residual cancer and obtain correct pathological staging.

Indications for proceeding to re-resection outlined in EAU 2024: [9]

- Incomplete initial TURBT
- If no muscle present in first resection (except Ta LG/G1 tumours and primary CIS)
- All T1 tumours (residual disease observed in 30% and upstaging noted in 30%)
- All high-grade/G3 tumours (residual disease observed in 40% + upstaging in 23%).

Re-resection is critical for staging accuracy because the management of T1 disease differs significantly from T2.

Re-resection has been shown to increase recurrence-free survival rates.

NICE recommends re-resection within 6 weeks of initial TURBT for all patients with high-risk NMIBC (HG/G3 tumours harbour residual disease in 40% + will be upstaged in 23% of cases).

GRADING

In 2004 ISUP published an updated histological classification of urothelial carcinoma (uptaken also in WHO 2022) which challenged the older 1973 WHO classification. [10]

All grades 1 became PUNLMP or LG; all grades 2 became LG or HG; all grades 3 became HG.

The prognostic value of both systems has been demonstrated and neither is superior to the other; therefore both can be used in current practice (EAU 2024).

Table 5 – WHO vs. ISUP classification of urothelial carcinoma of the bladder

1973 WHO Grading	2004 WHO Grading
Grade 1: well-differentiated	Papillary urothelial neoplasm of low malignant potential (PUNLMP)
	Low-Grade papillary urothelial carcinoma
Grade 2: moderately differentiated	Low-Grade papillary urothelial carcinoma
	High-Grade papillary urothelial carcinoma
Grade 3: poorly differentiated	High-Grade papillary urothelial carcinoma

The presence of LVI in TURBT specimens is associated with increased risk of pathological upstaging and worse prognosis.

STAGING

Table 6 – 2017 TNM Classification for the staging of bladder cancer [9]

T – Primary Tumour	
TX	Primary tumour cannot be assessed
T0	No evidence of primary tumour
Ta	Non-invasive papillary carcinoma
Tis	Carcinoma in situ: "flat tumour"
T1	Tumour invades sub-epithelial connective tissue
T2	Tumour invades muscle: T2a – Tumour invades superficial muscle (inner half) / T2b – Tumour invades deep muscle (outer half)
T3	Tumour invades peri-vesical tissue: T3a – Microscopically / T3b – Macroscopically (extra-vesical mass)
T4	Tumour invades other organs: T4a – Prostate, uterus or vagina / T4b – Pelvic wall or abdominal wall

N – Lymph Nodes	
NX	Regional lymph nodes cannot be assessed
N0	No regional lymph node metastasis
N1	Metastasis in single lymph node in the true pelvis (hypogastric, obturator, ext.iliac, presacral)
N2	Metastasis in multiple lymph nodes in true pelvis (hypogastric, obturator, ext.iliac, presacral)
N3	Metastasis in common iliac lymph node(s)
M – Distant Metastasis	
MX	Distant metastasis cannot be assessed
M0	No distant metastasis
M1	Distant metastasis: M1a – Non-regional lymph nodes M1b – Other distant metastasis

RISK STRATIFICATION

Both the NICE (Table 7) and EAU (Table 8) risk stratification for NMIBC can be used in clinical practice.

NICE currently remains at 2015 update; however, EAU updated their guidance in 2021 to add in a fourth subgroup *"Very High Risk"*.

EAU considers additional clinical risk factors as:

- Patient age > 70 years
- Multiple papillary tumours
- Tumour diameter > 3cm.

Table 7 – NICE 2015 risk classification in NMIBC [11]

Low Risk	Solitary G1/G2 (LG) pTa tumour < 3cm
	Any PUNLMP
Intermediate Risk	Solitary G1/G2 (LG) pTa tumour > 3cm
	Multi-focal G1/2 (LG) pTa tumours
	G2 pTa HG tumour
	Any low-risk recurring NMIBC within 12 months
High Risk	G3 disease
	G2/3 pT1 tumour
	CIS
	Any aggressive variant

Table 8 – EAU 2024 risk classification in NMIBC [9]

Low Risk	Primary, single Ta/T1 LG/G1 tumour < 3cm without CIS in patient ≤ 70 years
	Primary Ta LG/G1 tumour without CIS with ≤ 1 additional clinical risk factors
Intermediate Risk	Patients without CIS who are not included in any of the other groups
High Risk	All T1 HG/G3 without CIS, <u>except</u> those in very high risk group
	All CIS patients, <u>except</u> those in very high risk group
	Stage, grade with additional clinical risk factors
	Ta LG/G2 or T1 G1, no CIS with all 3 additional risk factors
	Ta HG/G3 or T1 LG, no CIS with ≥ 2 additional risk factors
	T1 G2 no CIS with ≥ 1 additional risk factors
Very High Risk	**Stage, grade with additional clinical risk factors**
	Ta HG/G3 and CIS with all 3 risk factors
	T1 G2 and CIS with ≥ 2 additional risk factors
	T1 HG/G3 and CIS with ≥ 1 additional risk factors
	T1 HG/G3 no CIS with all 3 risk factors

VIVA   You should learn both EAU and NICE NMIBC risk-stratification groups for the FRCS (Urol). However, as it is a rote-learning exercise and EAU groups have become more complicated to memorise, it is acceptable to have a broad idea of the EAU groups as long as you know the NICE groups inside out and state in your exam that you use NICE risk stratification in your clinical practice.

The EORTC and GUCG derived a scoring system from seven trials in NMIBC.

The scores can be applied to the EORTC table to calculate the percentage chance of progression and recurrence at 1 and 5 years.

These were derived from the six most significant clinical and pathological factors found.

Table 9 – EORTC–GUCG scoring system [9]

Factor	Score	
	Recurrence	Progression
Number of tumours		
Single	0	0
2–7	3	3
≥ 8	6	3
Tumour size		
< 3cm	0	0
≥ 3cm	3	3
Prior recurrence rate		
Primary	0	0
≤ 1 per year	2	2
> 1 per year	4	2
T classification		
Ta	0	0
T1	1	4

Carcinoma in situ		
No	0	0
Yes	1	6
Grade		
G1	0	0
G2	1	0
G3	2	5
Total score	0–17	0–23

Table 10 – Probabilities of recurrence and progression (after 1 year and 5 years) (95% CI)

Recurrence score	% Probability recurrence at 1 year	% Probability recurrence at 5 years
0	15	31
1–4	24	46
5–9	38	62
10–17	61	78
Progression score		
0	0.2	0.8
2–6	1	6
7–13	5	17
14–23	17	45

Prior disease recurrence rate and number of tumours are the most important prognostic factors for disease recurrence.

Stage and grade are the most important factors for disease progression and disease-specific survival.

Age and grade are the most important factors for overall survival.

MANAGEMENT

The first step of treatment in new bladder-cancer patient after full diagnostic work-up will be TURBT.

Following histology review at MDT, the patient is risk-stratified as per NICE (Table 11) and then seen in clinic to offer further treatment options accordingly.

Table 11 – NICE NMIBC management options per risk-stratification group

Risk Group	Investigation	Treatment
Low	Cystoscopy Cytology Histopathology	SI MMC
Intermediate	Cystoscopy Cytology Histopathology	SI MMC x6 maintenance MMC
High	Cystoscopy Cytology Histopathology	SI MMC Re-resection < 6 weeks BCG vs. RC

MITOMYCIN-C

MMC given as intra-vesical chemotherapy agent, which works as anti-tumour antibiotic causing DNA cross-linking in bladder tumour cells. [1]

Systemic toxicity is rare; however, if irritative LUTS or genito-palmar rash occur then halt treatment.

Given as single instillation (40mg in 40mL of saline over 1 hour) ideally immediately after TURBT to destroy circulating or residual tumour cells at resection site; however ≤ 24 hours is acceptable.

Delays > 24 hours imply tumour cells implant and are covered by extracellular matrix.

Alternative chemotherapy agents which also reduce recurrence rates include epirubicin or pirarubicin.

Single instillation chemotherapy should not be given if patient received this within last 12 months.

KEY PAPER | Sylvester et al. (2016) [12]

- Meta-analysis of 11 RCTs of (TURBT + single instillation chemotherapy) vs. (TURBT alone).
- Dose ≤ 24 hours of TURBT reduces risk of recurrence by 35%.
- Single instillation did not reduce recurrences in patients with prior recurrence rate < 1 year or with an EORTC recurrence score ≥ 5.
- No benefit to time to progression or death from bladder cancer.

MMC can be given in hyperthermic manner by a small microwave probe inserted via urethral catheterisation which heats the bladder wall.

The heat treatment is purported to make cancer cells more sensitive to the chemotherapy.

Hyperthermic MMC is given weekly for 4–8 weeks as adjuvant treatment to TURBT.

There are a series of HIVEC trials ongoing; however, currently hyperthermic MMC is not within NICE guidelines as there is insufficient evidence to support its widespread use

| KEY PAPER | HIVEC-1 Trial (2023) [13]

- Open-label, multi-centre RCT conducted in Spain across 13 centres for intermediate risk NMIBC.
- Patients received TURBT + single instillation MMC.
- Then randomised to four-weekly followed by three-monthly instillations of 40mg MMC at:
  normothermia (1) : 43°C for 30 minutes (1) : 43°C for 60 minutes (1).
- Primary outcome was recurrence-free survival at 24 months.
- Key finding was hyperthermic MMC was well tolerated but not superior to normothermic MMC.

BCG THERAPY

BCG (live attenuated vaccine form of Mycobacterium bovis) available strains include Connaught, OncoTICE® and RIVM with comparable efficacies.

Intra-vesical instillation, BCG attaches to bladder cell via fibronectin receptor and is internalised.

Mechanism of action poorly understood and likely multifactorial, including:

- Direct cytotoxic effect on bladder-cancer cells (induce apoptosis, generate cell necrosis)
- Induces immune response by up-regulating cytokine production (IL-6 and IL-8) within bladder wall and mediating macrophage chemotaxis
- Up-regulation of PD-L1 (an essential immune checkpoint expressed on surface of cancer cells).

Indications

High-risk NMIBC, usually after re-resection has confirmed detrusor muscle not involved (NICE).

Efficacy is comparable with MMC in low- and intermediate-risk NMIBC groups and therefore BCG is not recommended as first-line option due to added toxicity risk in these patients.

BCG can also be given second-line for patients with NMIBC recurrence after MMC regimen.

Maintenance BCG is mainstay for CIS (1 in 2 are disease-free at 5 years, 1 in 3 at 10 years) and good marker of response (1 in 10 responders progress to MIBC vs. 2 in 3 of non-responders).

Induction BCG is standard (weekly for 6 weeks) but different maintenance schedules have been used, e.g. Lamm's regime (27 instillations in total over 3 years).

Maintenance BCG only (not induction BCG) reduces progression risk in both papillary and CIS tumours.

Many patients do not complete the full maintenance regime, either due to inefficacy or intolerance.

| KEY PAPER | Sylvester et al. (2002) [14]

- Meta-analysis of 24 trials totalling 4,800 patients, comparing (TURBT + BCG) vs. (TURBT alone or TURBT + another treatment other than BCG)
- 27% RR reduction (4% ARR) progression to MIBC with maintenance BCG, 2.5-year follow-up

BCG Administration

Check for the following contraindications to intra-vesical BCG first:

- Immunosuppression
- Pregnant or breast-feeding women
- Known haematological malignancy
- Active TB
- Recent traumatic catheterisation/TURBT (concern of systemic absorption)
- Active heavy haematuria or UTI on the day of planned treatment
- Cirrhosis or liver disease (isoniazid cannot be given if they develop BCG-sepsis
- Severe incontinence (patient cannot retain BCG for the required 2 hours).

Administered via catheter which is removed, patient must retain BCG for 2 hours.

At end of session, sit down and pass urine to avoid splashing contamination, bleach toilet and wash hands immediately, drink plenty of fluids once home.

Risks and Toxicity

Cystitis symptoms are the most common side-effect of BCG treatment.

Low-grade fever and myalgia are also common and self-limiting symptoms.

BCGosis (sepsis) must be considered if patient on BCG therapy experiences fever/malaise:

- Admit as emergency, systematic A-to-E resuscitation and complete Sepsis-6 bundle
- Start treatment with anti-tuberculous therapy
- Treat in multi-disciplinary fashion with microbiology, respiratory and infectious diseases teams.

BCG Failure

A patient with a low-grade recurrence after BCG treatment does not constitute BCG failure.

High-grade recurrences after BCG imply that patient is unlikely to respond to further BCG. Radical cystectomy should be considered; however, further BCG remains an option (NICE).

Prompt re-discussion at the cancer MDT is recommended.

RE-RESECTION

NICE recommends re-resection for newly diagnosed NMIBC high-risk patients (Table 11).

Re-resection should be offered < 6 weeks after the first TURBT.

Residual disease after TURBT is found in 33–55% of pT1 tumours, and disease upstaging may occur in ≤ 30% after re-resection. [1]

Staging accuracy is paramount as management of T1 vs. T2 bladder cancer differs significantly.

RADICAL CYSTECTOMY

Covered in the MIBC section.

Recurrent NMIBC (Low Risk)

Consider fulguration without biopsy for patients with recurrent NMIBC provided (NICE): [11]

- No prior history of intermediate or high-risk NMIBC
- Disease-free interval of ≥ 6 months
- Solitary papillary recurrence
- Tumour diameter ≤ 3mm.

Follow-up Regime for NMIBC

Table 12 – NICE follow-up regime for NMIBC after treatment

Risk Group	Follow-up
Low	Cystoscopy 3 & 12 months If no recurrence, discharge at 12 months
Intermediate	Cystoscopy 3, 9 & 18 months Yearly thereafter Discharge after 5 years disease-free
High	Cystoscopy 3 monthly for 2 years Cystoscopy 6 monthly for 2 years Lifelong yearly cystoscopy thereafter

MUSCLE-INVASIVE BLADDER CANCER

OVERVIEW

Approximately 25% of new diagnoses of bladder cancer will be muscle-invasive at presentation.

For the 75% presenting with superficial disease, approximately 1 in 4 will progress to MIBC.

All MIBC cases are by definition high-grade urothelial carcinomas, and therefore grading MIBC does not provide additional prognostic value.

ASSESSMENT

As per "Haematuria" section.

Pelvic pain, urinary tract obstruction and fistulation are all symptoms of advanced disease.

Offer bi-manual (rectal–vaginal) examination in the presence of a chaperone to identify a palpable mass or mass fixed to the pelvic wall.

MIBC may be detected on re-resection TURBT for high-risk MIBC ($\leq$ 1 in 3 patients).

Patients with obvious bladder cancer on imaging can avoid flexible cystoscopy and proceed to TURBT.

Consider prostatic urethra biopsies during TURBT in suspected MIBC, particularly if tumour is near bladder neck, in view of planning orthotopic neobladder construction.

IMAGING

The goal of imaging bladder cancer patients is to:

- Differentiate between T1 and T2 disease, as their treatment differs considerably
- Evaluate for upper-tract obstruction
- Evaluate metachronous upper-tract cancer, locally advanced or metastatic disease.

In clinical practice, CT and MRI are the most commonly used modalities.

Use with caution if eGFR < 30mL/min – in cases of AKI due to MIBC obstructing the upper tract(s), consider nephrostomy insertion first to improve renal function prior to contrast scan.

CT Scanning

NICE and EAU recommend CT TAP with urographic phase for correct full staging of MIBC.

CT comparable to MRI for local staging and detecting extra-vesical extension (i.e. T2 vs. T3b disease).

CT is inferior to MRI in determining depth of bladder-wall involvement as it cannot discern the different wall layers (i.e. cannot differentiate between Ta to T3a tumours).

CTU is the most accurate imaging modality to detect upper-tract malignancy.

CT and MRI are comparable for lymph-node assessment – any equivocal cases can then be further evaluated with FDG PET-CT scan (NICE).

MRI Scanning

MRI has better soft-tissue resolution than CT, more accurate in determining T1 vs. T2 disease.

MRI pelvis prior to TURBT is desirable in cases suspicious for muscle-invasive disease.

VI-RADS is a structured reporting scheme for mpMRI of the bladder to assess risk of muscle invasion:

- Similar rationale of scores of 1–5 as in PI-RADS (1 – very unlikely, 5 – very likely)
- Not yet in use for routine clinical practice.

MRI can be also used as a tool to assess for response to systemic therapy (EAU 2024).

Lymph-node Imaging

LN assessment based solely on size is unreliable, as both CT and MRI are unable to confirm metastases in normal-sized or slightly enlarged LN.

Pelvic nodes > 8mm and abdominal nodes > 10mm are taken as significant.

Sensitivity and specificity of CT/MRI for LN involvement are relatively low.

PROGNOSTIC EVALUATION

Tumour and nodal staging are the main prognostic factors in the radical treatment of MIBC.

All factors that will predispose a patient to a poorer outcome from surgery (poor fitness, extremes of BMI, low albumin) are also relevant.

Evaluation of comorbidity is preferable as an indicator for life expectancy rather than patient age.

Charlson Comorbidity Index

The CCI score ranges from 0 to 30, and is calculated according to comorbidities of the patient (Table 13).

This index has been shown to be an independent prognostic factor for perioperative mortality and 5-year all-cause mortality after radical cystectomy.

Risk categories by score points include low (0), medium (1–3) and high (≥ 4). [15]

Alternative comorbidity indices include ECOG performance status and Clinical Frailty Scale. Use validated score to assess eligibility for radical treatment – do not use ASA score (EAU 2024).

Table 13 – Charlson Comorbidity Index [16]

Score	Condition
1	50–60 years, IHD, heart failure, COPD, PVD, dementia, diabetes, CVA, mild liver disease, peptic ulcer disease
2	61–70 years, localised tumour, leukaemia, lymphoma, moderate/end-stage renal failure
3	71–80 years, moderate/severe liver disease
4	81–90 years
5	> 90 years
6	Metastatic solid tumour, AIDS

WHO Performance Status

Performance status is a score estimating a patient's ability to perform certain activities of daily living.

Important factor for determining suitability of treatment as well as for selection criteria for clinical trials.

Table 14 – WHO (and ECOG) performance status [17]

Performance status	Description
0	Able to carry out all normal activity without restriction
1	Restricted in strenuous activity but ambulatory and able to carry out light work
2	Ambulatory, capable of all self-care but unable to carry out work; up and about > 50% waking hours
3	Symptomatic and in a chair or in bed for greater than 50% of the day but not bedridden
4	Completely disabled; cannot carry out any self-care; totally confined to bed or chair

Cardio-pulmonary Exercise Test

CPEX is an out-patient procedure. The patient sits on a bicycle or walks on a treadmill and is connected to a 12-lead ECG, blood-pressure cuff and pulse oximeter.

Three ventilatory variables are measured:

- Oxygen consumption
- Carbon-dioxide excretion
- Minute ventilation.

The exercise resistance is gradually increased over 10–15 minutes.

CPEX is a functional assessment of cardio-pulmonary reserve and is becoming routine in the pre-operative assessment of patients undergoing major surgery.

CPEX can evaluate via gas exchange analysis the *anaerobic threshold*, which is the point at which aerobic metabolism is no longer adequate and anaerobic supplementation begins.

Anaerobic threshold cut-off for major surgery $\geq$ 11mL/minute/kg. [18]

TREATMENT

Radical cystectomy is treatment of choice for localised MIBC in suitable-performance-status patients.

NICE and EAU 2024 endorse upfront radical cystectomy as alternative to BCG treatment, in NMIBC at highest risk of progression (e.g. T1, CIS, unusual histology, lympho-vascular invasion).

EBRT is an alternative treatment option for less-fit patients, but is less effective than surgery.

NEO-ADJUVANT CHEMOTHERAPY

KEY PAPER | ABC meta-analysis collaboration (2005) [19]

- Meta-analysis of 11 RCT comparing (local MIBC treatment) vs. (local MIBC treatment + NAC)
- > 3,000 patients included in ABC collaboration which periodically updates findings
- 5% absolute improvement in 5-year survival in treatment arm that includes NAC.

Cisplatin-based NAC should be offered prior to radical cystectomy or EBRT in fit patients (NICE). [20]

EAU 2024 recommends NAC should be offered for T2–T4a disease (i.e. not in NMIBC cases). [16]

Combination regimens includes GC (gemcitabine + cisplatin) or MVAV (methotrexate, vinblastine, Adriamycin, cisplatin).

Ensure the patient has an opportunity to discuss the risks and benefits of NAC with an oncologist.

Considerations regarding NAC include:

- Deliver at earliest time-point (lowest burden of micro-metastatic disease)
- Tolerability of chemotherapy is better before major surgery
- NAC does not affect risks of surgical morbidity
- Patients have to be fit for cisplatin-combination based therapy.

Adjuvant Chemotherapy

There is currently no evidence to support routinely giving adjuvant cisplatin-based chemotherapy to patients who have undergone radical surgery.

Consider adjuvant chemotherapy after radical cystectomy in patients with proven MIBC and/or LN positive disease, but that did not receive NAC as their TURBT histology was NMIBC. [20]

RADICAL CYSTECTOMY (RC)

The most effective treatment for localised MIBC.

Further indicated in SCCa, adenocarcinoma, G3T1 + CIS, BCG failures, obstructed upper tracts, high-volume recurrent papillary disease, select cases of EBRT failure.

Surgery should be expedited, as delays of > 12 weeks should be avoided as this has a negative impact on survival. (Consider the already added time required to treat with NAC.)

Do not offer pre-operative down-staging RTx as it does not improve survival (EAU 2024).

Prostate cancer is found incidentally in 25–40% of cysto-prostatectomy specimens. Such patients should undergo PSA monitoring as part of their follow-up plan.

Impact on overall survival of incidental prostate cancer in these cases is not known.

Operative Technique

Midline incision trans-peritoneal or extra-peritoneal approach.

Remove entire bladder and peri-vesical fat, prostate, seminal vesicles, distal ureters, regional lymph-node dissection, uterus and anterior vaginal wall and entire urethra in women.

Divide ureters close to bladder and anastomose to chosen technique of urinary diversion; protect these with ureteric stents.

There is no clear evidence to date to support a superior oncological outcome with any operative modality of radical cystectomy (open vs. robotic vs. laparoscopic).

Robotic-assisted has shorter hospital stay, longer operative time, increased costs, lower complication rates and less blood loss when compared to open cystectomy.

Surgeon experience and institution volume are considered the key factors for outcomes for both open and robot-assisted radical cystectomy, rather than the technique itself.

QOL outcomes appear to be comparable in the long term.

Lymph-node Dissection

The clinical importance of LND is controversial in terms of whether it should be considered a staging tool and/or a therapeutic procedure.

LN involvement is a strong predictor of 5-year CSS: N- 80% and N+ 40%.

There is currently no definitive consensus on the optimal extent of LND that should be undertaken: [16]

- *Standard*, up to common iliac bifurcation (internal iliac, pre-sacral, external iliac LN)
- *Extended (Level 1 and 2)*, includes standard + LN up to aortic bifurcation
- *Super-extended (Level 3)*, dissection reaches the inferior mesenteric artery level cranially.

Level 1 is likely adequate for most patients; Level 2 or 3 are an option if enlarged nodes on staging imaging.

EAU 2024 recommends that a LND should be performed as an integral part of radical cystectomy.

Primary Urethrectomy

Preserve the urethra if frozen section margins are negative (positive urethral margin is a contraindication to orthotopic neobladder formation).

Primary urethrectomy is advised if urethral margins are positive, primary tumour at bladder neck or within prostatic urethra, or with extensive CIS disease.

Risk of urethral recurrence is lower with the use of neobladder (4%) vs. ileal conduit (8%) (suggesting that urine is protective in this setting).

The risk of urethral recurrence rises to ≤ 18% in presence of prostatic urethral involvement.

Sexual Preserving Techniques

Different approaches for preserving sexual function in strongly motivated men have been described, but currently there is no consensus on which approach preserves function best.

Concern remains regarding their oncological outcome.

The MIBC must be localised, not invading the prostate or bladder neck. Approaches include:

- *Prostate sparing*, including vas, seminal vesicles and NVBs
- *Capsule sparing*, as for prostate sparing but prostate adenoma is removed
- *Seminal sparing*, preserving seminal vesicles, vas, NVBs
- *Nerve sparing*, the NVBs are the only tissue left in place.

Partial Cystectomy

Approximately 10% of patients with bladder cancer are potential candidates for partial cystectomy.

Suitable for those with small lesions and a lack of concurrent CIS (e.g. 1cm T2 lesion on the dome), tumour in diverticulum.

Multiple tumours, CIS, tumours close to ureteric orifices or on trigone are not suitable.

Palliative Cystectomy

Patients with locally advanced tumours (e.g. T4b) may experience debilitating symptoms such as intractable haematuria, pain and urinary obstruction.

Palliative cystectomy with urinary diversion is feasible. However, EAU 2024 recommends alternatives such as palliative RTx/TURBT or nephrostomy tube insertion if possible. [16]

URINARY DIVERSION

NICE recommends offering continent urinary diversion if no strong contraindications such as cognitive impairment, impaired renal function or significant bowel disease. [20]

Anatomically, there are three alternatives used for diversion after cystectomy:

- Abdominal e.g. ileal or colonic conduit
- Urethral, various forms of gastro-intestinal pouches attached to urethra (e.g. neobladder)
- Rectosigmoid diversions.

Ileal Conduit

The most common method of urinary diversion in the UK is the ileal conduit.

Additional complications of ileal conduit formation include:

- *Early* – bowel obstruction, anastomotic leak, conduit ischaemia
- *Late* – stomal stenosis, para-stomal herniation.

Metabolic acidosis is less common with ileal conduit when compared to neobladder.

Bricker technique – spatulate and anastomose each ureter to the serosa of the bowel separately.

Wallace 1 technique – both ureters spatulated to same length, medial walls anastomosed together and free edges of conjoined ureters are anastomosed to proximal end of open bowel segment.

Orthotopic Neobladder

The terminal ileum is the gastro-intestinal segment of choice for bladder substitution. However, a greater length (60cm) is required, thus increasing the risk of metabolic sequelae.

Emptying of the reservoir requires abdominal straining, intestinal peristalsis, sphincter relaxation.

90% are continent by day (slightly less by night).

The Studer neobladder is a commonly used technique in the UK.

Uretero-colonic Diversion

Procedure largely obsolete due to the risk of upper-tract infections and increased risk of colonic malignancy (≤ 29% risk at 20 years follow-up).

Pre-operatively the "porridge test" to assess suitability for uretero-colonic diversion involves flushing 500mL of liquid per rectum and asking patient to hold this in situ for ≥ 1 hour.

Avoids the use of stoma bag in countries where stoma care or community costs cannot be met.

Uretero-cutaneostomy

This is the simplest form of cutaneous diversion, reducing operative time, post-operative support and length of hospital stay when compared to ileal conduit.

Option for elderly and otherwise compromised patients.

Stoma stenosis is more common, however.

FOLLOW-UP AFTER RADICAL CYSTECTOMY

After RC consider a follow-up protocol comprising of: [20]

- Imaging for upper-tract monitoring for hydronephrosis/stones/cancer (annual)
- Imaging for local/distant recurrence using CT TAP (6, 12 and 24 months)
- Blood tests for metabolic acidosis, B12 and folate deficiency (annual), and
- Urethroscopy and/or urethral washing cytology in defunctioned urethras (annual for 5 years).

COMPLICATIONS OF RADICAL CYSTECTOMY

Radical cystectomy is associated with mortality within 90 days of ≤ 3% and very high morbidity rates.

Table 15 – Risks and complications after radical cystectomy

	Immediate	Early	Late
Risks	- Intra-operative death - Bleeding/blood transfusion	- DVT/PE - Infections: chest, wound, UTI - Ileo-ileal anastomotic leak - Uretero-ileal leak - CVA, MI, death	- Incisional/para-stomal hernias - Stomal stenosis - Anastomotic stricture - Hyperchloraemic metabolic acidosis - Cancer recurrence - Vaginal shortening

| **VIVA** | Questions around surgical complications in the FRCS (Urol) viva may arise; to score high marks you need structured, succinct answers. Different structures exist (e.g. local vs. systemic complications; or immediate vs. early vs. late); however, you should know the Clavien–Dindo classification of surgical complications (Table 16). |

Table 16 – Clavien–Dindo classification of surgical complications

Clavien–Dindo Grade	Nature of complication
1	Deviation from normal post-operative course without need for pharmacological/surgical/endoscopic/radiological treatment (i.e. anti-emetic/pyretic, analgesics or bedside wound opening are acceptable)
2	Requiring pharmacological treatment with drugs other than allowed for Grade 1 (e.g. blood transfusion, antibiotics, TPN)
3	Requiring surgical/endoscopic/radiological intervention: 3a – under regional/local anaesthesia 3b – under GA

4	Life-threatening complication requiring ITU:
	4a – single-organ dysfunction
	4b – multi-organ dysfunction
5	Patient death

Hyperchloraemic Metabolic Acidosis

Very common after ileal conduit formation, in most cases sub-clinical and in small proportion of patients it is observed long-term.

Bowel secretes sodium in exchange of hydrogen, and bicarbonate in exchange of chloride.

Bowel exposed to urine reabsorbs acid and chloride leading to chronic acid load (hyperchloraemic metabolic acidosis), worsened by lower kidney function and use of colonic vs. ileal segments.

This can be treated with oral sodium bicarbonate.

Other Metabolic Abnormalities

Low Potassium, intestinal secretory loss and renal wasting. Hypokalaemia can be exacerbated in the process of correcting the metabolic acidosis.

Low calcium, renal wasting and depletion of body calcium stores (the chronic metabolic acidosis is buffered by bone carbonate) and patient may require calcium supplementation.

Low magnesium

Macrocytic anaemia, as vitamin B12 absorption occurs in terminal ileum (B12 stores are sufficient for 3 years, so this deficiency may manifest late).

Bone Demineralisation

Bone calcium and carbonate mobilisation to buffer chronic metabolic acidosis can cause osteomalacia.

Furthermore metabolic acidosis impairs renal activation of vitamin D, which is essential for bone mineralisation, and activates osteoclast activity.

ADJUVANT TREATMENT AFTER SURGERY

Adjuvant cisplatin-based combination chemotherapy can be offered after radical cystectomy to patients with pT3/4 and/or N+ disease AND if NAC was not given.

Nivolumab is approved by NICE for patients not eligible for cisplatin-based chemotherapy.

EXTERNAL BEAM RADIOTHERAPY

Alternative to major surgery for those unfit or unwilling to have radical cystectomy.

There are no RCTs comparing the two modalities to date. However, 5-year survival rates reportedly better with surgery (possible bias as EBRT patients are likely less fit prior to treatment).

Typical curative dose is 66Gy over 6 weeks or alternatively moderately hypofractionated 55Gy.

Target field is bladder only; however, LN irradiation is an option on individual patient basis.

NAC is beneficial for patients undergoing EBRT and should be offered (NICE).

There is no benefit to survival in giving neo-adjuvant EBRT prior to radical cystectomy.

Contraindications to EBRT include:

- Severe LUTS
- Previous pelvic irradiation
- Inflammatory bowel disease
- Upper-tract obstruction
- CIS, SCC and adenocarcinoma (as these are poorly sensitive).

Salvage cystectomy is an option in select cases with 5-year survival rates < 50%.

Follow-up after EBRT

After EBRT consider a follow-up protocol comprising: [20]

- Rigid cystoscopy (3 months)
- Flexible cystoscopy (6 months and then 3 monthly for 2 years and then 6 monthly for 2 years)

- Imaging for upper-tract monitoring (annual)
- Imaging for local/distant recurrence using CT TAP (6, 12 and 24 months).

Recurrence after EBRT can be treated:

- Salvage cystectomy in fit patients with pT1/pT2+ (non-metastatic)
- Intra-vesical BCG for high-risk NMIBC recurrences
- TURBT for low-risk recurrences.

SURGERY VS. RADIOTHERAPY

Table 17 – Risks and benefits of radical cystectomy vs. EBRT as treatment for MIBC

	EBRT	Radical cystectomy
Benefits	Avoids major surgery Preserves bladder	Full staging available Better 5-year survival rates? Can treat CIS
Risks	LUTS Small bladder capacity Proctitis Second malignancy Does not treat CIS	Bleeding Infection DVT/PE Collection/anastomotic leak Stomal stenosis Hyperchloraemic metabolic acidosis

URACHAL TUMOUR

Very rare, usually adenocarcinoma (85%) but can also be SCCa or TCC, located at bladder dome.

Treatment is partial or radical cystectomy, 5-year survival ~50%.

Adenocarcinoma of bladder is more common in females, urachal tumours are more common in men.

METASTATIC DISEASE

10% of patients with bladder cancer present with metastases at diagnosis.

50% of radical cystectomy for MIBC patients will relapse; prognosis is poor (months).

MANAGEMENT

Consider debulking/palliative TURBT to obtain histology, treat haematuria and voiding symptoms.

MDT involvement of oncology and palliative care teams is essential.

TCC is a chemotherapy-sensitive cancer and this is first-line treatment:

- Patient has to be deemed fit and eligible for chemotherapy
- Combination (cisplatin-based + gemcitabine) therapy is more effective than single-agent
- Carboplatin-based may be an alternative in less-fit patients.

Immunotherapy (atezolizumab) can be given:

- Cisplatin-ineligible patients (e.g. GFR < 45mL/min) with high PD-L1 expression
- Second-line option after progression on chemotherapy.

Palliative RTx can be given for symptom control.

RENAL CANCER

EPIDEMIOLOGY

3% of all cancers worldwide; seventh most common cancer in the UK.

Highest incidence in Western countries (likely due to higher use of abdominal imaging detecting SRM).

Male to female ratio is 1.5:1.

RCC accounts for ~90% of all kidney malignancies.

Leiomyosarcoma is the most common type of renal sarcoma.

RISK FACTORS

Lifestyle factors – smoking, obesity, hypertension

Family history – first-degree affected relative

Hereditary – (5–8% of all cases) VHL, HPRC, HLRCC, BHD

Occupational – asbestos, cadmium

Other – horseshoe kidney, receiving dialysis with native kidneys in situ

HEREDITARY CONDITIONS

Von Hippel–Lindau Disease

Autosomal dominant genetic disorder affecting males and females equally, in 1/36,000 live births. [21]

VHL syndrome occurs due to loss of both copies of tumour suppressor gene at chromosome 3 (3p25-26), resulting in dysregulation of HIF 1 & 2.

Cells lacking VHL gene in hypoxic conditions accumulate HIF-1. This will over-express genes related to angiogenesis (VEGF and PDGF) and cell division.

Up-regulation of VEGF is the most prominent angiogenic factor in RCC.

VHL syndrome is characterised by phaeochromocytomas, visceral/ pancreatic cysts and neuroendocrine tumours, cerebellar haemangioblastomas and RCC (often multi-focal)

Most tumours in VHL share the characteristic of hyper-vascularity.

Loss of vision is common due to angiomatosis (nests of proliferating capillaries) in the retina.

RCC and cysts typically evolve in multiple sites in the kidney after 20 years of age (> 3cm in size is thought to be high risk for malignant transformation).

Treatment should focus on aim of maintaining nephrons. Monitor with US first and then intensive CT/MRI once lesions larger (> 2cm); consider ablative therapies or PN for smaller lesions.

Ultimately patient may require renal replacement therapy; role of transplantation is limited.

Main causes of death are related to complications of RCC and haemangioblastoma. [21]

Birt–Hogg–Dubé Syndrome

Autosomal dominant genetic condition that can cause susceptibility to kidney cancer, renal and pulmonary cysts, benign fibrofolliculomas of hair follicles.

BHD syndrome arises from mutations of the folliculin/FLCN gene on chromosome 17p. [22]

Fibrofolliculomas are mainly in the facial region and are the most common manifestation of BHD; pulmonary cysts may lead to spontaneous pneumothorax.

The most common renal tumour in BHD is mixed oncocytoma and chromophobe.

Hereditary Papillary Renal Cell Carcinoma

HPRC follows autosomal dominant inheritance, in familial cases is associated with mutation of *met* oncogene on chromosome 7.

Increases risk of type 1 papillary RCC (multiple/bilateral).

HPRC does not increase risk of tumours elsewhere, as for example noted in VHL. [23]

Hereditary Leiomyomatosis and Renal Cell Carcinoma (or Reed's Syndrome)

Autosomal dominant genetic condition.

Arises due to mutations of the fumarate hydratase gene (works in the Kreb's cycle).

HLRCC is the most aggressive form of hereditary RCC condition and tends to have an earlier age of onset and higher-grade cancers than HPRC.

Non-oncological manifestations include uterine fibroids and cutaneous leiomyomas. [23]

ANGIOMYOLIPOMA

Benign mesenchymal tumour composed of peri-vascular epithelioid cells containing blood vessels, immature smooth muscle and fat. Malignant transformation is rare.

Most commonly found in middle-aged women; only 5% of new patients present with multiple lesions.

Associated with tuberous sclerosis. [24]

Main risk of AML is spontaneous rupture causing bleeding into retro-peritoneum or collecting system.

Imaging

Most AML are incidentally diagnosed on routine imaging.

US shows echo-bright pattern as fat reflects US waves and there is no acoustic shadow (distinguishing it from calculus); CT has low Hounsfield units (< 10).

Treatment

AS is considered first-line option for most AML.

An AML > 4cm in size is considered cut-off for surveillance and treatment should be considered. [25]

Factors that should prompt consideration of treatment for AML include:

- > 4cm size and/or symptomatic AML
- Pregnant women with large AML (pose higher risk of bleeding)
- Patients in whom follow-up or access to emergency care may be inadequate.

Treatment options include selective arterial embolisation (first line), PN or RFA.

AML volume (e.g. multiple AML) can be reduced prior to intervention by the mTOR inhibitor everolimus.

Tuberous Sclerosis

Autosomal dominant condition, mapped to TSC1 (chromosome 9, coding for hamartin) and TSC2 (chromosome 16, coding for tuberin). [26]

Features the following manifestations:

- Hamartomas in the central nervous system (epilepsy, learning difficulty)
- AML and renal cysts
- Skin/facial angiofibromas
- Cardiac rhabdomyomas.

Wunderlich Syndrome

Rare condition of spontaneous acute renal haemorrhage into retro-peritoneal space. [27]

Presents with "Lenk's triad" of ipsilateral flank pain, palpable mass and hypovolaemic shock.

Ruptured AML is most common cause (others include renal cancer, rupture of renal artery aneurysm).

Wunderlich syndrome can be treated conservatively if the patient is haemodynamically stable, otherwise emergency embolisation or nephrectomy may be required.

DIAGNOSIS

PRESENTATION

Most renal tumours are incidentally diagnosed on routine imaging for other medical reasons.

For those presenting with symptoms, the most common one is visible haematuria.

The classic quoted triad of "loin pain, visible haematuria and palpable mass" is uncommon (< 10%) and correlates with aggressive histology and advanced disease.

Para-neoplastic manifestations occur in 30% (Table 18).

Table 18 – Para-neoplastic symptoms associated with RCC

Symptom	Aetiology
Hypertension	Renin production by the primary tumour (acting on the renin angiotensin aldosterone system)
Polycythaemia	Over-production of EPO
Hypercalcaemia	- Non-metastatic: PTH hormone-like peptide produced by RCC cells - Metastatic: osteolytic breakdown
Stauffer's syndrome	Signs/symptoms of liver abnormalities in absence of liver metastases e.g. raised LFTs, fever, weight loss, thrombocytopenia (IL-6 production)

IMAGING

Most common imaging modalities used are US, CT and MRI.

MRI/CT, however, cannot reliably distinguish oncocytoma and fat-free AML from RCC.

PET currently has no role in renal tumour diagnostics.

CT Urogram

Iodine-based contrast medium is used.

Phase 1 – non-contrast, for visualisation of calcifications/stones/fat as well as providing baseline attenuation (HU) for then assessing enhancement post-contrast

Phase 2 – nephrographic, (100 seconds post-contrast) highest sensitivity in detecting renal masses; comparison with unenhanced images is paramount to seek enhancement

Phase 3 – excretory, (10 minutes post-contrast) providing opacification of collecting systems, ureters and bladder, allowing evaluation of urothelium

If CTU is inconclusive, contrast-enhanced US is an alternative to further characterise renal lesions.

Split-bolus technique can be used to reduce radiation dose (local protocols vary):

- 75mL (IV) contrast administered at start
- Wait for 5–8 minutes
- Administer a further 75mL (IV) contrast
- Start scanning after ~60 seconds.

Aims to put together in a single image acquisition both the nephrographic and excretory phases, thus reducing the radiation dose to the patient. [28]

CT thorax should be undertaken simultaneously for evaluation of metastases.

Enhancement

The most important criterion for differentiating malignant lesions from benign ones is enhancement.

Enhancement suggests the presence of vascular tissue or communication with the collecting system.

A *change of > 15HU* between pre- and post-contrast images is considered significant in pointing toward a malignant diagnosis. [29]

MR-Urogram

MRU uses gadolinium-based contrast medium.

Indicated in patients allergic to IV contrast, pregnant or in renal failure, and option for limiting radiation exposure in patients with hereditary conditions needing long-term surveillance.

MRU may also provide additional information on venous involvement if this is a concern.

BOSNIAK CLASSIFICATION OF RENAL CYSTS

This is a classification based on CT that is used to determine follow-up and predict risk of underlying malignancy:

- *Type 1*, benign and can be discharged
- *Type 2*, benign and can be discharged
- *Type 2F*, follow-up advised for ≤ 5 years (10% risk of transformation)

- *Type 3*, 50+% will be malignant – consider intervention or long-term surveillance
- *Type 4*, > 90% will be malignant – consider intervention.

Table 19 – 2019 Bosniak classification of renal cysts

Bosniak Cyst	Features	Follow-up
I	Well-defined, thin (≤ 2mm) smooth wall Homogenous simple fluid (-9 to -20HU) No septa, no calcifications, wall may enhance	Benign
II	Thin wall (≤ 2mm) and ≤ 3 septa which may enhance Homogenous hyperattenuating (≥ 70HU) masses at non-contrast CT Homogenous non-enhancing masses, 20HU at renal mass protocol Homogenous masses -9 to -20HU at non-contrast CT Homogenous masses 21 to 30HU at portal venous phase CT Homogenous low-attenuation masses that are too small to characterise	Benign
IIF	Smooth minimally thickened (3mm) enhancing wall Or smooth minimal thickening (3mm) of ≥ 1 enhancing septa Or ≥ 4 smooth thin (≤ 2mm) enhancing septa	Follow-up (10% are malignant)
III	≥ 1 walls or septa that are enhancing thick (≥ 4mm width) Or enhancing irregular	Surgery or surveillance (50+% are malignant)
IV	≥ 1 enhancing nodules (≥ 4mm convex protrusion with obtuse margins) Or convex protrusion of any size that has acute margins	Surgery (Most are malignant)

PATHOLOGY

There are three main types of RCC: *clear cell, papillary* and *chromophobe*.

Clear-cell RCC is the most common sub-type (70% of RCC).

Papillary RCC is second most common, and formerly was divided into types 1 and 2.

Chromophobe RCC currently cannot be graded by the WHO/ISUP system because of innate nuclear atypia; however, prognosis in this sub-type is more favourable.

5-year OS for non-metastatic RCC is: 91% (chromophobe), 82% (papillary) and 81% (clear cell).

Sarcomatoid RCC is not a specific sub-type, but rather represents a de-differentiation associated with adverse outcomes/survival irrespective of RCC sub-type, and should be graded as G4.

Grading system for RCC is detailed in "Prognostic Factors" below.

Oncocytoma is covered below in "Benign Renal Masses" along with other benign renal tumours.

Renal Tumour Biopsy

RTB via US- or CT-guided imaging can be used for the following reasons:

- Uncertainty regarding nature of the lesion (e.g. lipid-poor AML), provided patient is fit
- Prior to systemic therapy (e.g. metastatic RCC)
- Prior to cryotherapy or RFA
- Prior to tumour surveillance.

An evidently enhancing and radiologically convincing tumour does not require RTB prior to intervention.

In large/aggressive tumours, avoid sampling the central area, which may be necrotic and inconclusive.

RTB is not indicated in frail/comorbid patients unfit for intervention.

Risk of seeding is a historical concern and extremely low.

| KEY PAPER | Marconi et al. in *European Urology* (2016) [30] |

- Systematic review of > 50 studies and > 5,000 patients undergoing RTB to determine safety and accuracy of the procedure
- 92% median diagnostic rate with percutaneous core biopsy sensitivity/ specificity > 99%
- Very low rate of Clavien–Dindo ≥ 2 complications
- Concluded that RTB is accurate and safe diagnostic procedure in renal cancer.

STAGING

Table 20 – TNM classification for staging of renal cell carcinoma [31]

T – Primary Tumour	
TX	Primary tumour cannot be assessed
T0	No evidence of primary tumour
T1	Tumour ≤ 7cm in greatest dimension, limited to the kidney: T1a – Tumour ≤ 4cm T1b – Tumour > 4cm but ≤ 7cm
T2	Tumour > 7cm in greatest dimension, limited to the kidney: T2a – Tumour > 7cm but ≤ 10cm T2b – Tumour > 10cm, limited to the kidney
T3	Tumour extends into major veins or perinephric tissues, but not ipsilateral adrenal gland and not beyond Gerota's fascia T3a – Extends into renal vein or segmental branches or tumour invades perirenal/sinus fat but not beyond Gerota's T3b – Tumour grossly extends into the IVC below the diaphragm T3c – Tumour grossly extends into the IVC above the diaphragm or invades IVC wall
T4	Tumour invades beyond Gerota's fascia (including into ipsilateral adrenal gland)
N – Lymph Nodes	
NX	Regional lymph nodes cannot be assessed
N0	No regional lymph node metastasis
N1	Metastasis in regional lymph node(s)

M – Metastasis	
M0	No distant metastasis
M1	Distant metastasis (includes contra-lateral adrenal gland involvement)

Staging of IVC Involvement

RCC associated with IVC involvement in ≤ 10% of cases; surgery is the only curative option. [32]

The different stages of IVC involvement of renal tumour are shown in Image 1. [33]

- Level I – tumour thrombus extending to renal vein and < 2cm above renal vein orifice
- Level II – tumour thrombus extending > 2cm above renal vein orifice but below hepatic veins
- Level III – tumour thrombus extending above hepatic veins but below the diaphragm
- Level IV – tumour thrombus extending above the diaphragm.

Image 1 – Stages of IVC involvement of renal tumour

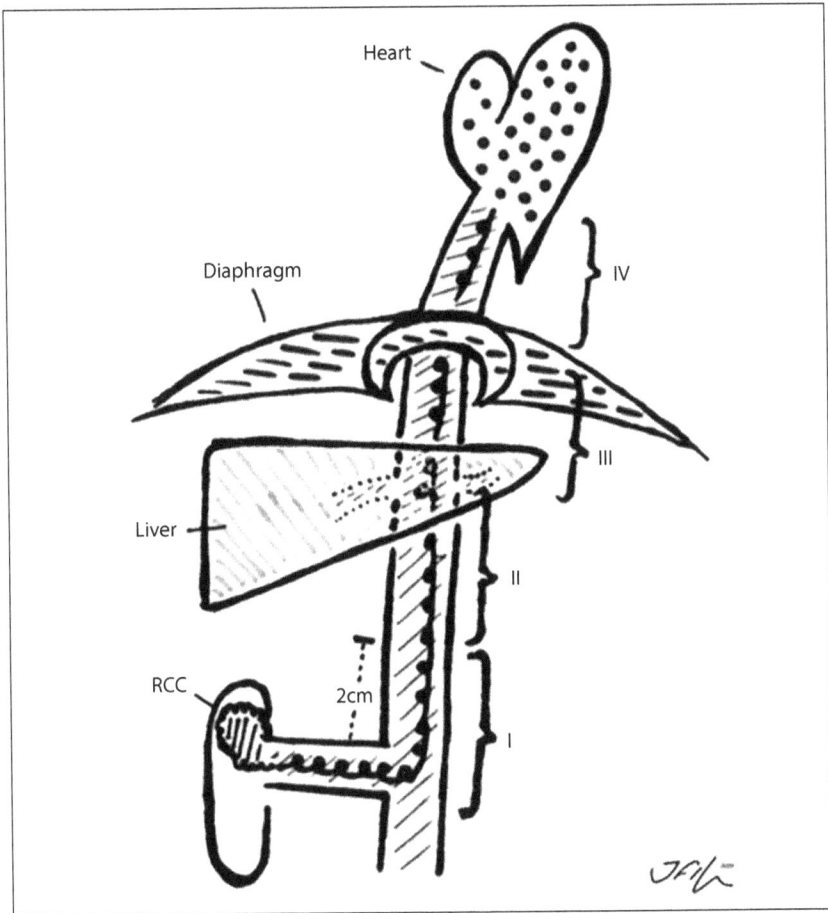

PROGNOSTIC FACTORS

Anatomical factors (TNM staging), histology grading and clinical factors (e.g. performance status, comorbidities, anaemia) all have an impact on prognosis in RCC.

Tumour grade is one of the most important prognostic factors.

WHO/ISUP Grading Classification

The former *Fuhrman* RCC grading system has been replaced by WHO/ISUP grading.

ISUP RCC grading system developed in 2012 and subsequently adopted by the WHO in 2016, validated for prognostication of RCC. [34]

Based on nucleolar prominence and eosinophilia.

Applies currently only to clear cell and papillary RCC sub-types (not chromophobe).

Table 21 – WHO/ISUP grading classification for renal tumours [35]

Grade	Description
1	Nucleoli absent or inconspicuous at x400 magnification
2	Nucleoli conspicuous and eosinophilic at x400 magnification but not prominent at x100 magnification
3	Nucleoli are conspicuous and eosinophilic at x100 magnification
4	Extreme nuclear pleomorphism, multi-nucleate giant cells and/or rhabdoid and/or sarcomatoid differentiation

Leibovich Scoring System

Leibovich scoring system used to predict an RCC patient's risk of developing metastases after RN. [36]

The risk categories are stratified as follows:

- *Low* risk: 0–2 points
- *Intermediate* risk: 3–5 points
- *High* risk: ≥ 6 points.

Metastasis-free survival at 10 years is 90% (low risk), 60% (intermediate risk) and 25% (high risk).

Table 22 – Leibovich scoring system for risk stratification of RCC after RN

	Score
T – stage	
pT1a	0
pT1b	2
pT2	3
pT3–4	4
Tumour size (cm)	
< 10cm	0
> 10cm	1
Regional lymph node(s)	
No nodes	0
Node(s) positive	2
Nuclear grade	
Grade 1–2	0
Grade 3	1
Grade 4	3
Tumour necrosis	
None	0
Present	1

TREATMENT

NEPHRON-SPARING SURGERY

There are various indications for undergoing partial nephrectomy (PN):

- *Absolute*, single kidney, bilateral synchronous RCC
- *Relative*, unilateral RCC with poorly functioning contra-lateral kidney and/or comorbid conditions predisposing to kidney disease (e.g. diabetes)
- Increased lifetime risk of further future renal cancers (e.g. VHL)
- *Elective*, localised unilateral RCC with normal contra-lateral kidney (T1 < 7cm).

Tumours near the hilum may make a patient unsuitable for PN.

Informed consent for PN must discuss risk of open conversion ($\leq$ 2%), conversion to RN ($\leq$ 10%), bleeding requiring embolisation ($\leq$ 10%), urine leak (0.5–2%) and positive margin ($\leq$ 8%).

Most common complication after PN for endophytic tumours is urine leak – this can be managed with antibiotics, stent insertion and leaving drain in situ.

EAU recommends PN should be offered to all suitable patients with T1 tumours. [31]

PN has been shown to better preserve kidney function but higher risk of bleeding than RN.

PN positive surgical margin $\leq$ 8% (higher than for RN), unclear whether any adverse impact on CSS (only $\leq$ 16% will have a recurrence) hence re-resection is not routinely indicated.

Oncological outcomes of open vs. laparoscopic vs. robot-assisted PN are comparable.

Open technique has shorter operative time, longer in-patient stay, greater blood loss.

Partial Nephrectomy Steps

The key steps for performing PN are:

- Patient is prepped and draped in lateral position and upward arc and WHO checklist complete
- Mobilise bowel, free up upper and lower poles and de-fat the kidney
- Identify and delineate the tumour, identify hilum
- Clamp vessels and start timer
- Excise tumour > 1mm margin, close any collecting system injury with absorbable sutures, drain placement (+/- stent).

Warm ischaemia time should be < 25 minutes.

Cold ischaemia (i.e. addition of ice) can mitigate this but challenging to employ in robotic surgery.

RENAL/PADUA Scores

PN is a challenging operation and scoring systems have been devised to predict the peri-operative complications of this procedure. [37]

Both RENAL and/or PADUA scores can be used, as they both broadly focus on radiological anatomical features and tumour size.

The PADUA score is detailed in Table 23 and Image 2.

The renal sinus was defined as the cavity surrounded by kidney parenchyma, lined by capsule and almost filled by renal vessels and pelvis with the remaining space filled by fat. [38]

Table 23 – PADUA scoring system for predicting peri-operative complications during PN

	1 point	2 points	3 points
Maximum radius (cm)	≤ 4	4–7	≥ 7
Exo-/endophytic	≥ 50% exophytic	< 50% exophytic	Entirely endophytic
Location to sinus line	Entirely above/ below or < 50% crossing	> 50% crossing or entirely between lines	
Renal rim	Lateral	Medial	
Renal sinus	No relationship	Renal sinus location	
Collecting system	Not involved	Infiltrated	

Image 2 – PADUA scoring system for peri-operative complications in PN

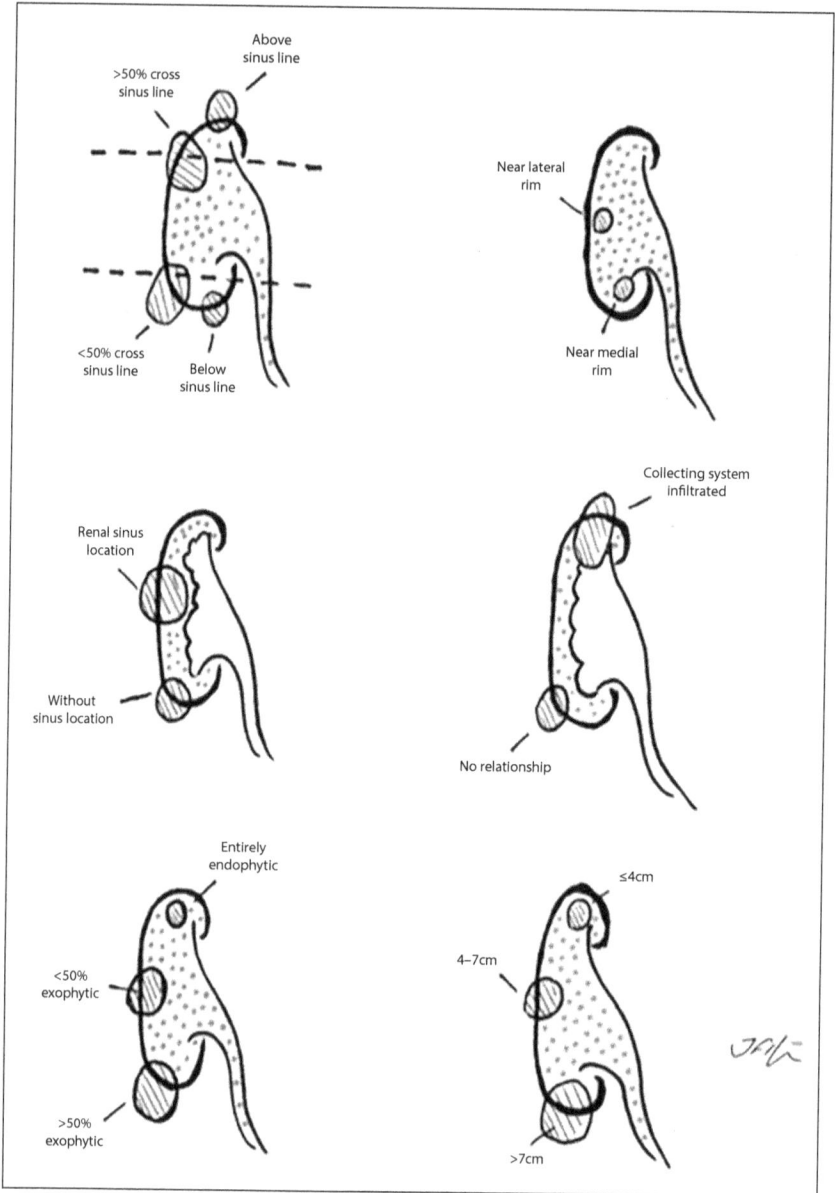

RADICAL NEPHRECTOMY

RN remains the gold-standard operation to treat T2–4 RCC and T1 unsuitable for PN.

Involves excising the kidney with all the tumour, Gerota's fascia +/- adrenalectomy +/- LND.

Laparoscopic vs. open RN have comparable oncological outcomes; however, laparoscopic has shorter in-patient stay, lower blood loss and morbidity, and greater operative time.

Retro- or intra-peritoneal approaches have similar oncological outcomes and QOL variables.

Retro-peritoneal approach allows early visualisation of the renal artery, reduced risk of injury to organs in peritoneal cavity and any bleeding is contained within retro-peritoneal cavity.

Trans-peritoneal allows more space for operative working field.

There is currently no role for any neo-adjuvant treatment prior to surgical intervention for RCC.

Adrenalectomy

Ipsilateral adrenalectomy in the absence of radiological/intra-operatively evident adrenal gland involvement has no survival advantage and is not indicated.

Only perform if pre-operative imaging suggests adrenal involvement (or found intra-operatively).

Lymph-node Dissection

The indication for LND together with PN or RN remains controversial.

If clinically enlarged then LND may be considered for staging purposes.

CT/MRI cannot distinguish metastatic vs. normal LN if node size is normal, and < 20% of dissected suspicious nodes during RN are positive for metastatic disease on histology anyway.

Currently in patients with localised disease without evidence of LN metastasis, performing LND in conjunction with RN confers no benefit to CSS or OS.

Adjuvant Treatment

NICE has approved use of pembrolizumab for adjuvant treatment of RCC after surgery in cases at high risk of recurrence.

There are several conditions that need to be met for eligibility:

- No more than 12 weeks must have elapsed from surgery
- Complete resection achieved (R0) and any M1 disease must have been completely resected (usually an up-to-date CT TAP is required prior to pembrolizumab treatment)
- Patient is at increased risk of recurrence (pT2N0M0 with G4 or sarcomatoid, pT3N0M0 with any grade, pT4N0M0 any grade, pTN1M0 any grade).

Pembrolizumab given as 400mg IV infusion every 6 weeks (NICE) – can be given 200mg every 3 weeks.

Given for maximum 1 year, treatment interrupted if not tolerated or recurrence occurs within the year.

> **KEY PAPER**   Choueiri et al. (2024) in *New England Journal of Medicine* [39]

- Double-blind trial of clear-cell RCC patients at an increased risk of recurrence after surgery
- 496 patients randomised 1:1 to receive (adjuvant pembrolizumab) vs. (adjuvant placebo)
- DFS and OS were primary and secondary key end-points respectively
- Found adjuvant pembrolizumab associated with significant improvement in OS (median follow-up 57.2 months) and is basis of subsequent NICE approval of its use.

Renal Artery Embolisation

Embolisation of the renal artery can be undertaken just before RN operation commences.

Embolisation reduces blood loss and may be indicated prior to operating on very large aggressive tumours.

"Post-infarction syndrome" is the most common complication – pain, nausea, fever.

ACTIVE SURVEILLANCE

AS is the initial monitoring of tumour size/features by serial abdominal imaging (US, CT, MRI) with delayed intervention reserved for tumours showing radiological progression.

Most renal tumours are slow growing.

Largest series of AS found growth of renal tumours was low and metastatic progression 1–2%. [40]

Overall, both short- and intermediate-term oncological outcomes indicate that in selected frail/comorbid patients, AS is initially appropriate to monitor small renal masses.

Lower long-term cancer-specific mortality for patients undergoing surgery.

CRYOTHERAPY

Cryotherapy of renal masses is generally reserved for tumours < 4cm in size.

Usually performed under GA, the kidney can be accessed CT-guided (percutaneous), loin incision (open) or laparoscopically +/- concurrent renal biopsy.

Involves direct insertion of freezing probes into tumour and two separate freeze–thaw cycles resulting in the formation of an "ice-ball".

Complication rates are comparable for percutaneous vs. laparoscopic techniques.

Complications of cryotherapy include:

- Infection, pain and bleeding requiring transfusion
- Need for further treatment
- Pneumothorax requiring insertion of chest drain
- Injury to liver, spleen, pancreas, bowel, major vessels.

Cryotherapy vs. RFA are comparable in oncological outcomes (OS, CSS, RFS) and complication rates.

Cryotherapy vs. PN have mixed results in terms of oncological outcomes and complication rates.

AS, RFA or cryotherapy should all be offered to elderly/comorbid patients with SRM.

RADIO-FREQUENCY ABLATION

Should be offered only to tumours < 4cm in size (EAU 2024).

Usually performed percutaneously under local anaesthetic (+/- sedation); however, occasionally under GA if laparoscopic RFA is performed.

Similar technical principles to cryotherapy; however, CT-guided imaging is used to place the electrode probes which create radio-frequency energy to heat the tumour and kill cancer cells.

Complications are similar to those listed for cryotherapy.

The most reliable method of determining treatment success after RFA is via CT/MRI with contrast, which should show a shrinkage in size and decrease in degree of tumour enhancement.

FOLLOW-UP

There is no consensus on radiological follow-up strategies after RCC treatment, as survival benefit of early recurrence detection during follow-up has yet to be proven.

No surveillance regimens have been validated or defined for ablative therapies.

Risk stratification after PN/RN is required to predict prognosis and determine follow-up schedule, which is the same whether patient had PN or RN.

For clear-cell RCC, the Leibovich scoring system is used.

EAU 2024 currently proposes lifelong surveillance following surgery for RCC.

Table 24 – EAU 2024 surveillance schedule following treatment for RCC

Risk Profile	Follow-up Date after Surgery								
	3 mo	6 mo	12 mo	18 mo	24 mo	30 mo	36 mo	> 3 years	> 5 years
Low risk									
(clear cell: Leibovich ≤ 2) (non-clear cell: pT1a–T1b pNX–0 M0 and grade ≤ 2)	-	CT	-	CT	-	CT	-	CT every 2 years	
Intermediate risk									
(clear cell: Leibovich 3–5)	-	CT	CT	-	CT	-	CT	CT once year	CT every 2 years
(non-clear cell: pT1b pNX–0 and/or grade 3–4)									
High risk									
(clear cell: Leibovich ≥ 6)	CT	CT	CT	CT	CT	-	CT	CT once year	CT every 2 years
(non-clear cell: pT2–4 any grade or pT any with pN1)									

METASTATIC RCC

25% of patients have mRCC at presentation, a further 30% progress to metastases after nephrectomy.

Patients will require MDT approach with input from oncology and palliative care teams.

The International Metastatic RCC Database Consortium may be used as prognostic risk stratification in mRCC and determining available treatment options.

Table 25 – International Metastatic RCC Database Consortium prognostic factors and risk categories for mRCC [41]

Prognostic Factor	Cut-off Point
Karnofsky performance status	< 80
Time from diagnosis to treatment	< 12 months
Haemoglobin	< LLN
Neutrophil	> ULN
Corrected serum calcium	> ULN
Platelet	> ULN

Risk Category	Factors Present
Good prognosis	0–1
Intermediate prognosis	2
Poor prognosis	> 2

MANAGEMENT

Cytoreductive Nephrectomy

For most patients with mRCC, CN is palliative and systemic treatments will be necessary if patient is fit; CN does not confer survival benefit in poor prognosis patients.

For select patients with oligo-metastases, CN can be curative if all deposits are excised.

Pre-operative embolisation can be used to reduce bleeding.

Sunitinib

Sunitinib is a targeted therapy drug and a TKI.

Tyrosine kinases are enzymes responsible for the activation of proteins by signal transduction cascades (phosphorylation – adding a phosphate group to the protein).

Sunitinib is an anti-angiogenic agent that targets the VEGF pathway.

Usual dosage is 50mg (PO) daily for 4 weeks followed by 2 weeks rest (i.e. a cycle is 6 weeks) and can be continued for as long as it is working and/or tolerated.

Sunitinib can be used in mRCC provided histological proof of renal cancer has been confirmed.

The renal cancer sub-type most likely to benefit from TKI therapy is clear-cell RCC.

KEY PAPER | CARMENA Trial [42]

- Trial of patients with confirmed mRCC (clear cell) who were fit for CN
- 450 patients randomised 1:1 to (CN + adjuvant sunitinib) vs. (sunitinib alone)
- Primary end-point was OS
- (Sunitinib alone) non-inferior to (CN + sunitinib) when used for intermediate- and poor-risk mRCC.

KEY PAPER | SURTIME Trial [43]

- Trial of patients with confirmed mRCC (clear cell) with resectable disease and fit for surgery
- 99 patients randomised 1:1 to (immediate CN + adjuvant sunitinib) vs. (3 cycles sunitinib, then CN if no progression on medication, then more sunitinib)
- Primary end-point was PFS, whilst OS and adverse events were secondary end-points
- Finding that deferred CN did not improve PFS at 28 weeks.

Other Oncological Options

Alternative TKI drugs for mRCC include pazopanib and axitinib.

mTOR inhibitors (e.g. everolimus) are drugs that inhibit the rapamycin target and can be considered in patients who are intolerant/failed targeted therapies.

Immunotherapy agents (e.g. pembrolizumab, nivolumab) can be used in appropriately experienced centres for patients who are intolerant/failed targeted therapies.

Do not offer chemotherapy to patients with mRCC (EAU 2024).

> **VIVA** | Oncological management of mRCC is complex and evolving, and you will not be expected to know all the finer details of medications for your FRCS (Urol) viva as this comes under the domain of the oncologist. However, you may be expected to discuss the use of TKI drugs and how this relates to CN, hence the trials I have included above.

BENIGN RENAL MASSES

Oncocytoma

Oncocytoma is the most common benign renal tumour (5% of all tumours) and tends to affect the elderly.

Most are diagnosed incidentally; however, can present with flank pain, VH, palpable mass.

Oncocytomas cannot reliably be distinguished radiologically from RCC. Signs for oncocytoma:

- Central stellate scar (CT/MRI)
- Spoke-wheel pattern of feeding arteries (angiography).

Macroscopically, they are spherical, homogenous, tan-coloured lesions.

Microscopically, they do not have any malignant features (e.g. invasion, metastases, lymphadenopathy) and are uniform eosinophilic cells packed with mitochondria.

RTB is not recommended because oncocytoma and RCC can co-exist, and eosinophilic variant of chromophobe RCC can be difficult to distinguish from oncocytoma on biopsy.

Treatment is PN or RN; however, after histological confirmation, patients do not need to be followed up.

Polycystic Kidney Disease

Autosomal dominant

- Associated with development of multiple expanding bilateral parenchymal cysts
- Commonly presents 30–40 years and leads to 10% of all cases of ESRF
- Associated with Berry aneurysms, hepatic cysts, diverticulosis and mitral valve prolapse
- Genetic defect located on short arm of chromosome 16 and PKD2 gene on chromosome 4

Autosomal recessive

- Much rarer and distinct from ADPKD as it presents in utero or in childhood
- Bilateral renal parenchyma enlargement replaced by radially orientated cysts
- Associated with biliary dysgenesis, pulmonary hypoplasia, oligo-hydramnios

Acquired Renal Cystic Disease

Condition occurring in patients with ESRF (particularly those on dialysis) as a result of prolonged high levels of nitrogen-containing compounds in the blood (azotaemia).

It is a feature of ESRF rather than being caused by its treatment.

Cysts that burst can result in pain and VH requiring embolisation.

The association of RCC and dialysis treatment is due to the malignant transformation of cysts; cut-off of 3cm in size raises suspicion of underlying RCC.

Multi-cystic Dysplastic Kidney

Can be sporadic or inherited in an autosomal dominant manner.

More common unilaterally; bilateral disease is lethal. Associated with contra-lateral PUJO and reflux.

Features irregular collection of tense non-communicating cysts lined with cuboidal tubular epithelium and dysplastic renal parenchyma.

Confers 4x increased risk of malignancy (Wilms' tumour, not RCC); however, prophylactic nephrectomy is not routinely recommended unless for treating refractory hypertension.

Almost always associated with ureteric atresia/obstruction.

Multi-locular Cyst (Cystic Nephroma)

More common in females and demonstrates bi-modal age distribution.

Benign bulky cysts, with thick capsules and highly echogenic septa – aspiration yields yellow fluid.

They range from being benign to Wilms' tumour to cystic RCC – surgical excision recommended.

UPPER-TRACT UROTHELIAL CANCER

EPIDEMIOLOGY

UTUC is uncommon, constituting approximately 5–10% of all urothelial cancers, and ≤ 10% of all renal malignancies, incidence increasing likely due to ageing population. [1]

Pelvi-calyceal TCC twice as common as ureteric TCC.

17% of patients with new diagnosis of UTUC also present with metachronous tumour(s) in the bladder.

Recurrences in the bladder after UTUC treatment occur in ≤ 29%; however, recurrences in the contra-lateral kidney are much less common (≤ 5%).

Lynch syndrome has familial links to UTUC; urinary tract should be screened for this at diagnosis.

UTUC are almost always urothelial carcinomas – sub-types are rare, but may include squamous or sarcomatoid differentiations, which worsen prognosis.

RISK FACTORS

Age	- Peak incidence age 70–90 years
Gender	- More common in men (70% of cases)
Smoking	- 2.5–7x increased RR [43]
Occupation	- Aromatic amine exposure (rubber and dye manufacturing, pesticides)
HNPCC	- (Lynch syndrome) is a cancer syndrome associated with UTUC
Drugs	- Phenacetin (NSAID no longer in use), aristolochic acid (Chinese herbal medicine)
Genetic	- Chromosome 9, 17 (p53 loci) and 13 (retinoblastoma gene), Lynch syndrome

DIAGNOSIS

The most common symptom is painless visible haematuria.

Other symptoms may include flank pain (clot colic or obstruction), weight loss, anorexia, malaise and night sweats which raise concern regarding possibility of metastatic disease.

Cystoscopy should be performed if VH – but also without VH if UTUC found on imaging, due to the risk of metachronous bladder cancer.

Imaging

CTU has the highest accuracy for detecting UTUC of all the imaging techniques:

- Radiological finding of hydronephrosis is a poor prognostic sign
- Enlarged local LN is highly predictive of metastasis.

MRU (gadolinium-based contrast) is an alternative to CTU for patients contraindicated to radiation or iodinated contrast media; however, not suitable if eGFR < 30mL/min.

Cytology

Should preferably be performed "selectively" in situ, with a ureteric catheter collecting during URS (prior to performing retrograde study, which can cause deterioration of sample).

Voided urine cytology is alternative option but less sensitive than selective urine.

Diagnostic Ureteroscopy

This should be used in scenarios of clinical uncertainty or when kidney-sparing surgery is considered, such as single kidney.

BAUS review found 80% of nephroureterectomies did not have prior histological diagnosis (and almost all specimens confirmed malignancy). [1]

Under-staging with ureteroscopic biopsies is common.

EAU 2024 accepts upfront RNU in cases where imaging/cytology supports UTUC diagnosis.

STAGING

The majority of UTUCs are invasive at diagnosis (60%) when compared to bladder tumours (15%).

Concurrent bladder tumours with UTUC are common (17%) and recurrences in the bladder after UTUC treatment occur in 22–47%.

Synchronous and metachronous UTUCs occur in 3% approximately, highlighting the importance of surveillance (cystoscopic, radiological and cytological) for these patients.

Table 26 – TNM staging classification for UTUC [44]

T – Primary Tumour	
TX	Primary tumour cannot be assessed
T0	No evidence of primary tumour
Ta	Non-invasive papillary carcinoma
Tis	Carcinoma in situ
T1	Tumour invades sub-epithelial connective tissue
T2	Tumour invades muscularis
T3	(Renal pelvis) – tumour invades beyond muscularis into peripelvic fat or renal parenchyma
	(Ureter) – tumour invades beyond muscularis into periureteric fat
T4	Tumour invades adjacent organs or through the kidney into perinephric
N – Lymph Nodes	
NX	Regional lymph nodes cannot be assessed
N0	No regional lymph node metastasis
N1	Metastasis in single lymph node $\leq$ 2cm in greatest dimension
N2	Metastasis in single lymph node > 2cm in greatest dimension or multiple lymph nodes
M – Metastasis	
M0	No distant metastasis
M1	Distant metastasis

PROGNOSTIC FACTORS

Many prognostic factors have been identified and can be used to risk-stratify patients.

Patient-related factors which worsen prognosis include:

- Increasing age
- Genetic predisposition (e.g. Lynch syndrome)
- Smoking history
- Increasing comorbidities, WHO performance status.

Tumour-related factors which worsen prognosis include:

- Increasing T-stage (muscle-invasive disease carries poor prognosis) and grade
- Multi-focality of tumours
- Presence of hydro-ureteronephrosis
- Increasing tumour size
- Tumour necrosis, lympho-vascular invasion and/or LN involvement.

To date there is not a validated score/nomogram/model that can be used for UTUC risk stratification.

Risk should therefore be assessed and discussed on a case-by-case basis.

TREATMENT

LOCALISED LOW-RISK UTUC

KSS for low-risk UTUC spares the patient from the morbidity of major surgery, without compromising renal function or oncological outcome.

In low-risk disease, survival is similar between KSS and RNU. [44]

KSS should be considered as primary approach in all low-risk tumours, and in imperative cases for high-risk disease (e.g. single kidney, chronic renal impairment). [44]

PN is not routinely considered as an option for treating low-risk UTUC.

An isolated distal ureteric tumour should be treated with excision of cuff of bladder; however, a ureteric segmental resection has a role where renal preservation is paramount (e.g. single kidney).

Ureteroscopy

Ablation of UTUC via rigid/flexible URS using Ho:YAG or Nd:YAG LASER (retrograde stenting required) can be used in low-risk disease provided complete tumour destruction achievable.

Patient needs to be informed of likely need of early second re-look and the need for stringent follow-up.

Percutaneous Access

Disrupts urothelial integrity and is more invasive; however, it allows excellent access to renal pelvis with 30Fr sheath to ablate/resect tumour.

Allows delivery of adjuvant therapy such as MMC or BCG.

Potential risk of tumour seeding.

Adjuvant Instillations

BCG or MMC can be instilled in antegrade fashion via PCN (after KSS management), provided there is no ureteric obstruction or leakage.

Single adjuvant MMC dose may reduce risk of recurrence, although clear benefit remains to be proven.

LOCALISED HIGH-RISK UTUC

Radical Nephroureterectomy

Cystoscopy prior to RNU must be undertaken to rule out bladder tumour.

RNU with bladder cuff excision is the standard treatment for UTUC regardless of its location.

Open RNU can be done entirely through a midline incision, or with a loin incision and a second Pfannensteil or lower midline incision for the cuff.

Laparoscopic/open/robotic RNU have similar oncological outcomes.

Distal ureter can be mobilised via *"rip and pluck"*, whereby it is cystoscopically resected to peri-vesical fat and then plucked during dissection. Avoids second incision but risks tumour cell spillage.

LND should not be performed for TaT1 disease.

Adjuvant Therapy

Radiotherapy has no role in the management of UTUC.

Due to risk of bladder TCC recurrence after UTUC treatment (≤ 47%), single-instillation MMC should be given soon after RNU (EAU 2024). [44]

Adjuvant platinum-based systemic chemotherapy should be given to pT2–4 patients if fit.

| **KEY PAPER** | POUT Trial [45] |

- Multi-centre UK-based RCT evaluating role of chemotherapy after RNU in UTUC
- 261 patients with WHO performance status 0–1
- Randomised 1:1 to (post-operative surveillance) vs. (x4 cycles adjuvant cisplatin chemotherapy)
- Primary end-point was DFS at 3 years
- Found benefit of adjuvant chemotherapy (DFS of 71% treatment arm vs. 46% surveillance)

FOLLOW-UP

Close follow-up of UTUC is essential to monitor for metachronous bladder and contra-lateral recurrences (diagnostic tools include flexible cystoscopy, cytology, CTU, URS).

There is no defined validated follow-up scheme recognised in clinical practice.

After RNU a follow-up regimen could include:

- (*Low-risk*) cystoscopy at 3 months, 12 months and then yearly for 5 years
- (*High-risk*) cystoscopy + cytology 3-monthly for 2 years, then 6-monthly for 3 years and then annually thereafter, and CT TAP with urographic phase every 6 months.

For patients who have undergone KSS, the follow-up should be more intense and therefore relies on significant patient compliance.

After KSS a follow-up regimen could include:

- (*Low-risk*) cystoscopy + CTU at 3 and 6 months, then yearly for 5 years, re-look URS at 3 months
- (*High-risk*) early second look URS + cytology; if clear then follow principles for high-risk follow-up as per post-RNU patients.

METASTATIC DISEASE

Approximately 1 in 10 patients present with metastatic disease, which carries a poor prognosis.

MDT discussion should include input from oncology and palliative care teams.

Platinum-based chemotherapy remained standard of care for advanced or metastatic UTUC – cisplatin is preferred agent, carboplatin can be used if patient unfit for cisplatin.

Evidence supports using enfortumab + pembrolizumab to improve PFS and OS [46], but this is currently not recommended by NICE.

RNU may have a role in symptomatic patients for palliative purposes, role of metastasectomy is limited.

REFERENCES

1. Mak D, Khan MJ, Fernando HS (2018). Urothelial cancer. In: Arya M, Shergill IS, Fernando HS, et al., *Viva Practice for the FRCS (Urol) and Postgraduate Urology Examinations*, second edition, CRC Press, London.
2. Pareek G, Shevchuk M, Armenakas NA, et al. (2003). The effect of finasteride on the expression of vascular endothelial growth factor and microvessel density: a possible mechanism for decreased prostatic bleeding in treated patients. *Journal of Urology*, *169*(1), 20–23.
3. Britton JP, Dowell AC, Whelan P (1992). A community study of bladder cancer screening by the detection of occult urinary bleeding. *Journal of Urology*, *148*(3 Part 1), 788–790.
4. Messing EM, Madeb RR, Golijanin D (2006). 881: Long-Term Outcome of Hematuria Home Screening for Bladder Cancer (BC). *Journal of Urology*, *175*(4S), 284–285.
5. Khadra MH, Pickard RS, Charlton M (2000). A prospective analysis of 1,930 patients with hematuria to evaluate current diagnostic practice. *Journal of Urology*, *163*(2), 524–527.
6. NICE 2023 guideline: Suspected cancer: recognition and referral. Available at: https://www.nice.org.uk/guidance/ng12/resources/suspected-cancer-recognition-and-referral-pdf-1837268071621 [last accessed 28 July 2024].
7. Price SJ, Shephard EA, Stapley SA, et al. (2014). Non-visible versus visible haematuria and bladder cancer risk: a study of electronic records in primary care. *British Journal of General Practice*, *64*(626), e584–e589.
8. Heer R, Lewis R, Vadiveloo T, et al. (2022). A Randomized Trial of PHOTOdynamic Surgery in Non-Muscle-Invasive Bladder Cancer. *NEJM Evidence*, 1(10), 1–10.
9. Pontero P, Birtle A, Comperat E, et al. (2024). EAU Guidelines on Non-muscle-invasive Bladder Cancer (TaT1 and CIS). Available at: https://d56bochluxqnz.cloudfront.net/documents/full-guideline/EAU-Guidelines-on-Non-muscle-Invasive-Bladder-Cancer-2024.pdf [last accessed 28 July 2024].
10. Montironi R, Lopez-Beltran A (2005). The 2004 WHO classification of bladder tumors: a summary and commentary. *International Journal of Surgical Pathology*, *13*(2), 143–153.
11. NICE: Managing non-muscle-invasive bladder cancer (2020). Available at: https://pathways.nice.org.uk/pathways/bladder-cancer/managing-muscle-invasive-bladder-cancer [last accessed 29 May 2020].

12. Sylvester RJ, Oosterlinck W, Holmang S, et al. (2016). Systematic review and individual patient data meta-analysis of randomised trials comparing a single immediate instillation of chemotherapy after transurethral resection with transurethral resection alone in patients with stage pTa-pT1 urothelial carcinoma of the bladder: which patients benefit from the instillation. *European Urology, 69*(2), 231–244.

13. Angulo JC, Alvarez-Ossorio JL, Dominguez-Escrig JL, et al. (2023). Hyperthermic Mitomycin C in intermediate-risk non-muscle-invasive Bladder Cancer: Results of HIVEC-1 Trial. *European Urology Oncology, 6*(1), 58–66.

14. Sylvester RJ, van der Meijden AP, Lamm DL (2002). Intravesical bacillus Calmette–Guerin reduces the risk of progression in patients with superficial bladder cancer: a meta-analysis of the published results of randomized clinical trials. *Journal of Urology, 168*(5), 1,964–1,970.

15. Johnston MC, Marks A, Crilly MA (2015). Charlson index scores from administrative data and case-note review compared favourably in a renal disease cohort. *European Journal of Public Health, 25*(3), 391–396.

16. Witjes JA, Bruins M, Carrion A, et al. (2024). EAU Guidelines on Muscle-invasive and Metastatic Bladder Cancer. Available at: https://d56bochluxqnz.cloudfront.net/documents/full-guideline/EAU-Guidelines-on-Muscle-Invasive-and-Metastatic-Bladder-Cancer-2024.pdf [last accessed on 30 July 2024].

17. NICE: Appendix C, WHO performance status classification. Available at: https://www.nice.org.uk/guidance/ta121/chapter/Appendix-C-WHO-performance-status-classification [last accessed 30 May 2020].

18. Agnew N (2010). Preoperative cardiopulmonary exercise testing. *Continuing Education in Anaesthesia, Critical Care & Pain, 10*(2), 33–37.

19. Vale CL (2005). Neoadjuvant chemotherapy in invasive bladder cancer: update of a systematic review and meta-analysis of individual patient data: Advanced Bladder Cancer (ABC) Meta-analysis Collaboration. *European Urology, 48*(2), 202–206.

20. NICE: Managing muscle-invasive bladder cancer (2020). Available at: https://pathways.nice.org.uk/pathways/bladder-cancer/managing-muscle-invasive-bladder-cancer [last accessed 30 May 2020].

21. Lonser RR, Glenn GM, Walther M (2003). von Hippel–Lindau disease. *Lancet, 361*(9,374), 2,059–2,067.

22. Menko FH, Van Steensel MA, Giraud S, et al. (2009). Birt–Hogg–Dubé syndrome: diagnosis and management. *Lancet Oncology, 10*(12), 1,199–1,206.

23. Haas NB, Nathanson KL (2014). Hereditary kidney cancer syndromes. *Advances in Chronic Kidney Disease, 21*(1), 81–90.
24. Koo KC, Won TK, Won SH (2010). Trends of presentation and clinical outcome of treated renal angiomyolipoma. *Yonsei Medical Journal, 51*(5), 728–734.
25. Luca D, Rossetti R (1999). Management of renal angiomyolipoma: a report of 53 cases. *BJU International, 83*(3), 215–218.
26. Crino PB, Nathanson KL, Henske EP (2006). The tuberous sclerosis complex. *New England Journal of Medicine, 355*(13), 1,345–1,356.
27. Medda M, Picozzi SC, Bozzini G (2009). Wunderlich's syndrome and hemorrhagic shock. *Journal of Emergencies, Trauma and Shock, 2*(3), 203.
28. Maheshwari E, O'Malley ME, Ghai S (2010). Split-bolus MDCT urography: upper tract opacification and performance for upper tract tumors in patients with hematuria. *American Journal of Roentgenology, 194*(2), 453–458.
29. Bromwich E, Qteishat A, Fernando HS, et al. (2018). In: *Viva Practice for the FRCS (Urol) and Postgraduate Urology Examinations*, second edition, CRC Press, London.
30. Marconi L, Dabestani S, Lam TB (2016). Systematic review and meta-analysis of diagnostic accuracy of percutaneous renal tumour biopsy. *European Urology, 69*(4), 660–673.
31. Ljungberg B, Bex A, Albiges L, et al. (2024). EAU Guidelines on Renal Cell Carcinoma. Available at: https://d56bochluxqnz.cloudfront.net/documents/full-guideline/EAU-Guidelines-on-Renal-Cell-Carcinoma-2024.pdf [last accessed 10 July 2024].
32. Adams LC, Ralla B, Bender YNY, et al. (2018). Renal cell carcinoma with venous extension: prediction of inferior vena cava wall invasion by MRI. *Cancer Imaging, 18*(1), 17.
33. Sweeney P, Wood CG, Pisters LL, et al. (2003). Surgical management of renal cell carcinoma associated with complex inferior vena caval thrombi. *Urol Oncol, 21*, 327–333.
34. Delahunt B, Eble JN, Egevad L (2019). Grading of renal cell carcinoma. *Histopathology, 74*(1), 4–17.
35. Moch H (2016). The WHO/ISUP grading system for renal carcinoma. *Der Pathologe, 37*(4), 355–360.
36. Leibovich BC, Blute ML, Cheville JC, et al. (2003). Prediction of progression after radical nephrectomy for patients with clear cell renal cell carcinoma: a stratification tool for prospective clinical trials. *Cancer: Interdisciplinary International Journal of the American Cancer Society, 97*(7), 1,663–1,671.

37. Hew MN, Baseskioglu B, Barwari K, et al. (2011). Critical appraisal of the PADUA classification and assessment of the RENAL nephrometry score in patients undergoing partial nephrectomy. *Journal of Urology, 186*(1), 42–46.

38. Ficarra V, Novara G, Secco S, et al. (2009). Preoperative aspects and dimensions used for an anatomical (PADUA) classification of renal tumours in patients who are candidates for nephron-sparing surgery. *European Urology, 56*(5), 786–793.

39. Choueiri TK, Tomczak P, Park SH, et al. (2024). Overall Survival with Adjuvant Pembrolizumab in Renal-Cell Carcinoma. *New England Journal of Medicine, 390*(15), 1,359–1,371.

40. Jewett MA, Mattar K, Basiuk J (2011). Active surveillance of small renal masses: progression patterns of early stage kidney cancer. *European Urology, 60*(1), 39–44.

41. Ko JJ, Xie W, Kroeger N, et al. (2015). The International Metastatic Renal Cell Carcinoma Database Consortium model as a prognostic tool in patients with metastatic renal cell carcinoma previously treated with first-line targeted therapy: a population-based study. *Lancet Oncology, 16*(3), 293–300.

42. Méjean A, Ravaud A, Thezenas S, et al. (2018). Sunitinib alone or after nephrectomy in metastatic renal-cell carcinoma. *New England Journal of Medicine, 379*(5), 417–427.

43. Bex A, Mulders P, Jewett M, et al. (2019). Comparison of Immediate vs Deferred Cytoreductive Nephrectomy in Patients with Synchronous Metastatic Renal Cell Carcinoma Receiving Sunitinib: The SURTIME Randomised Clinical Trial. *JAMA Oncology, 5*(2), 164–170.

44. Masson-Lecomte A, Gontero P, Birtle A, et al. (2024). EAU Guidelines on Upper Urinary Tract Urothelial Carcinoma. Available at: https://d56bochluxqnz.cloudfront.net/documents/full-guideline/EAU-Guidelines-on-Upper-Urinary-Tract-Urothelial-Carcinoma-2024.pdf [last accessed 10 August 2024].

45. Birtle A, Johnson M, Chester J, et al. (2020). Adjuvant chemotherapy in upper tract urothelial carcinoma (the POUT trial): a phase 3, open-label, randomised controlled trial. *Lancet, 395*(10,232), 1,268–1,277.

46. Powles T, Valderrama BP, Gupta S, et al. (2024). Enfortumab Vedotin and Pembrolizumab in Untreated Advanced Urothelial Cancer. *New England Journal of Medicine, 390*(10), 875–888.

UROLOGICAL ONCOLOGY 1 MCQS

1. Which of the following statements regarding the use of finasteride to treat BPH-related visible haematuria is false?

    A) Half-life of oral finasteride is 6 hours in adults
    B) Finasteride is a highly lipophilic compound
    C) Finasteride prevents the formation of neurosteroids
    D) Cases of finasteride overdose can be treated with inclisiran
    E) Finasteride reduces GABAA activity

2. What is the correct range of wavelength of blue light utilised in PDD cystoscopy?

    A) 280–350nm
    B) 380–450nm
    C) 480–550nm
    D) 580–650nm
    E) 680–750nm

3. As an alternative to 5-ALA, what other prodrug can be instilled into the bladder to perform PDD cystoscopy?

    A) Pentaminolevulinate
    B) Hexaminolevulinate
    C) Heptaminolevulinate
    D) Octaminolevulinate
    E) Nonaminolevulinate

4. What is the chemical component in tobacco-based cigarettes that is linked to the increased risk of developing bladder cancer?

    A) Acetalaldehyde
    B) Polycyclic aromatic hydrocarbons
    C) Nicotine-derived nitrosamine ketone
    D) Cumene
    E) Arylamines

5. What is the correct TNM 2017 staging for a newly diagnosed patient with bladder cancer, whose tumour invades the deep muscle and staging CT TAP reveals metastatic disease in three obturator nodes and two axillary nodes?

    A) T2aN1M1
    B) T2bN2M1b
    C) T2aN2M1a
    D) T2bN2M1a
    E) T2bN1M1b

6. What is the correct TNM 2017 staging for a newly diagnosed patient with
    bladder cancer, whose tumour invades the uterus and staging CT TAP
    reveals metastatic disease in one common iliac node?

    A) T4aN1M0
    B) T4aN0M1a
    C) T4aN3M0
    D) T4bN1M0
    E) T4bN1M1a

7. Which of the following NMIBC histologies would put the patient in the
    intermediate risk group based on NICE 2015 guidelines?

    A) Multi-focal G2pTa LG
    B) Solitary G2pTa LG, 2cm in size, which is a recurrence after 18 months
    C) Solitary G3pTa, 1cm in size
    D) Solitary G2pT1
    E) G1pTa + CIS

8. Which of the following is not a BCG strain which has been developed for
    intra-vesical instillation in the treatment of bladder cancer?

    A) BCG-cyst
    B) Connaught strain
    C) Pasteur strain
    D) Oncotice
    E) Immunobladder

9. Which of the following is not a routinely measured value given by CPEX
    testing?

    A) VO2
    B) VCO2
    C) Lactate
    D) Anaerobic threshold
    E) Work rate

10. What is the correct absolute improvement in survival in MIBC if patients are
     given NAC prior to local therapy (radical cystectomy or EBRT)?

    A) 2.5%
    B) 5%
    C) 7.5%
    D) 10%
    E) 12.5%

11. *What is the approximate length of ileum used for ileal conduit formation as urinary diversion technique in radical cystectomy?*

   A) 5–10cm
   B) 15–20cm
   C) 20–25cm
   D) 25–30cm
   E) 35–40cm

12. *What structure forms the lateral border of a standard lymph-node dissection in radical cystectomy?*

   A) Obturator internus
   B) Circumflex iliac vein
   C) Lacunar ligament
   D) Cloquet's node
   E) Genitofemoral nerve

13. *To which structure does a super-extended lymph-node dissection reach cranially during radical cystectomy?*

   A) Coeliac trunk
   B) Internal iliac bifurcation
   C) Common iliac bifurcation
   D) Inferior mesenteric artery
   E) Aortic bifurcation

14. *What is the typical curative dose of moderately hypofractionated EBRT given to treat MIBC?*

   A) 25Gy
   B) 35Gy
   C) 45Gy
   D) 55Gy
   E) 65Gy

15. *Histology from recent radical cystectomy has confirmed pT3 N1 M0 TCC bladder; however, the patient is ineligible for cisplatin-based chemotherapy. Which agent would you consider prescribing?*

   A) Atezolizumab
   B) Penbrolizumab
   C) Nivolumab
   D) Adalimumab
   E) Bevacizumab

16. *On which chromosome is the VHL tumour suppressor gene located?*

    A) 3
    B) 5
    C) 7
    D) 9
    E) 11

17. *Which of the following are not typically associated with VHL syndrome?*

    A) Serous cystadenoma of pancreas
    B) Papillary cystadenoma of epididymis
    C) Spinal cord haemangioblastoma
    D) Neuroendocrine tumour of pancreas
    E) Cerebellar medulloblastoma

18. *The mutation of which gene on chromosome 17 is associated with BHD syndrome?*

    A) RHEB
    B) FCLN
    C) APOL1
    D) MGP
    E) BHD

19. *On which chromosome is the TSC1 abnormality located in tuberous sclerosis?*

    A) 5
    B) 7
    C) 9
    D) 11
    E) 13

20. *Which of the following regarding AML is false?*

    A) They appear as hyper-echoic on US
    B) They are mesenchymal tumours
    C) Epithelioid variant is more commonly associated with malignancy
    D) They belong to a group of tumours called PEComa
    E) They are not associated with phakomatoses

21. Which of the following is not a factor used in the calculation of Leibovich Score in RCC?

    A) Dimension
    B) N-stage
    C) M-stage
    D) Tumour necrosis
    E) T-stage

22. A patient has undergone radical nephrectomy, with full staging imaging and histology available, the tumour was extending into the renal sinus fat, involvement of contra-lateral adrenal gland and no lymph nodes were involved. What is the correct TNM stage?

    A) T3aN0M0
    B) T3aN0M1
    C) T3bN0M0
    D) T3bN0M1
    E) T4N0M0

23. What is the correct IV infusion dose and regime for adjuvant pembrolizumab after patient surgery for RCC?

    A) 400mg (IV) every 3 weeks
    B) 600mg (IV) every 3 weeks
    C) 200mg (IV) every 6 weeks
    D) 400mg (IV) every 6 weeks
    E) 600mg (IV) every 6 weeks

24. Which of the following is not associated with autosomal dominant polycystic kidney disease?

    A) Mitral valve prolapse
    B) Aortic valve stenosis
    C) Liver cysts
    D) Berry aneurysms
    E) Abdominal wall hernias

25. Which of the following is not a factor used in the International mRCC Database Consortium to predict survival with systemic therapy?

    A) Karnovsky performance status < 60%
    B) < 1 year from time of diagnosis to systemic therapy
    C) Platelets > upper limit of normal
    D) Neutrophils > upper limit of normal
    E) Corrected calcium > upper limit of normal

26. *Which plant extract used in Chinese traditional medicine is associated with an increased risk of developing UTUC?*

    A) Icariin
    B) Coptis chinensis
    C) Isatis indigotica
    D) Astralagus
    E) Aristolochic acid

27. *A patient's RNU specimen histology has shown UTUC invading the muscularis and involvement of multiple regional lymph nodes, full staging imaging confirms enlarged regional lymph nodes. What is the correct TNM staging?*

    A) T2N2M0
    B) T2N0M1
    C) T3aN1M0
    D) T3aN2M0
    E) T3bN0M1

PROSTATE CANCER

EPIDEMIOLOGY

PCa is the second most common cancer in men diagnosed worldwide (14% of all cancers); however, it is the most common cancer in men in the UK.

51,000+ cases diagnosed in UK yearly – more prevalent in developed countries (disease of old age) and greater incidence in countries with highest rates of screening.

Post-mortem studies – evidence of PCa in 30% of 50 year olds, ≤ 71% of > 79 year olds.

Lifetime risk 1 in 8 in the UK. (However, only 3% of all male deaths will be due to PCa.)

The most common age for men to be diagnosed with prostate cancer is between 70 and 74 years.

71% of PCa deaths occur > 75 years.

Late-stage diagnosis is more common in aged > 80 years (56% stage 3–4 at time of diagnosis). [1]

RISK FACTORS

Age
- 75% of all cancers diagnosed in men > 65 years. (However, vitamin-D deficiency is more common in elderly.)

Ethnicity
- Afro-Caribbean > White > Asians (their migration west increases risk). [2]

- Higher risk in Scandinavia and countries adopting a Westernised diet; proposed association with reduced sunlight exposure + vitamin D.

- Afro-Caribbean men have relative incidence of 1.6 compared to white men.

- In UK, 1 in 4 black men will get prostate cancer in their lifetime.

Hereditary (true only in 9%)

- Defined as (3+ affected relatives) and/or (3+ successive generations) and/or (2+ with early onset disease i.e. < 55 years).

- > 100 common susceptibility loci (including BRCA) identified contributing to risk of (aggressive) prostate cancer (~15% of all cases harbour any germline mutation).

- RRx2 (x1 first-degree rel.), RRx4 (x2 first-degree rel.), RRx5 if hereditary.

- BRCA1/2 carriers more frequently associated with ISUP ≥ 4, T3/4 stage, nodal or mPca compared to non-carriers.

Obesity	- Lower risk of low-grade PCa, higher risk of high-grade PCa (REDUCE study).
	- Cholesterol/HDLs/LDLs no risk association, statins do not confer protection against PCa (REDUCE study). [3]
	- Lower circulating androgens (causing lower PSA) and higher free IGF-1 levels.
Exercise	- Confers protection vs. PCa.
	- Proposed mechanism by reducing IGF-1, insulin, testosterone.
	- Stimulates antioxidant pathways to reduce harmful reactive oxygen species.
Diet	- Current evidence will not support a causal relationship between any dietary factor and development of PCa (lack of high-quality evidence).
	- Proposed increase risk: dairy (high calcium which suppresses vitamin D), excess or abstinence from alcohol (i.e. J-shape), vitamin E (SELECT Trial). [4]
	- Proposed decrease risk: lycopene (carotene) in tomato (cooked tomato-based foods).
Vitamin D	- U-shaped relationship with PCa.
	- Polymorphisms result in vitamin-D receptors with lower activity increasing PCa risk.
Testosterone	- No reported increased risk when given to hypogonadal men. [5]
5ARIs	- Not approved by EMA for the role of chemoprevention (but you should be able to discuss the theory of chemoprevention if asked i.e. PCPT and REDUCE).

- Proposed lower incidence of PCa but slightly higher risk of high-grade PCa, albeit not impacting mortality (PCPT). [6]

Prostatitis   - Chronic prostatitis or inflammation, IBD, gonorrhoea, CMV, HPV – impaired ability to combat oxidative stress.

GENETIC PREDISPOSITIONS

Gene fusions are common in PCa and are fundamental for cancer growth and progression.

Most commonly involves fusion of TMPRSS2 to members of ETS family.

Promotes genes under androgenic control (fusion found in up to 50% cases of primary PCa). [7]

TMPRSS2-related gene fusions are highly specific for PCa.

The TMPRSS2 is prostate specific and expressed in both benign and malignant prostatic epithelium.

A variety of other genes are implicated in PCa:

- Cell-cycle genes: cyclinD2, 14-3-3
- DNA repair genes: GSTpi, GPX3 and GSTM1
- Tumour suppressor genes: APC, RASSF1alpha, DKK3, E-cadherin
- Hormonal response genes: ERalphaA, ERbeta, RARbeta.

| KEY PAPER | PCPT Trial (2003) [6]

PCPT – Prostate Cancer Prevention Trial

Recruited 18,000 men with no known evidence of PCa and PSA < 3ng/mL.

Randomised to placebo vs. finasteride 5mg OD for < 7 years.

TRUS biopsy was performed if: rising PSA > 4, new abnormal DRE or once end of study.

Placebo arm (24% had PCa) vs. finasteride arm (18% had PCa) – reduce risk by 25%.

Higher incidence of high-grade PCa with finasteride (6.4%) vs. placebo (5.1%).

KEY PAPER | REDUCE Trial (2010) [3]

REDUCE – Reduction of Dutasteride of Prostate Cancer Events

International, multi-centre, double-blind, placebo-controlled chemo-prevention study.

Inclusion: negative prostate biopsy within 6 months of entry and PSA 2.5–10 (50–60 years) and PSA 3–10 (> 60 years), total of 6,700+ patients.

TRUS biopsy repeated at 2 and 4 years after entry into trial.

Relative risk reduction of PCa by 22% in dutasteride arm (but higher incidence of high-grade PCa).

KEY PAPER | SELECT Trial (2011) [4]

SELECT – Selenium and Vitamin E Cancer Prevention Trial

Multi-centre trial from North America of 35,000 men.

Inclusion: PSA < 4, no PCa suggested by DRE, age > 50 years (black) and > 55 years (all others).

Randomly assigned to 4 groups: (selenium) vs. (vitamin E) vs. (vitamin E + selenium) vs. (placebo).

Main outcome measure: PCa incidence.

Finding: <u>vitamin E significantly increased PCa incidence</u>. (However, combination treatment had no effect.)

SCREENING

VIVA | You should be prepared to discuss PSA screening in a viva station, which should include firstly a mention of Wilson and Jungner criteria followed by overview of evidence (e.g. ProtecT and ERSPC).

EAU 2023 recommends not to subject men to PSA testing without counselling them on risks vs. benefits (*strong*).

PSA screening for PCa is controversial and does not fulfil all Wilson and Jungner's criteria for a screening programme, as listed below: [8]

Table 1 – Wilson and Jungner classic screening criteria

Condition should be an important health problem.

There should be an accepted treatment for patients with disease.

Facilities for diagnosis and treatment should be available.

There should be a recognisable latent or early symptomatic stage.

There should be a suitable test for the disease.

The test should be acceptable to the population.

The natural history of the condition should be adequately understood.

There should be an agreed policy on whom to treat as patients.

The cost of case-finding should be balanced in relation to medical care cost as a whole.

Case-finding should be a continuing process and not a "once and for all" project.

PSA lacks specificity (only 40%) and sensitivity.

PCa has long latent period allowing patient to die from other causes.

The incidence of PCa is highest in countries with the highest uptake of PCa screening.

| KEY PAPER | PLCO Trial (2009) [9] |

PLCO – Prostate, Lung, Colon and Ovary

76,000+ men (aged 55–74 years) enrolled in multi-centre trial in the USA.

Randomly assigned to intervention (organised annual PSA testing for 6 years and annual DRE for 4 years) vs. control (usual care including opportunistic screening).

No difference in PCa mortality in organised systematic annual PSA testing vs. opportunistic PSA testing (although 52% of control arm had ad-hoc screening).

| KEY PAPER | ProtecT Trial (2017) [10] |

ProtecT – Prostate Testing for Cancer and Treatment

Obtained men from "PCa study" – 82,000 recruited (aged 50–69 years) between 1999 and 2009 via PSA test, of which 2,664 received diagnosis of localised PCa.

Patients then randomised equally between radiotherapy (RTx) vs. radical prostatectomy (RP) vs. active surveillance (AS).

Primary outcome – PCa mortality at 10 years follow-up. No significant difference was found between treatment modalities.

KEY PAPER   ERSPC Study (2013) [11]

ERSPC – European Randomised Study of Screening for Prostate Cancer

Multi-national European study group which publishes their ongoing results of meta-analysis of RCTs. Screening arm vs. observation arm.

The 2013 results reported 13-year median follow-up: NNT = 27 (1 PCa death averted per 27 additional PCa detected), NNS = 781 (1 PCa death averted per 781 men invited for PSA screen).

PSA screening reduced cancer-specific death rates by 20%; no difference in OS.

Extended follow-up (16 years) has since been reported. Again no change in mortality reduction; however, the NNT and NNS decreased (reflecting slow nature of PCa as a disease).

PATHOLOGY

> 95% of PCa arises from the prostatic acinar or ductal epithelium (adenocarcinoma).

The critical feature in prostate adenocarcinoma is <u>absence of the basal cell layer</u> (including absence of staining for basal cell markers p63 and cytokeratin 34BE12).

The basement membrane is breached by malignant cells (small glandular acini) which invade into prostatic fibromuscular stroma.

75% of cases originate in peripheral zone – more frequently associated with extra-capsular extension, seminal vesicle extension, lymph node (LN) metastases.

20% in transitional zone – arise near foci of BPH and are usually smaller in size and better differentiated at cellular level.

5% arise in embryologically distinct central zone.

Prostatic sarcomas – rare, mainly in childhood, usually as rhabdomyosarcoma.

Local spread is often along course of autonomic nerves (peri-neural invasion). Rarely does PCa extend beyond Denonvillier's fascia into the rectum.

Bony metastases are characteristically *sclerotic* (rarely lytic) – most commonly occur in axial skeleton (ribs, spine, pelvis) followed by proximal long bones, skull.

Lymph nodal spread – most commonly to obturator fossae, iliac (common/internal/external).

HIGH-GRADE PROSTATIC INTRA-EPITHELIAL NEOPLASIA

Consists of architecturally benign prostatic acini and ducts lined by cytologically atypical cells:

- The basal cell layer is present although basement membrane may be fragmented
- High- vs. low-grade depending on prominence of the nucleoli.

HGPIN is a proposed precursor to PCa but definitive evidence of this remains unproven. The site of HGPIN does not correlate with future site of detection of PCa.

Exists in 4 grades (tufting, micropapillary, cribriform, flat); however, 97% are tufting and there are no known clinically relevant differences between the different architectural patterns.

HGPIN does not secrete PSA. [13]

If 1 biopsy core features PIN – chance of PCa on repeat biopsy is 20% (i.e. do not repeat biopsy), if > 1 core – chance can be 70%.

EAU 2023 does not routinely recommend repeat biopsy if HGPIN detected. [14]

ATYPICAL SMALL ACINAR PROLIFERATION

Acini are lined with cytologically abnormal epithelial cells and may exhibit atrophic features. Basal layer is focally absent, columnar cells have prominent nuclei.

EAU 2023 does not routinely recommend repeat biopsy if HGPIN detected. [14]

The rate of Gleason 7+ cancers on subsequent biopsies is very low, so patients with ASAP could alternatively be managed with PSA surveillance alone. [15]

OTHER PROSTATE CANCER SUB-TYPES

Intra-ductal (0.5% of cases), defined as an extension of cancer cells into pre-existing prostatic ducts/acini, are typically aggressive (Gleason 8 or more) with unfavourable prognosis.

Mucinous adenocarcinoma is rare, aggressive, associated with early metastases, high PSA + ALP.

Small cell carcinoma (occasionally secretes ADH, ACTH), leiomyosarcoma (mesenchymal tumour).

GLEASON GRADING

VIVA | You may be shown histology slides of prostate cancer and be asked which Gleason grade they pertain to, so spend some time revising this via online images/examples.

Developed in 1966 by pathologist Donald Gleason.

Adenocarcinoma is graded 1–5 according to its gland forming differentiation (see Table 2):

2–6 (well differentiated), 7 (moderately differentiated) and 8–10 (poorly differentiated).

Table 2 – Gleason grading system for prostate cancer

Grade 1	Well-demarcated nodule
Grade 2	Irregular spacing between glands and irregular outline
Grade 3	Variability in gland shape and spacing
Grade 4	Gland fusion
Grade 5	Diffuse solid sheet of undifferentiated cells

The scoring process:

- 2 most dominant types added to give score
- If only 1 pattern is observed, double the grade to give the score
- If 3 grades observed, score the most common plus highest grade (irrespective of extent)
- If predominantly G4/5, do not incorporate G3 if this is < 5%.

Gleason scoring correlates well with prognosis and crude survival, significant predictor of time to recurrence after RP.

Most important prognostic indicator following radical treatment. [17]

Good inter-observer reproducibility. However, the scoring can be affected by RTx and 5ARIs (to exhibit score 8–10) and as such pathologist may not wish to report.

Cytological features do not play a part in Gleason grading.

Under-estimation of score is more common (30–40% after RP specimens are analysed) whilst over-estimation is uncommon (5%).

INTERNATIONAL SOCIETY OF UROLOGICAL PATHOLOGY (2014)

ISUP modified the Gleason score of biopsy detected PCa to align PCa grading with other cancers and to further qualify the highly significant distinction between G3+4 and G4+3 (see Table 3). [18]

Table 3 – ISUP grading of biopsy proven prostate cancer

Gleason Score	ISUP Grade	
2–6	1	
7 (3+4)	2	
7 (4+3)	3	
8 (4+4) or (5+3) or (3+5)	4	Consider full staging scans at diagnosis
9–10	5	(i.e. bone scan and CT TAP)

PROSTATE-SPECIFIC ANTIGEN (PSA)

PSA is a 34kD serine protease, an organ-specific (not cancer-specific) glycoprotein, and is produced by the columnar acinar and ductal prostatic epithelial cells.

Encoded on chromosome 19.

PSA also known as hk3 (member of kallikrein family) and its function is to liquefy the seminal coagulum within the ejaculate to facilitate fertilisation.

PSA exists in 3 forms within serum:

1. *Unbound* (half-life 2 hours) – small fraction of total [cleared by kidney]
2. (Majority) *bound to ACT* – (half-life 4 days) [cleared by liver]
3. *Bound to AMG* (half-life 4 days) – not used for measuring purposes.

PCa patients have a greater fraction of PSA complexed to ACT (i.e. lower free PSA in PCa). [19]

Overall PSA half-life is 2–3 days.

PSA is a million times more concentrated in semen compared to serum.

1g BPH produces 0.15–0.3ng/mL of PSA.

5ARIs will lower PSA levels by 50% after 6 months of treatment; however, the ratio of free to bound PSA remains unchanged. [20]

Cancer cells produce less PSA (mRNA and protein) than normal prostate or BPH cells. The reason for PSA elevation in cancer (and inflammation) is architectural glandular disruption.

In benign epithelium PSA is intensely expressed compared to hK2, in contrast to cancerous tissue in which more intense expression of hK2 is seen.

PSA measurement: Total PSA = Free PSA + Complexed PSA (only ACT bound)

There is no absolute cut-off PSA below which prostate cancer cannot be present.

Table 4 – Oesterling age-specific reference ranges for PSA [21] also used in NICE "Suspected cancer: recognition and referral" (NG12) which adds the "Below 40" and "Above 79" sections

Age	PSA (ng/mL)
Below 40	Use clinical judgement
40–49	2.5
50–59	3.5
60–69	4.5
70–79	6.5
Above 79	Use clinical judgement

80% of men with PCa and PSA < 4 have organ-confined disease.
66% of men with PCa and PSA 4–10 have organ-confined disease.
> 50% of men with PCa and PSA > 10 have disease beyond the prostate.

Consider using the ERSPC risk calculator for PCa (based on PSA, prostate volume, age, etc.).

PSA Velocity

Defined as the rise in PSA per year (in ng/mL/year).

PSAV should be calculated with at least 3 separate PSAs, and a rise of > 0.6–0.75ng/mL/year in PSA is associated with increased risk of PCa. [22]

PSAV = 0.5 x ((PSA 2 – PSA 1 / time 1 in years) + (PSA 3 – PSA 2 / time 2 in years))

PSA Doubling Time

Defined as length of time for PSA to double in months or years (calculated using regression analysis of recorded PSA tests).

PSADT can help in patients with high PSA but negative biopsy, monitoring low-risk disease, or rising PSA following radical treatment. [23]

Generally a PSADT > 1 year is considered favourable.

PSA Density

Defined by the serum PSA per millilitre of prostate tissue (PSA/volume in mL). [24]

Prostate volume (ellipsoid formula) = height x width x length x 0.52

PSA density > 0.15ng/mL/mL is predictive of cancer; however, it is difficult to quantify volume of prostate.

Alternatively use PSATZD (amount of PSA/mL of transitional zone tissue).

Free to Total PSA

Defined as ratio of free (f) PSA to total (t) serum PSA. [25]

In BPH the f/t PSA ratio is significantly higher; however, this is not currently used as diagnostic test for PCa and its clinical value is limited (EAU 2023).

Super-sensitive PSA

Allows PSA to be detected to a threshold of 0.003ng/mL.

Potential application for the early detection of biochemical relapse after RP. [26]

uPM3 Test

Detects prostate cancer antigen 3 (PCA3) which is a gene produced by prostate epithelial cells 60–100 times more in PCa vs. Benign disease. [27]

Collect first 20mL of urine after prostatic massage for analysis.

STAGING [1]

Table 5 – TNM staging for prostate cancer

T – Primary Tumour
TX   Primary tumour cannot be assessed
T0   No evidence of primary tumour
T1   *Clinically inapparent tumour that is non-palpable*
T1a – Tumour incidental histological finding in ≤ 5% of tissue resected
T1b – Tumour incidental histological finding in > 5% of tissue resected
T1c – Tumour identified by needle biopsy (e.g. patient with elevated PSA)
T2   *Tumour that is palpable and confined within the prostate*
T2a – Tumour involves one half of one lobe or less
T2b – Tumour involves more than half of one lobe, but not both lobes
T2c – Tumour involves both lobes
T3   *Tumour extends through the prostatic capsule*
T3a – Extra-capsular extension (unilateral or bilateral) including microscopic bladder neck involvement
T3b – Tumour invades seminal vesicle(s)
T4   Tumour is fixed or invades adjacent structures other than seminal vesicles: external sphincter, rectum, levator muscles, and/or pelvic wall
N – Regional Lymph Nodes
NX   Regional lymph nodes cannot be assessed
N0   No regional lymph node metastasis
N1   Regional lymph node metastasis (regional include true pelvic nodes i.e. pelvic nodes below the bifurcation of common iliac arteries)

M – Distant Metastasis

M0   No distant metastasis

M1   Distant metastasis

   M1a Non-regional lymph node(s)

   M1b Bone(s)

   M1c Other site(s)

N-STAGING

Pelvic lymphadenectomy is the gold-standard assessment of N-stage in PCa. [28]

It increases operative time during RP and associated with higher morbidity whilst not conferring an overall survival benefit.

This should be undertaken bilaterally even if prostate biopsy is positive unilaterally (contra-lateral LN involvement in 1/3 cases).

Low-risk patients (e.g. predicted risk of nodal involvement on Briganti nomogram < 7%) should be spared from pelvic lymphadenectomy, although 70% of dissections will return clear anyway and the 7% risk cut-off will still result in missing 1.5% of patients with nodal invasion.

PSA alone is unhelpful for predicting LN metastasis.

CT and MRI have low sensitivity and specificity – as microscopic LN invasion does not enlarge nodes, and size of non-metastatic LNs vary and overlap with size of metastatic nodes. [29]

Choline PET/CT

11C or 18F choline PET can be used as alternative for LN assessment; however, sensitivity and specificity do not match pelvic lymphadenectomy. [30]

Roach formula – 2/3 PSA + (10 x [Gleason – 6]) = % likelihood of LN mets

Partin's Tables

Use Gleason score, PSA, clinical PCa stage to predict risk of seminal vesicle involvement, extra-capsular extension, lymph nodal involvement. [31]

Derived from RP specimens (EPLND rarely performed so nomograms prone to under-estimation).

M-STAGING

Tc-99m isotope bone scan is most widely used imaging technique for detecting bony metastases in PCa. Sensitivity and specificity approximately 80%.

Do **not** routinely offer bone scan in CPG 1 or 2 patients (NICE 2023).

MDP is taken up by areas of bone with increased blood supply and osteoblastic activity.

Confounding lesions include old fractures, osteomyelitis, TB, benign bone lesions (e.g. osteoma).

Independent predictors of bone-scan positivity include PSA, Gleason score and clinical stage. [32]

- PSA 20–50 will feature positive bone scan in 16%;
- PSA 10–20 will feature positive bone scan in 5%.

18F-sodium fluoride PET has highest sensitivity for detecting metastases, but is less cost-effective. It does not detect LN metastases as well as choline PET does.

Whole-body MRI is more sensitive and specific than bone scan or CT.

Choline PET has higher specificity for metastases than Tc-99m bone scan.

> **KEY PAPER** | Pro-PSMA Study (*Lancet* 2020)

RCT evaluating whether using PSMA PET-CT to assess for metastases in patients with high-risk prostate cancer before curative-intent surgery or radiotherapy, improved accuracy with respect to conventional CT and NM bone scan.

302 men included – randomised to PSMA PET-CT (n=150) or conventional imaging (n=152).

Primary outcome – accuracy of first-line imaging finding either pelvic nodal or distant metastatic disease.

Key finding was PET-CT had higher accuracy, sensitivity (85% vs. 38%) and specificity (98% vs. 91%) when compared to CT + NM bone scan.

MRI IN PCA

Requires 1.5 or 3 Tesla scanner, a dedicated uro-radiologist, multi-parametric (T2-weighting, diffusion weighting (DWI/ADC), dynamic contrast enhancement (T1 DCE)).

Gadolinium is used for contrast enhancement.

T2-weighted imaging remains the most useful method for local staging on mpMRI.

T2 – water is bright (peripheral zone bright as high water content) and PCa will appear as low signal (dark) abnormality on MRI; provides good anatomical delineation.

False negative rate 5–25%.

Endo-rectal MRI appears more accurate for T-staging compared to surface MRI; [33] however, patients find this uncomfortable and it has not gained wide acceptance.

DWI-MRI relies on Brownian motion of water molecules. In areas with densely packed tumour cells, diffusion of the molecules is impeded (i.e. restricted diffusion) and thus they appear bright.

DCE imaging relies on fast T1 images after gadolinium contrast, to assess tumour angiogenesis (rapid wash-in/wash-out).

EAU 2023 recommends to perform MRI before prostate biopsy (*strong*).

Do not offer mpMRI to patients unsuitable for radical treatment (NICE 2023).

KEY PAPER | PROMIS Study (2017) [34]

PROMIS – (Prostate MRI Imaging Study)

Multi-centre study published in 2017.

Inclusion criteria: PSA < 15, no previous biopsy (n = 576 patients)

All patients underwent mpMRI, TRUS and template biopsy (chosen as reference test). Conduct of tests all blinded to other results. Clinically significant PCa defined as Gleason 4+3 or above.

MRI could detect higher-risk disease with greater sensitivity than TRUS biopsy. Allowed greatest detection of clinically significant PCa in conjunction with biopsy.

mpMRI when added to TRUS diagnosed 18% more cases than TRUS alone.

NPV of mpMRI was 89% and could have avoided 1 in 4 biopsies; however, a negative MRI missed 10% of men with clinically significant cancer.

mpMRI sensitivity 93%, TRUS sensitivity 48%.

VIVA | I recommend reading the PROMIS trial paper in full and familiarising yourself with how and why the study was conducted, and its key findings, as you may be expected to describe this in your viva section.

KEY PAPER | PRECISION Study (2018)

Multi-centre randomised trial of 500 men with clinical suspicion of PCa, no previous biopsy.

Assigned at random to either upfront TRUS group (n=248) vs. MRI group (n=252) who then had targeted TRUS (n=175 of 252) if MRI was suspicious.

Outcome – more clinically significant PCA found in MRI+TRUS group vs. TRUS alone.

PI-RADS Scoring

Standardised system of reporting level of suspicion the reporting radiologist has for presence of a clinically significant PCa on MRI. [35]

MRI prostate inter-reader reproducibility is moderate, limiting use by general (non-uro) radiologists.

Table 6 – PI-RADS (version 2.1) scoring system for prostate cancer (2019)

PI-RADS 1	Very low likelihood
	Highly unlikely to be present
PI-RADS 2	Low likelihood
	Unlikely to be present
PI-RADS 3	Intermediate
	Presence is equivocal
PI-RADS 4	High likelihood
	Highly likely to be present
PI-RADS 5	Very high likelihood
	Highly likely to be present

MRI Risk Stratification to Avoid Biopsy

Prostate biopsies are invasive, often poorly tolerated and ≤ 20% of men would not accept a repeat biopsy (if clinically indicated) – important to be selective in listing patients.

MRI is often explored as a potential diagnostic tool to avert biopsy.

VIVA | You may be asked whether you would offer a biopsy to a given patient. Your Area Network guidelines may vary, but as an example Schoots and Padhani (*BJU Int* 2021) in EAU 2023 proposed a risk-adapted biopsy decision based on MRI and PSAD which you could utilise to answer the question.

Risk-adapted matrix for biopsy decision management

	Low PSAD (< 0.10)	Intermed– Low PSAD (0.10–0.15)	Intermed– High PSAD (0.15–0.20)	High PSAD (> 0.20)
PI-RADS 1–2	No biopsy	No biopsy	No biopsy	Consider biopsy
PI-RADS 3	No biopsy	Consider biopsy	Highly consider biopsy	Biopsy
PI-RADS 4–5	Biopsy	Biopsy	Biopsy	Biopsy

PROSTATE BIOPSY

Performed with 7.5MHz trans-rectal US probe and 18G Trucut biopsy needle.

Indications for performing a prostate biopsy:

- Abnormal DRE and/or elevated PSA and/or abnormal mpMRI prostate finding
- Previous negative biopsy but rising PSA and/or abnormal DRE
- As part of active surveillance programme.

Trans-rectal approach sepsis risk (1–2%) [36] – give IV gentamicin, PR metronidazole, PO quinolone.

Trans-perineal approach is currently the recommended approach by EAU 2023:

- Has much lower infection risk – antibiotic prophylaxis not required
- Provides better access to the anterior zone of the prostate.

Template-mapping approach uses grid applied to perineum to take a biopsy every 5mm (30–50 cores):

- 95% accurate and considered gold standard
- Higher rate of side-effects, need for GA, increased procedural time and burden on histopathologist limit its routine use outside of research setting
- Enhances identification of PCa not detected by previous biopsy in patients at high risk of it [38]
- NICE do <u>not</u> recommend offering template-mapping biopsy as part of initial assessment.

Obtain informed consent – risks of sepsis, bleeding, urinary retention, pain. Perform DRE. Measure prostate volume using ellipsoid formula.

For standard biopsies – 12 cores accepted compromise – length of biopsy significantly correlates with PCa detection.

Use 10mL of 2% lignocaine using long spinal needle.

The *Vienna nomogram* is a tool to guide number of cores to be taken, taking into account age and prostate volume in mL. [37]

If PSA 4–10ng/mL and patient has negative TRUS biopsy, the chance of positive second biopsy (22%) or third (10%).

Hypo-echoic lesions include granulomatous prostatitis, BPH nodules, PCa; however, haematological malignancies are *iso-echoic*.

Corpora amylacea are calcifications most commonly seen between transitional and peripheral zones of prostate.

- Diffuse calcifications across prostate occur naturally with age;
- Large calcifications could be calculi which may be relevant in context of infection.

The finding of peri-neural invasion on biopsy suggests higher risk of capsular penetration. [39]

Peri-neural invasion in radical prostatectomy specimens has no prognostic value.

RISK STRATIFICATION

Establishing a patient's risk group allows you to determine the appropriate staging tests and treatment.

Table 7 – NICE 2023 Cambridge Prognostic Group risk stratification for localised and locally advanced PCa [40]

Cambridge Prognostic Group	Criteria
1	Gleason score 6 (grade group 1) **and** PSA < 10µg/L **and** Stages T1–2
2	Gleason score 3 + 4 = 7 (grade group 2) or PSA 10–20 µg/L **and** Stages T1–2
3	Gleason score 3 + 4 = 7 (grade group 2) and PSA 10–20 µg/L and Stages T1–2 **or** Gleason 4 + 3 = 7 (grade group 3) and Stages T1–2
4	One of: Gleason score 8 (grade group 4), PSA > 20µg/L, Stage T3
5	Two or more of: Gleason score 8 (grade group 4), PSA > 20µg/L, Stage T3 **or** Gleason score 9–10 (grade group 5) **or** Stage T4

NICE 2019 used a 3-tier model for risk stratification; however, newer evidence suggests a 5-tier risk-stratification model is better at predicting cancer-specific mortality.

The 3-tier model included *low-*, *intermediate-* and *high-*risk categories (D'Amico risk stratification).

VIVA You should be aware of both the 5-tier and 3-tier risk-
stratification models; however, if asked in your viva about how
to manage a given prostate cancer patient, consider saying *"as
per the Cambridge Prognostic Groups in NICE 2023 guidelines, this
patient is in Group X and therefore I would recommend treatment
options Y or Z..."*

*Table 8 – D'Amico risk stratification for prostate cancer, used in former NICE
guidelines*

Level of Risk	PSA		Gleason Score		Clinical Stage
Low risk	< 10ng/mL	and	≤ 6	and	T1–T2a
Intermediate risk	10–20ng/mL	or	7	or	T2b
High risk1	> 20ng/mL	or	8–10	or	≥T2c

1 – High-risk localised prostate cancer is also included in the definition of locally advanced prostate cancer

(Locally advanced)	Any PSA		Any		cT3–4 or
			(Any ISUP)		N+

TREATMENT

*Table 9 – Treatment options recommended by NICE guidelines [40] according to risk
group*

	CPG 1	CPG 2	CPG 3	CPG 4 and 5
Watchful waiting	Option	Option	Option	Option
Active surveillance	Offer	Offer	Consider	Not recommended
RP	Consider	Offer	Offer	Offer
Radical DXT	Consider	Offer	Offer	Offer
Brachytherapy	Not recommended	Consider (combined with EBRT)	Consider (combined with EBRT)	Consider (combined with EBRT)
Cryotherapy	Not recommended	Not recommended	Not recommended	Not recommended
HIFU	Not recommended	Not recommended	Not recommended	Not recommended

Consider using measures other than age or performance status when assessing PCa treatment options.

Examples include *Clinical Frailty Scale* or *mini-COG* tools.

Charlson Comorbidity Index is method of predicting mortality by classifying comorbidities. [41]

- A score of 2+ implies patient will most likely die from other causes by 10 years follow-up.
- Check the CCI before proceeding to TRUS biopsy.

WATCHFUL WAITING

Defined as the conscious decision to avoid treatment until required when symptoms of progressive disease develop.

Considerations for selecting WW as management strategy:

- Life expectancy < 10 years
- Significant comorbidities which preclude radical treatment (treatment intent is palliative)
- WW can apply to all patient stages; aims to minimise side-effects of treatment.

The 10-year cancer-specific mortality for WW patients is 15% and risk of metastases is 20%.

ACTIVE SURVEILLANCE

Management option for men who have potentially curable PCa but wish to avoid the complications associated with intervention.

The aim is to avoid treatment in those men with indolent cancers by only treating those with signs of progression (AS may avoid radical intervention in 60–80% of patients).

There are numerous criteria for selecting AS, for example the Royal Marsden Criteria: [42]

- Age 50–80
- Fit for radical treatment
- PSA < 15ng/mL
- Stage T1/2
- Gleason 3+4 or less
- < 50% positive cores.

There is no established consensus on a standardised AS protocol – NICE 2023 proposes:

- 0–12 months from starting AS:
  > PSA every 3–4 months (to include PSA kinetics calculations)
- At the 12-month check-point after starting AS:
  > DRE
  > mpMRI (at 12–18 months)
- After 12 months from starting AS:
  > DRE every 12 months
  > PSA every 6 months (monitoring PSA kinetics)
  > Consider repeat mpMRI or prostate biopsy if clinical scenario changes.

Switching to active treatment should be considered:

- Upon patient request
- Radiological progression on mpMRI
- Histological progression: Gleason score, number of involved cores, length core involvement
- Biochemical progression (e.g. short PSADT).

Canadian study by Klotz et al. (2009) of 450 low-risk AS patients – a third came off AS, at 8 years the cancer specific survival was 99%. [43]

Table 10 – EAU 2023 Summary of the differences between AS and WW

	Watchful Waiting	Active Surveillance
Treatment intent	Palliative	Curative
Follow-up	Patient-specific	Pre-determined schedule
Aim	Minimise treatment-related toxicity	Minimise treatment-related toxicity without affecting survival
Protocol	Occasional PSA, no biopsies	Regular PSA, repeat mpMRI/biopsy/DRE
Life expectancy	< 10 years	> 10 years
Eligibility	Patients with all disease stages	Mostly low-risk patients

RADICAL PROSTATECTOMY (RP)

RP may be performed open, laparoscopic or robot-assisted (introduced in 2002). No surgical approach has clearly shown superiority in terms of functional or oncological outcomes.

Patient > 10-year life expectancy pre-operatively is paramount.

Increasing surgeon volume is associated with lower positive margin and complication rates.

Robot-assisted RP (now preferred minimally invasive approach) when compared to open approach:

- Reduced EBL and transfusion rates
- Reduced LOS and complication rates.

The most common site of positive margins on RP specimen is at the apex.

Complications for robot-assisted RP include:

- Early – bleeding requiring transfusion, pain, infection, DVT/PE, urine leak, rectal injury (0.5%), ileus, mortality
- Late – impotence, incontinence, penile shortening, port-site hernia, bladder neck contracture.

Incontinence mild in 50% at one year, 5% severe long term which may benefit from intervention after 12 months: bulking agents, sling or AUS (only surgery recommended by NICE). Patients should be taught PFEs prior to surgery.

Impotence – age and pre-operative potency are the most important predictors of post-RP erectile function, consider PDEi usage prior to RP or early post-op as penile rehabilitation plan.

Vesico-urethral anastomosis should be aligned, water-tight, tension-free. A variety of approaches exist (e.g. Van Velthoven) and chosen method should be based on surgeon's experience.

Preservation of seminal vesicles does not improve potency, incontinence or margin status.

The 10-year survival figures following RP are:

OS (> 95%), metastasis free (90%), PSA free (70%).

Therefore almost 1 in 3 patients experience PSA failure after RP, the majority within first 3 years.

Biochemical recurrence after RP is defined as 2 PSA readings > 0.2ng/mL and rising.

KEY PAPER | PIVOT (Prostate cancer Intervention Versus Observation Trial) [44]

- USA study comparing observation vs. RP in men with localised PCa.
- Primary outcome was overall mortality, secondary outcome PCa-specific mortality.
- RP did not significantly reduce overall- or PCa-specific mortality.
- Sub-group analyses revealed RP may reduce mortality if PSA > 10 and/or higher-risk tumours.

KEY PAPER | SPCG-4 (Scandinavian PCa Group) [45]

- 695 patients (≤T2 stage, PSA < 50, negative bone scan) randomly assigned to WW vs. RP.
- Primary end-points were overall death, death from PCa, risk of metastases.
- Study found reduction in mortality after RP.

Nerve-Sparing

NVB are located in lateral pelvic fascia between prostatic and elevator fasciae.

Preservation of NVB can spare erectile function; however, balancing risk of positive margins.

Potential contraindications to NS surgery should take into account:

- Palpable disease (if unilaterally palpable, can potentially preserve other side)
- High ISUP grade, high PSA, high PI-RADS score
- Capsular breach on mpMRI, EPE.

Unilateral NS (50% potent), bilateral NS (60% potent).

Pelvic LN Dissection

EPLND during RP does not improve oncological outcomes; however, it provides the most accurate information for staging and prognosis.

EPLND significantly increases morbidity in RP, lymphocoeles being the most common adverse event.

The individual risk of patients harbouring positive LNs, to guide whether EPLND should be undertaken or not, can be estimated using validated nomograms, such as the *2019 Briganti nomogram*. [46]

Using this nomogram, EPLND could be spared if risk of involvement < 7%; however:

- 1.5% of patients with nodal involvement would be missed
- 70% of patients would still undergo unnecessary EPLND. [47]

Frozen section LN analysis to determine whether to perform EPLND or not should not be performed.

An EPLND should be performed in high-risk and locally advanced PCa (EAU 2023).

Neo-adjuvant Treatment

Hormone treatment prior to RP has been shown to reduce prostate volume and positive surgical margin rate; however, no evidence of improved CSS and therefore not recommended.

Adjuvant Treatment

Do not offer adjuvant hormonal therapy after RP for pN0 disease.

(EAU 2023) In cN1 disease, long-term ADT can be offered as adjuvant treatment after RP (or after RTx).

RADICAL RADIOTHERAPY

RTx is the use of ionising radiation to achieve fatal damage to neoplastic cells.

In external beam RTx, x-rays (photons) are produced by a linear accelerator which accelerates electrons, abruptly stopping them with a metal target (kinetic energy converted into x-rays).

The energies required to generate XRs capable of penetrating human tissue are in the megavoltage range (typically > 8MV).

The inverse square law of electromagnetic radiation states that as distance from radiation source doubles, the intensity falls to one quarter (principle exploited by brachytherapy).

RTx works by a proportion of the XR energy being absorbed by proliferating tissues, generating free radicals which result in DNA damage and irreparable double-strand breakage.

Radiobiology promotes the "four 'R's" of the radiation response:

Repair – DNA repair occurs after RTx, cells are more radio-sensitive in G2 or S phase of cell division, fractionation allows more cells to be in sensitive phase.

Reoxygenation – O2 required for free radical formation, as more cells die then more O2 becomes available.

Reassortment – cells in G0 (rest) phase will not express damage immediately until cell division occurs; however, G2 + S phase are radiosensitive, so ideally RTx should be given to catch the opportune moment of cell division.

Repopulation – viable tumour cells continue to divide, which compromises efficacy.

The energy absorbed is measured in Gray (1J of energy per kg of tissue = 1Gy).

NICE 2023 recommends:

- Offer hypofractionated RTx (60Gy in 20 fractions) using IMRT unless contraindicated, or
- Offer conventional RTx (74Gy in 37 fractions) to people who cannot have hypofractionated RTx.

Intensity Modulated Radiotherapy (IMRT) – technique using computer technology to deliver precise tailored radiation doses which conform to patient's 3D-shape of tumour/prostate (analysed by pre-treatment CT/MRI), reducing toxicity to surrounding tissues.

> **KEY PAPER** CHHiP trial (Conventional vs. hypofractionated high-dose IMRT for PCa) [48]

- RCT comparing conventional RTx (74Gy in 37 fractions) with two hypofractionated schedules.
- Found the hypofractionated schedules were non-inferior in terms of time to biochemical failure.
- No significant differences in side-effects after 5 years.
- Hypofractionated RTx 60Gy in 20 fractions thus recommended as new standard of care.

Linear Quadratic Model

Uses two co-efficients, alpha (A) and beta (B), to describe dose response relationship. A is probability lethal damage by single event (e.g. ds-DNA break), B is by two separate events.

The A/B ratio of a tissue will determine how it behaves to changes in fractionation.

Early responding tissues (skin, marrow and tumour) are triggered to respond and proliferate within weeks of RTx and tend to have A/B ratio (10–30Gy), the cells have little time to repair photon-induced DNA damage.

Late-responding tissues (spinal cord, CNS tissue) have low cell renewal and thus good opportunity for repair between RTx fractions. The ratio here is lower (< 3Gy) and thus sensitive to change in fractionation dose (i.e. late onset of complications).

The A/B ratio for PCa is 1.5Gy (due to its slow growth) suggesting benefit of hypofractionation.

Radiotherapy Planning

The patient attends a planning session before actually starting the RTx treatment.

Patient will have a planning CT – preferably with full bladder to stabilise prostate by reducing its movement, and empty rectum which may require enema.

Small metal (fiducial) markers may be inserted by needle near the prostate cancer for accurate targeting.

A pre-treatment permanent skin tattoo is marked on the patient.

Contraindications to RTx:

• Severe LUTS, previous pelvic irradiation, inflammatory bowel disease.

Table 11 – Complications after RTx for prostate cancer

	Early	Late
Urinary	Urgency, frequency, dysuria	Incontinence, bleeding (radiation haemorrhagic cystitis), storage LUTS, strictures
Bowel	Diarrhoea, flatulence, cramps, PR bleeding	May be similar to immediate side-effects; rare incontinence
Sexual		Erectile dysfunction (wide variation in reported rates, up to 80% men)
Fertility		Infertility (consider sperm banking prior to treatment)
Secondary cancer		Increased risk of bladder + bowel cancer (extra 0.5–1 cases per 100 treated patients)

PSA Bounce – refers to benign rise in PSA that occurs after initial fall following RTx/BTx typically after 9 months (the PSA level should not exceed 1.5ng/mL).

Neo-adjuvant + Adjuvant Therapy with RTx

RTx should be used in conjunction with ADT in select cases.

NICE 2023 recommends:

- Short-term neo-adjuvant ADT for 3–6 months for all CPG 2–5 and locally advanced PCa
- Consider continuing adjuvant hormones for 3 years for CPG 4–5 and locally advanced PCa.

| KEY PAPER | EORTC 22863 – [49]

- RCT (by Bolla) comparing EBRT alone vs. EBRT + 3 year of hormones (LHRH analogue).
- Disease-free survival (40% vs. 74%) and OS (62% vs. 78%).
- Basis of the combination of RTx + hormones which is standard practice today.

Relapse Post-RTx:

There is no single PSA reading after RTx that can define biochemical recurrence.

Relapse post RTx is defined as any PSA increase ≥ 2ng/mL above the nadir value reached during RTx treatment ("Phoenix criteria").

Sequential rise in PSA can prompt investigations for recurrence such as mpMRI, PSMA PET or CT.

Hormone therapy is mainstay. These do not offer further chance of cure and the time to castrate resistance is 18–24 months.

Salvage therapy is an option if there are no metastases. Salvage RP is technically challenging, salvage cryotherapy or HIFU have a potential role but lack long-term data.

Proton Beam Therapy

Proton beams are an attractive alternative to photon beams as they deposit almost all their radiation dose at the end of the particle's path in the tissue (Bragg Peak) with a sharp fall-off after this which minimises involvement of normal tissues.

(*Bragg Peak* – this is a pronounced peak on the Bragg curve which plots the energy loss of ionising radiation during its travel through matter.)

This is promising but currently experimental.

BRACHYTHERAPY

Involves the implantation of BTx seeds (usually 125 iodine) under general anaesthetic in the lithotomy position.

Two stages required:

1. *Planning* (TRUS study in relation to perineal template to plan seeds) and
2. *Treatment* (60–120 seeds implanted via trans-perineal route) to deliver 150Gy approx.

BTx can be used as a single modality of treatment or in combination with EBRT (boost treatment).

Boost treatment has 15-year biochemical progression free survival (bPFS) of 85% (low-risk PCa), 80% (intermediate-risk PCa) and 68% (high-risk PCa).

NICE 2023 recommends:

- Consider BTx in combination with RTx for CPG 2–5
- Do not offer BTx alone to CPG 4–5 or locally advanced PCa.

Contraindications:

- Life expectancy < 5 years
- Recent TURP in the last 3 months (risk of incontinence)
- Large prostate (> 50cc) or large median lobe (difficult to implant seeds)
- Coagulation disorder
- Previous pelvic irradiation
- Moderate–severe LUTS (risk of retention) IPSS > 12, Qmax < 15mL/s

Complications:

- Irritative LUTS, urinary retention, urinary incontinence, ED, proctitis

If local recurrence is suspected, then RP/EBRT/cryotherapy/HIFU are all options provided there are no metastases. Morbidity is greater for all these options when used secondarily.

High-dose Brachytherapy

Uses a radioactive source temporarily introduced into prostate to deliver radiation, as monotherapy or combined with EBRT.

Note that iridium-192 is isotope of choice.

Results are limited from very experienced centres and patients should be counselled accordingly.

Table 12 – Differences between low-dose and high-dose rate brachytherapy techniques

Low-dose Rate	Permanent seeds implanted I-125 used Dose delivered over weeks/months Acute side-effects resolve over months Radiation protection issues for family
High-dose Rate	Temporary implantation Ir-192 used Dose delivered in minutes Acute side-effects resolve over weeks No radiation issues for family

CRYOTHERAPY

A *whole-gland therapy* utilising freezing techniques to induce cell death by:

- Dehydration resulting in protein denaturation
- Direct rupture of cellular membranes by ice crystals
- Vascular stasis/micro thrombi, resulting in ischaemic apoptosis.

Done using TRUS guidance placing liquid argon or nitrogen via cryo-needles. Two freeze–thaw cycles are used at -40°C. Day-case anaesthetic.

Number of cycles is the most important parameter for tissue ablation.

Frozen tissue appears hypo-echoic on US.

EAU 2023 recommends cryotherapy be used only in context of clinical trial (not in high-risk PCa).

Complications – ED, urinary incontinence, LUTS, proctitis, recto-urethral fistula

HIFU

A *whole-gland therapy* utilising focused US waves emitted from a transducer whilst patient under GA/spinal and in lateral position.

Tissue damage achieved by mechanical, thermal (> 65°) and cavitation, and the heating causes coagulative necrosis without damaging rectal wall (maximum depth 4cm).

EAU 2023 recommends HIFU be used only in context of clinical trial (not in high-risk PCa).

Complications are comparable to cryotherapy, most common is urinary retention.

Patients should be informed regarding lack of outcome data > 10 years and in the PCa salvage setting the available data is scarce.

HORMONE THERAPY

Androgen deprivation therapy (ADT) refers to any treatment that lowers androgen activity.

Prostate epithelial cells are physiologically dependent on androgens to function, grow, proliferate. When androgen deprivation occurs, androgen-sensitive prostate cells undergo apoptosis.

Bcl-2 (anti-apoptotic protein) is normally expressed in the prostate; however, over-expression is associated with development of hormone refractory disease.

p53 (facilitates apoptosis) and mutations also correlate with hormone refractory disease.

Physiology of Androgen Secretion

The hypothalamo–pituitary–gonadal (HPG) axis is described:

-> Hypothalamus secretes GnRH

-> Stimulates anterior pituitary LH + FSH

-> LH stimulates Leydig cells to make testosterone.

Testosterone is then converted to DHT (10x more active biologically) by 5AR enzymes 1 and 2.

Once bound to the receptor in the cytoplasm, the androgen-receptor complex enters the nucleus where it interacts with DNA to influence cell growth and division.

95% of androgens are produced by the Leydig cells of testes (5% from adrenal cortex which is stimulated by ACTH).

| VIVA | You may be asked to draw the HPG axis to explain to the examiner how each medication or hormonal treatment works. Please familiarise yourself with Figure 1 later on in the chapter.

Different Mechanisms of Inducing Androgen Deprivation

Medical and surgical forms of castration have equivalent efficacy.

Castrate serum testosterone defined as < 20ng/dL (although in trials < 50 is still used as marker).

General side-effects of ADT:

- Loss of libido, ED
- Weight gain, lethargy, gynaecomastia, hot flushes
- Altered mood, cognitive changes, memory loss
- Osteoporosis and pathological fractures

Intermittent Hormone Therapy

IHT can be used in localised disease to limit side-effects of ADT treatment, reduce the cost and preserve patient's bone density.

IHT must not cycle on/off for less than 9 months at a time as this is the interval required for testosterone to restore normal levels again.

IHT is not suitable if PSA rising – currently no threshold of PSA to stop/start ADT again.

IHT aims to delay to development of castrate resistance – if ADT is stopped prior to androgen-dependent cells becoming androgen-independent, any subsequent tumour growth may remain androgen-dependent.

BILATERAL ORCHIECTOMY

Each testis tunica albuginea is incised, seminiferous tubules excised and then defect closed. Can be done under LA. Irreversible.

Serum testosterone falls within 12 hours to < 50ng/dL (quickest intervention to achieve this).

LHRH AGONISTS

Synthetic long-acting analogues of GnRH given by subcutaneous depot injection on 1–2–3–6–12-monthly basis, e.g. goserelin acetate (brand name Zoladex).

Chronic exposure and over-stimulation of the anterior pituitary by these drugs will down-regulate the GnRH receptors and thus suppress LH, FSH production and therefore testosterone.

Castrate levels are reached within 2–4 weeks.

Tumour Flare

Occurs on first administration of LHRH analogue featuring a transient surge in testosterone as the drug stimulates the anterior pituitary LHRH receptors.

Complications can include spinal-cord compression, fatal cardiovascular events due to hyper-coagulation, increased bony pain, bladder outlet or ureteric obstruction.

Risk reduced by giving anti-androgens 1 week pre- and 2 weeks post- first dose of LHRH agonist, although flare can still occur despite this strategy.

Higher risk of tumour flare happening is in patients who have very high metastatic burden.

LHRH ANTAGONISTS

Bind immediately to LHRH receptors leading to rapid decrease in LH, FSH and testosterone (without flare) to achieve castrate level by day 3.

Degarelix is only such drug licensed in Europe, only available as monthly depot. Definitive superiority over LHRH analogues remains to be proven.

Standard dosage of degarelix is 240mg stat, followed by monthly injections of 80mg.

ANTI-ANDROGENS

There are two classes of anti-androgens: *steroidal* and *non-steroidal*.

Both compete with androgens at the receptor level.

Non-steroidal anti-androgens (e.g. bicalutamide) act purely as competitors and do not affect testosterone levels, i.e. preserving libido, bone density, cognition.

Side-effects: gynaecomastia common (70%) (gynaecomastia may be treated with RTx to breasts 8–10Gy, or tamoxifen, or bilateral mastectomy), potential liver toxicity (must monitor LFTs)

Dosage: 150mg/day as monotherapy, 50mg/day for MAB or flare-prevention

Steroidal anti-androgens (e.g. cyproterone acetate) block androgen receptors as well as down-regulating LHRH secretion by central action.

MAB is achieved for example with zoladex + bicalutamide.

EAU 2023 does not recommend using anti-androgens monotherapy alone in M1 disease.

OESTROGENS

Suppress testosterone and preserve bone density.

Their side-effect profile and thrombo-embolic risk imply oestrogens not considered first line.

Table 13 – A summary of the different modalities of delivering ADT

Reduced androgen production	
Surgical castration	Removes Leydig cells
Medical castration	Reduces LH production
LHRH agonists	Down-regulate pituitary GnRH receptors e.g. goserelin (zoladex)
LHRH antagonists	Inhibits GnRH receptors e.g. degarelix

Blocks androgen effect	
Non-steroidal anti-androgens	Blocks androgen at receptor level e.g. bicalutamide

Combined effect	
Oestrogen	Suppresses Leydig cells
	Inactivates androgen
	Down-regulates LHRH secretion
Steroidal anti-androgens	Down-regulates LHRH secretion
	Blocks androgen at receptor level e.g. cyproterone

CASTRATE-RESISTANT PCA (CRPC) TREATMENT

CRPC is defined by disease progression despite ADT and may present as serial PSA rise or development of new metastases. Inevitable eventual consequence of ADT.

EAU 2023 still define CRPC as testosterone < 50ng/dL, and:

- Radiological progression (appearance of new lesions), or
- Biochemical progression (3 consecutive rises in PSA one week apart resulting in x2 50% increases over nadir and PSA > 2).

Androgen-independence may result from:

- Development of androgen-independent clones
- Over-expression of the androgen receptor
- Intracellular synthesis of testosterone by cancer cells (targeted by abiraterone).

Treated initially with second-line hormonal therapy (maximal androgen blockade).

Third-line therapy may include cortico-steroids or oestrogens (with aspirin 75mg OD as cover).

METASTATIC PCA TREATMENT

The mainstay of treatment for mPCa is immediate ADT (medical or surgical castration) and these are best delivered at diagnosis rather than onset of symptoms (EAU 2023).

There is no evidence to support use of any particular modality of ADT over another – the fastest treatments to achieve castration are surgical orchiectomy and LHRH antagonists.

> **VIVA** You may be asked in your viva to describe the options to treat a clinically well patient presenting with mPCa. Always consider mentioning presence of CNS and MDT discussion having taken place, and then list the following:

- ADT as hormones +/- upfront docetaxel (followed by eventually MAB)
- Surgical castration by bilateral orchiectomy
- LHRH antagonists (i.e. degarelix)
- Consider deferred treatment (only asymptomatic patients with strong wish to avoid treatment-related side-effects).

Clinical disease progression after ADT will occur after 12–18 months.

If PCa progresses the following options can be considered:

- First line: abiraterone, enzalutamide, docetaxel
- Second line: abiraterone, enzalutamide.

Median survival of patients with newly diagnosed mPCa is 42 months with ADT alone.

Chemotherapy

Systemic chemotherapy is indicated in men with mCRPC (providing they have adequate renal function and good performance status).

Docetaxel upfront can increase survival by median survival by 10 months (but only 2 months if used at the time of castrate resistance). [51]

Chemotherapy should be commenced within 12 weeks of starting ADT (NICE 2023).

Docetaxel can be given IV via cannula (alternatively central line may be required):

- Given once every 3 weeks (i.e. each cycle lasts 3 weeks) and treatment takes ~1 hour
- Dosage is 75mg/m2
- Prednisolone may be given day before therapy and for 2 days after to reduce allergic reactions
- Total of 6 cycles are given as standard (can go up to 10 cycles)
- Side-effects include: (common) infections, allergy, bleeding/bruising, fatigue, loss of appetite, hair loss, peripheral neuropathy, (rare) heart failure, VTE, liver toxicity.

In mCRPC, cabazetaxel can be used as second-line chemotherapy agent.

| KEY PAPER | STAMPEDE (Systemic Therapy in Advancing or Metastatic PCa: Evaluation of Drug Efficacy) [52] |

Multi-centre RCT for high-risk, locally advanced or mPCa, evaluating standard of care (SOC – hormone therapy for > 2 years) plus additional medication.

2,900 patients randomised between 2005 and 2013.

Randomisation ratios: 2 (SOC) : 1 (SOC + ZA) : 1 (SOC + docetaxel) : 1 (SOC + docetaxel + ZA)

No reported significant survival benefit for (SOC + ZA) or (ZA + docetaxel).

Recommended upfront docetaxel at start of hormone therapy should become standard of care.

| KEY PAPER | CHAARTED Trial (Chemohormonal Therapy in Metastatic Hormone-sensitive PCa) [53] |

RCT of 790 patients randomised in 1:1 fashion to receive ADT + docetaxel vs. ADT alone, to evaluate whether combination therapy would result in longer OS than ADT alone.

Median time to disease progression in combination arm (20.2 months) vs. ADT alone arm (11.7 months).

Trial concluded that ADT + 6 cycles of docetaxel resulted in significantly longer OS than ADT alone.

Abiraterone and Enzalutamide

Abiraterone acetate is CYP17 inhibitor which decreases intracellular testosterone level seen in CRPC by suppressing production in cells (intra-crine) and at adrenal level.

Abiraterone must be given along with prednisolone to prevent drug-induced hyper-aldosteronism.

Enzalutamide blocks androgen-receptor transfer and compared to bicalutamide it will suppress any possible agonist-like activity.

Both are licensed for mCRPC only.

Figure 1 – Summary of different strategies of ADT for prostate cancer]

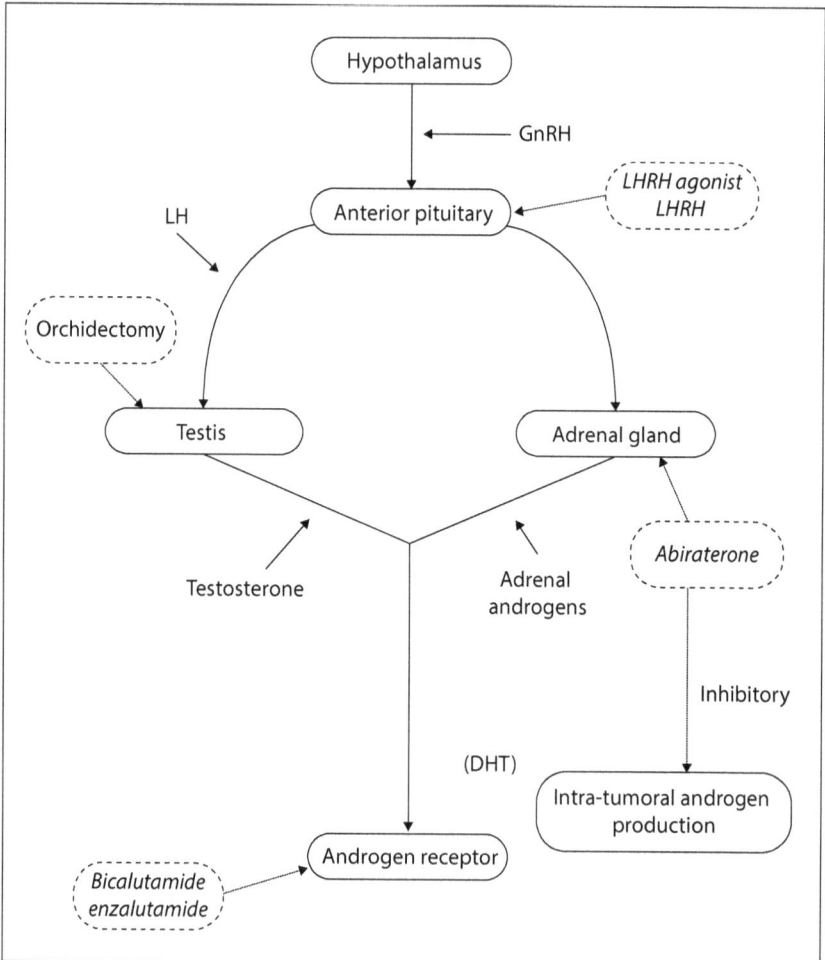

mPCa Symptom Palliation

Early involvement of MDT to include palliative care, oncologist and cancer nurse specialist.

Bisphosphonates (ZA) have been shown to reduce skeletal-related events and reduce bony pain in 80% of patients with mPCa and should be considered (NICE 2023).

NSAIDs are best oral option to target bone pain.

EBRT can target painful bone lesions as a single dose.

NICE Guidelines mPCa

Offer bilateral orchiectomy to all men with mPCa as alternative to hormone therapy.

Do not offer MAB as first-line treatment.

Can offer bicalutamide monotherapy, if sexual function preservation is priority and patient counselled regarding adverse impact on OS and gynaecomastia (if sexual function becomes unsatisfactory, stop bicalutamide and start ADT).

Offer cortico-steroid (e.g. dexamethasone) if MAB fails, as third line and consider concomitant docetaxel chemotherapy.

SALVAGE TREATMENT

PSA monitoring is cornerstone of follow-up after PCa treatment (thresholds for recurrence depend on local treatment used), and PSA recurrence almost always precedes clinical recurrence.

The timing and modality of salvage treatment after RP/RTx remain controversial.

After RP/RTx, the following salvage treatment options are available:

- Salvage RTx (if previous RP) or RP (if previous RTx)
- ADT
- Cryotherapy/HIFU.

Observation of the patient is another option.

Although biochemical recurrence is defined as PSA > 0.2ng/mL, many advocate to wait until PSA > 0.5ng/dL before proceeding to radiological investigations (e.g. PSMA PET, MRI, CT).

This is to increase the yield of positive findings.

NHS TARGET

The NHS 62-day cancer target applies to the process of prostate cancer referral, diagnosis and treatment as per the following timeline.

Figure 2 – NHS cancer pathway timeline for prostate cancer]

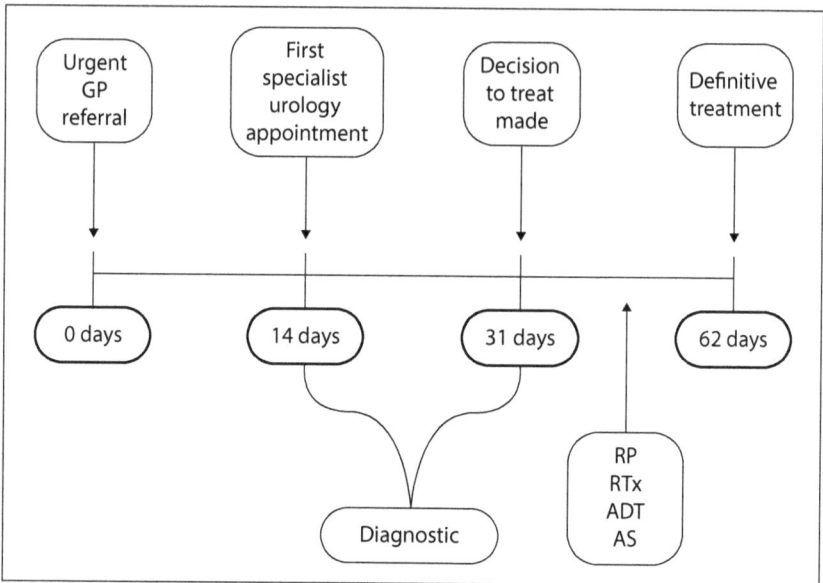

TESTICULAR CANCER

EPIDEMIOLOGY

TC constitutes 1% of all new male cancers in UK and approximately 5% of urological tumours. [54]

Most common solid cancer in men aged 15–49 years.

Lifetime risk is approximately 1 in 220.

At diagnosis 1–2% are bilateral and > 90% are germ cell tumours.

Peak incidence for non-seminoma is 20–30 years, and 30–40 years for seminoma.

20% can present with testicular pain as their first symptom (10% of men presenting with testicular pain will have a tumour). [55]

96+% of patients survive TC for ≥ 10 years in the UK.

Risk Factors

Age	- If age > 60 years, more than half of men with TC will have lymphoma.
	- Half of all TC cases occur < 35 years.
	- Infants and young boys tend to develop yolk-sac tumours.
Race	- White Caucasian highest risk (also Maoris in New Zealand) > black.
Previous TC	- 12–18x increased risk of metachronous TC.
UDT	- 10% of TC patients have history of cryptorchidism (risk of TC 4–6x higher). [56]
	- Ultra-structural testicular changes by UDT occur by age 3 (i.e. early orchidopexy).
	- Risk of TC: 1/500 (normal), 1/125 (unilateral UDT), 1/45 (bilateral UDT).
HIV	- Increased risk of seminoma. [57]
ITGCN	- Synonymous with CIS of the testis.
	- 50% of cases will progress to invasive germ cell TC within 5 years.

Family Hx   - Father (6x higher risk) and brother (8x higher risk).

Sub-fertility - Poor semen analysis parameters increases risk of TC.

  - 25% of men diagnosed with TC have oligospermia at presentation. [58]

Genetic Factors

Iso-chromosome of short arm of chromosome 12 has been described in all histological types of germ cell tumours. [59]

p53 locus alterations have been identified in 66% of cases of GCNIS.

Klinefelter – (47XXY)

Kallman's syndrome – defective GnRH release (hypogonadotropic hypogonadism); most commonly presents with delayed puberty, anosmia, high risk of infertility; mainstay of treatment is hormone replacement

PATHOLOGY

Germ cell tumours (GCT) are a heterogenous group of neoplasms that arise mainly in gonads and rarely extra-gonadal sites along the midline (e.g. sacrum, retro-peritoneum).

95% of TC are malignant GCT – clinically and histologically split into seminomatous (most common) and non-seminomatous, both originating from germ cells.

Most malignant post-pubertal GCT originate from GCNIS.

The specimen should be stored in Bouin's solution (rather than formalin) to preserve morphology.

From the pathologist's report one would require the following information:

- Histological type and pathological stage
- Size and multiplicity
- Rete testis involvement
- Presence of GCNIS (formerly known as ITGCN)
- Microvascular invasion
- If seminoma, are there any non-seminomatous elements.

Testicular Epidermoid Cyst

Accounts for 1% of all testicular tumours, has an onion-ring appearance on US (well-circumscribed hypo-echoic lesion with hyper-echoic margins). [60]

Not associated with GCNIS.

Only perform radical orchidectomy if diagnostic uncertainty; organ-preserving surgery is possible if intra-operative biopsies are negative. [61]

Table 14 – WHO (2022 update) pathological classification of testicular cancer (summary – full list online) [62]

1. GCT (derived from GCNIS)	
Non-invasive germ cell neoplasia	GCNIS, gonadoblastoma
Germinoma family of tumours	Seminoma
Non-seminomatous GCT	Teratoma (mature / post-pubertal) Embryonal carcinoma, yolk-sac tumour, Choriocarcinoma
Mixed GCT	Mixed GCT
GCT of unknown type	Regressed GCT
2. GCT (unrelated to GCNIS)	
	Spermatocytic tumour Pre-pubertal type teratoma / yolk sac / neuroendocrine tumour
3. Sex cord stromal tumours	
Leydig cell tumour	Leydig cell tumour
Sertoli cell tumour	Sertoli cell tumour, large cell calcifying Sertoli cell tumour
Granulosa cell tumour	Adult or juvenile granulosa cell tumour
4. Tumours of testicular adnexa	
Ovarian-type tumours	Serous / mucinous cystoadenomas or cystoadenocarcinomas
Tumours of collecting ducts / rete testis	Adenoma / adenocarcinoma of collecting ducts and rete testis
Para-testicular mesothelial tumours	Mesothelioma
Tumours of epididymis	Cystadenoma / adenocarcinoma / SCC of the epididymis

Seminoma

Germ cells can differentiate into spermatocytic tissue (seminoma) (40–45% of TC cases).

Seminomas have a lower metastatic potential compared to NSGCT, predominantly metastasising to the para-aortic region.

Seminomatous types of cancer are more sensitive to radiation.

Divided into classic (homogenous, lymphocytic infiltrate), spermatocytic (older men, usually benign, no GCNIS) and anaplastic (no infiltrate).

Only 10% of seminomas have raised tumour markers (always βhCG), 10% have raised LDH.

Non-seminomatous Germ Cell Tumour

Pluripotent germ cells can divide into somatic elements (teratoma) or trophoblast or yolk sac – e.g. choriocarcinoma (only makes ßhCG), embryonal.

80% of NSGCTs will have raised tumour markers (60% will have raised AFP).

Leydig Cell Tumour

1–3% of TCs, 3% are bilateral, 10% are malignant.

Not associated with history of UDT.

Most commonly spreads to the retro-peritoneum – radical orchidectomy is the initial treatment, considered refractory to chemotherapy and RTx.

Tend to produce hormones and therefore create para-neoplastic syndromes, for example: [63]

- Early virilisation in children due to testosterone production
- Gynaecomastia in adults due to oestrogen production.

Germ Cell Neoplasia in Situ (GCNIS)

Formerly known as ITGCN, GCNIS is a precursor lesion for most post-pubertal GCT and present in contra-lateral testis in 5% of TC patients (consider contra-lateral biopsy in all cases).

Histologically appears as malignant germ cells lining seminiferous tubules containing Sertoli cells in a single row, with nuclear pleomorphism and an intact basement membrane.

- Tubules are usually of smaller diameter than normal.
- Show decreased/absent spermatogenesis.
- Atypical cells are usually aligned along the basement membrane.

Overall population incidence is 0.8%.

GCNIS is the common precursor for all types of adult male GCT except spermatocytic seminoma. (Paediatric GCT do not typically arise from GCNIS.)

GCNIS does not raise tumour markers.

Risk of progression to invasive GCT is 50% in 5 years. [64]

Increased risk for GCNIS includes small testis (< 12mL), history of cryptorchidism and young age. [65]

Treatment options for biopsy positive GCNIS is local RTx (16–20Gy) which causes infertility and need for testosterone replacement; alternative options are US surveillance or orchidectomy.

Chemotherapy is not reliably effective to eradicate GCNIS.

Presence of GCNIS in addition to TC-bearing testicle does not affect the prognosis.

Choriocarcinoma

This is the only GCT which will disseminate haematogenously.

Uniformly associated with elevated βhCG levels but it does not produce AFP.

These patients should always have a CT head to exclude metastases.

Caution administering chemotherapy in patients with brain metastases as these tumours are highly vascular and can bleed. [66]

Figure 3 – Summary of pathology of different testicular tumours]

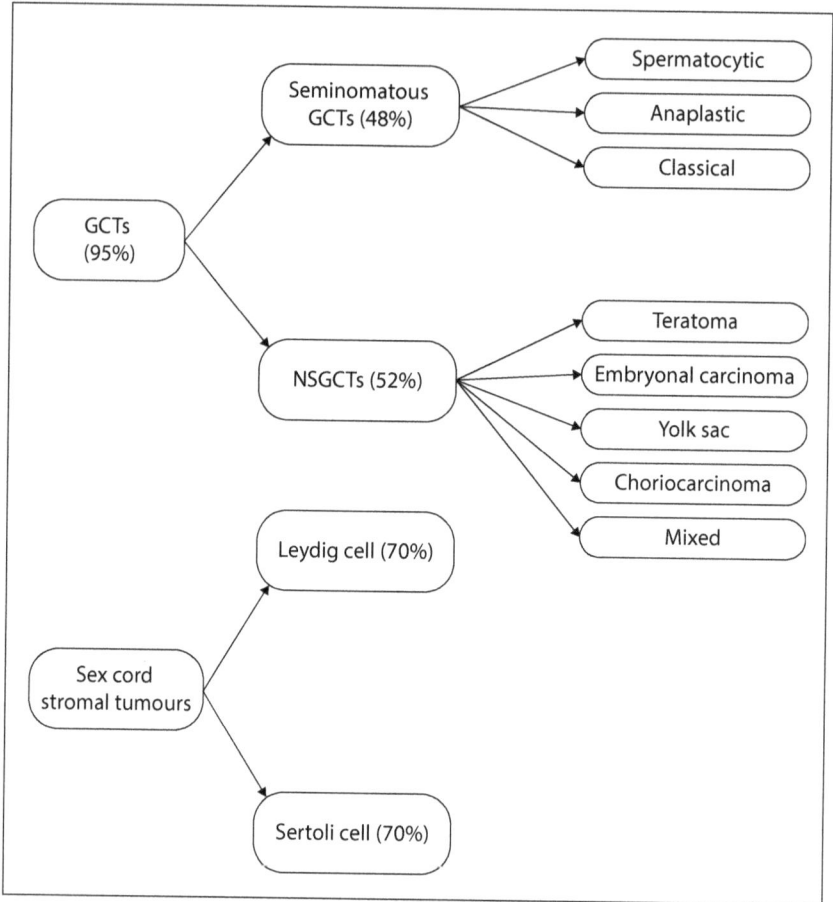

TUMOUR MARKERS

Serum tumour markers are prognostic factors and contribute to diagnosis and staging.

The following should be measured before and 5–7 days after radical orchidectomy:

- Lactate dehydrogenase (LDH)
- Alpha-fetoprotein (AFP)
- Beta-HCG (βhCG).

Across the board, 50% of all TCs will have raised tumour markers, varying with the tumour type.

Presence of normal markers before orchidectomy does not exclude metastatic disease, and likewise normalisation of markers after surgery does not rule out distant disease.

90% of all NSGCTs will have a rise in tumour markers (if all measured simultaneously). [67]

Alpha-fetoprotein (Oncofetal Protein)

In 50–70% of NSGCTs there is raised AFP.

Pure seminomas do not secrete AFP – if AFP is raised in the context of seminoma this suggests that a mixed element to the tumour is likely.

Serum half-life is 5 days.

Other conditions can also raise AFP – liver/pancreatic/stomach/lung malignancies and benign liver pathology.

Beta-human Chorionic Gonadotrophin (Oncofetal Protein)

Expressed by syncytio-trophoblastic elements of:

- Choriocarcinomas (100%)
- Teratomas (40%)
- Seminomas (10%).

Serum half-life is 36 hours.

Other conditions can raise βhCG – liver/pancreas/stomach/lung/breast/bladder/kidney cancers and in marijuana smokers.

High levels of LH in hypogonadal patients can interfere with βhCG measurements and yield spuriously high readings.

Lactate Dehydrogenase (Cellular Enzyme)

Less specific marker due to elevation by other cause.

Elevated in 10% of seminomas, correlating to tumour burden and a useful measure of response.

Placental Alkaline Phosphatase (Cellular Enzyme)

Elevated in 40% of patients with advanced GCTs – not widely used as non-specific and can be artificially raised in smokers.

Can be histologically useful in determining the germ cell origin of a tumour.

IMAGING

US sensitivity reaches almost 100% (lesions are hypo-echoic) (7–10MHz transducer).

These should be performed for any palpable testicular mass or retro-peritoneal mass with elevated tumour markers in the absence of palpable testicular abnormality.

Sonographic appearance of seminoma is smooth, homogenous, hypo-echoic.

Sonographic appearance of a teratoma is irregular, calcifications present and necrosis.

MRI provides higher sensitivity and specificity than US in diagnosing TC, but cost does not justify its use – consider only when US is inconclusive.

CT TAP is imaging of choice for staging.

PET has no role in the initial staging.

Testicular Microlithiasis

Features widespread calcifications throughout the testicular parenchyma and is present in 5% of the general population.

Defined as the presence of ≥ 5 calcifications (each < 2mm) per image field on US.

Incidence of TC in microlithiasis is no different to rate of population as a whole, and therefore patients can be discharged with advice to regularly self-examine. [68]

In those with significant risk factors (e.g. UDT, family history) an annual US can be considered as follow-up regime along with review with urologist.

STAGING

Staging is a process by which clinically, radiologically and pathologically the extent of disease is defined to allow prognosis for relapse and survival.

The mainstay of radiological staging is abdominal CT (sensitivity 70% for retro-peritoneal nodes) with threshold of 3mm to define metastatic nodes.

MRI yields comparable results to CT, though cost and availability are limitations; however, has a role in iodine contrast-allergy, radiation reduction or poor kidney function.

The American Joint Committee on Cancer (AJCC) staging classification of TNM and serum markers is shown below. The use of tumour markers in the TNM staging is unique to TC.

VIVA | Unfortunately, you have to know the TNM staging for all urological cancers inside out, as you can expect to be given clinical details for a patient and asked to determine their full staging, in both the MCQ and viva exams. This is one of the few areas of the FRCS (Urol) exam where you just have to employ rote learning until it becomes second nature to you.

Table 15 – TNM staging for testicular cancer

pT – Primary Tumour	
pTX	Primary tumour cannot be assessed
pT0	No evidence of primary tumour
pTis	Intratubular germ cell neoplasia (carcinoma in situ)
pT1	Tumour limited to testis and epididymis without vascular/lymphatic invasion; may invade tunica albuginea but not vaginalis
pT2	Tumour limited to testis and epididymis with vascular/lymphatic invasion; or tumour extending through tunica albuginea and vaginalis
pT3	Tumour invades spermatic cord with or without vascular/lymphatic invasion
pT4	Tumour invades scrotum with or without vascular/lymphatic invasion
N – Regional Lymph Nodes – Clinical	
NX	Regional lymph nodes cannot be assessed
N0	No regional lymph node metastasis
N1	Metastasis with a lymph node mass ≤ 2cm in greatest dimension or multiple lymph nodes, none > 2cm in greatest dimension
N2	Metastasis with a lymph node mass > 2cm but ≤ 5cm in greatest dimension; or > 5 nodes positive, none > 5cm; or evidence of extra-nodal extension of tumour
N3	Metastasis with a lymph node mass > 5cm in greatest dimension

pN – Regional Lymph Nodes – Pathological	
pNX	Regional lymph nodes cannot be assessed
pN0	No regional lymph node metastasis
pN1	Metastasis with a lymph node mass ≤ 2cm in greatest dimension and ≤ 5 positive nodes, none > 2cm in greatest dimension
pN2	Metastasis with a lymph node mass > 2cm but ≤ 5cm in greatest dimension; or > 5 positive nodes, none > 5cm; or evidence of extra-nodal extension of tumour
pN3	Metastasis with a lymph node mass > 5cm in greatest dimension
M – Distant Metastasis	
MX	Distant metastasis cannot be assessed
M0	No distant metastasis
M1	(M1a) – Distant metastasis: non-regional lymph node(s) or lung (M1b) – Distant metastasis: other sites
Serum Tumour Markers	
SX	Serum markers not available
S0	Serum markers within normal limits

	LDH (U/l)	hCG (mIU/mL)	AFP (ng/mL)
S1	< 1.5 x N, and	< 5,000, and	< 1,000
S2	1.5–10 x N, or	5,000–50,000, or	1,000–10,000
S3	> 10 x N, or	> 50,000, or	> 10,000

An alternative system is the *Royal Marsden Staging System*:

- Stage 1 – TC isolated to the testicle
- Stage 2 – Spread to retro-peritoneal lymph nodes
- Stage 3 – Spread to the lymph nodes above the diaphragm
- Stage 4 – Metastasised to other organs.

RADICAL ORCHIDECTOMY

This should be performed urgently on next available elective operative list (within 7 days).

Only if widespread metastasis/respiratory compromise at presentation, refer for emergency chemotherapy first and then operate subsequently.

Performed through an inguinal incision.

Prior to manipulating the testis the cord should be isolated and clamped, to allow control of draining lymphatics to minimise tumour spill.

The cord should be dissected up to the deep inguinal ring and transected. The testis, epididymis and spermatic cord are excised en-bloc.

This is curative in 75% of patients.

Tumour markers should be repeated 7 and 14 days after surgery.

The ilio-inguinal nerve is at risk of damage during the operation.

If during surgery the cord is unexpectedly involved, go as high as possible on it and transect; leave non-absorbable suture on cord as a marker, as patient likely to have RPLND + chemotherapy.

Contra-lateral Testicular Biopsy

Performed through scrotal incision, delivery of testicle and 5mm incision into tunica at each pole (double-biopsy open technique) to extrude seminiferous tubules (99% sensitivity).

Note: these must sent in Bouin's solution (not formalin).

Alternatively biopsy gun Trucut needle can be performed providing similar-quality biopsy.

There is no consensus as to which patients should undergo biopsy; however, recommended: [67]

- Age < 40 years
- Contra-lateral testicular volume < 12mL
- History of cryptorchidism
- History of sub-fertility/poor spermatogenesis (Johnsen score 1–3).

GCNIS present in 5% of contra-lateral cases of TC (34% with all above risk factors).

Prostheses Insertion

EAU 2023 recommends testicular prosthesis should be offered to all patients receiving orchidectomy.

Can be made of silicone or alternatively saline-filled. Should be matched to size contra-lateral testis.

Complications include extrusion (5%), migration (5%), chronic pain and infection (1%). [69]

If suspected metastases (raised markers and/or imaging), option to defer prosthesis insertion as patient may need chemotherapy post-operatively which could be delayed if graft infection.

| KEY PAPER | Robinson et al. (2016) – testicular prosthesis insertion safety at radical orchidectomy [70]

Retrospective audit of 900+ men in north-west UK undergoing radical orchidectomy for TC, collecting data for post-operative complications.

No significant difference in complication rates between those receiving prosthesis vs. those not.

Organ-sparing Surgery

This is not routinely indicated if the contra-lateral testis is healthy.

There are certain circumstances which may warrant this:

- Contra-lateral TC
- Single testicle (with normal testosterone levels) with tumour
- Tumour volume < 30% of testicular volume
- Strong suspicion of a benign tumour.

Sperm Banking

Semen parameters commonly drop following orchidectomy (particularly in seminoma) and approximately 5% of patients develop azoospermia.

EAU 2023 recommends discussing sperm banking with all men prior to starting treatment for TC, which should be offered before orchidectomy if possible.

2–3 separate semen samples required after ideally at least 3 days of abstinence. Frozen in liquid nitrogen at -196°C.

Screened for hepatitis B/C, HIV, syphilis, CMV.

Illness at time of banking can compromise sperm quality.

Spermatogenesis can recover 1+ years after chemotherapy.

Cost – free on NHS usually for initial assessment and storage; subsequent cover varies across UK but can cost approximately £300/year, usually stored for 10 years, but this can be extended.

Estimated that 10% or less of those who chose to bank their sperm actually end up using this.

STAGE 1 GCT TREATMENT

STAGE 1 SEMINOMA

Of all seminomas, 75% are confined to the testis at presentation. Only 15% will have regional nodal metastases and 10% have more advanced disease.

Following radical orchidectomy, the patient is staged and then managed by the oncologist.

Surveillance

Cure rate with orchidectomy alone is 80–85% – hence approximately 16% will relapse over a 5-year period, implying surveillance is an option. [71]

The important risk factors are: [72]

1. Tumour size > 4cm
2. Rete testis involvement.

If both factors present (*high risk*) (relapse 32%), one factor (16%) or neither (*low risk*) (12%).

Risk-adapted approach has been developed whereby patients at higher risk of relapse are encouraged to undergo adjuvant treatment (e.g. chemotherapy/RTx).

Surveillance protocols vary; however, one should consider:

- Yearly CT of the retro-peritoneum for the first 4 years after diagnosis
- 6-monthly CXR
- 3-monthly tumour marker assessment.

20% of later relapses occur > 4 years, suggesting potential lifelong follow-up is required.

Adjuvant Chemotherapy

Single-dose carboplatin is the chemotherapy regime if patient wishes to have adjuvant treatment. This has an equal efficacy to radiotherapy but is easier and quicker to deliver.

Carboplatin is much less nephrotoxic than cisplatin. [73]

Cisplatin carries a risk of ototoxicity, nephrotoxicity, sensory nerve impairment.

Adjuvant Radiotherapy

Prescribed as 20Gy dose over 10 fractions – will reduce relapse rate to 1%.

Acute GI toxicity is common (60%) and chronic GI sequelae in 5%.

Scrotal shield should be used to protect the contra-lateral testicle.

Figure 4 – Schematic approach to stage 1 seminoma management]

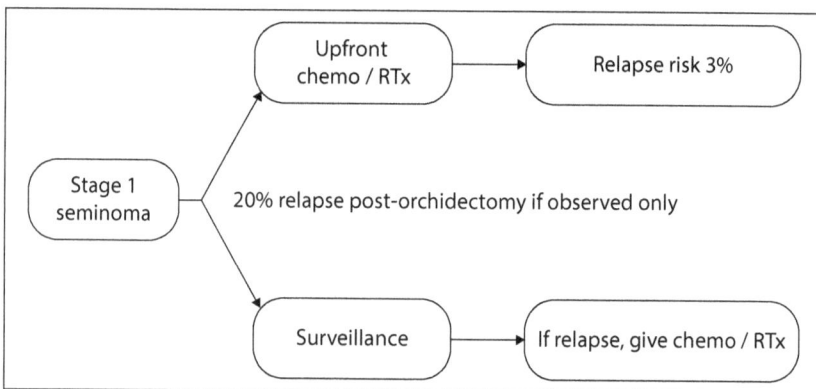

STAGE 1 NSGCT

Following orchidectomy, the risk of relapse is <u>higher</u> than for seminomas.

Up to 30% of patients with CS-1 NSGCT will have sub-clinical metastases at presentation and will thus relapse during surveillance (majority in lungs and retro-peritoneum).

The important risk factor is <u>vascular invasion</u>:

- If present there is 48% risk of relapse (high risk) and therefore chemotherapy is advised
- If absent the relapse risk is < 20% (low risk) and therefore surveillance is advised.

Embryonal component and absence of yolk-sac component are adverse factors.

The overall survival rate bearing in mind the available treatment options is close to 100%.

Surveillance

This remains an option; however, patients need careful counselling as to risks/benefits of strategy.

CT advised at 0, 3 and 12 months.

80% of recurrences will occur within 12 months (1/3 will have normal tumour markers).

Salvage chemotherapy yields excellent survival rates (> 99%) hence why surveillance can be adopted with a good back-up treatment option.

Adjuvant Chemotherapy

One cycle BEP (bleomycin + etoposide + cisplatin) is recommended protocol by EAU 2023.

Poorly compliant patients may benefit from this treatment rather than surveillance CT, as would high-risk patients with vascular invasion.

One cycle of BEP does not appear to adversely affect fertility or sexual activity.

If relapse occurs after x1 BEP, then a x3 cycle is recommended.

A cycle of BEP lasts 3 weeks, consisting of 2 weeks of chemotherapy drugs, one week rest, and recommencement of the next cycle.

RPLND

In view of the high cancer-specific survival rates of surveillance, the low relapse rate when adjuvant chemotherapy is given and excellent salvage chemotherapy option, the role of primary diagnostic RPLND has diminished.

In the UK first-line treatment is surveillance or chemotherapy.

If patient is unwilling to have surveillance or chemotherapy then RPLND can be offered.

RPLND is primarily used for de-bulking any residual tumour after chemotherapy.

RPLND in itself will diagnose 30% of patients with LN+ disease which upstages their disease to Stage II which will then require x2 BEP.

It is estimated that half the patients undergoing RPLND would not have relapsed in the first place.

Figure 5 – Schematic approach to stage 1 NSGCT management]

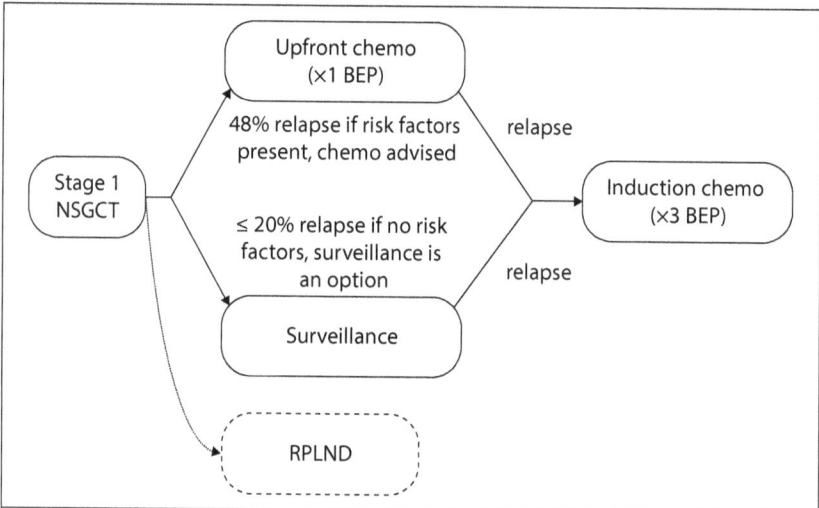

STAGE II A/B SEMINOMA TREATMENT

Metastatic seminomatous disease can be classified into:

- Low-volume disease including Stages IIA (< 2cm nodal mass) + IIB (2–5cm nodal mass)
- Advanced metastatic disease including Stage IIC (nodal mass > 5cm) + Stage III (supra-diaphragmatic metastases).

RPLNs < 2cm with normal tumour markers pose a diagnostic challenge and observation for 8 weeks with repeat staging is recommended.

Chemotherapy

Mainstay UK treatment for Stage II A/B seminoma is chemotherapy (x3 BEP or x4 EP for those unsuitable for bleomycin e.g. smokers).

Chemo- and radiotherapy are equally effective. European urologists favour the use of RTx.

The major limitation of bleomycin is pulmonary toxicity.

Radiotherapy

Alternative to chemotherapy.

Dosage is 30Gy (Stage IIA) and 36Gy (Stage IIB).

Distribution in IIA is further lateral compared to Stage I (to include ipsilateral iliac field) and in IIB should include an additional boost to para-aortic LNs.

STAGE II A/B NON-SEMINOMA TREATMENT

Initial chemotherapy should be given to all advanced NSGCT with raised tumour markers (except IIA with negative markers – can be managed with RPLND or surveillance).

If surveillance is chosen, repeat CT at 6 weeks and re-evaluation of size is indicated. Progression can warrant RPLND or chemotherapy.

CT- or US- guided biopsy may be warranted as an alternative to the surveillance group.

Figure 6 – Schematic approach to stage 2a NSGCT management]

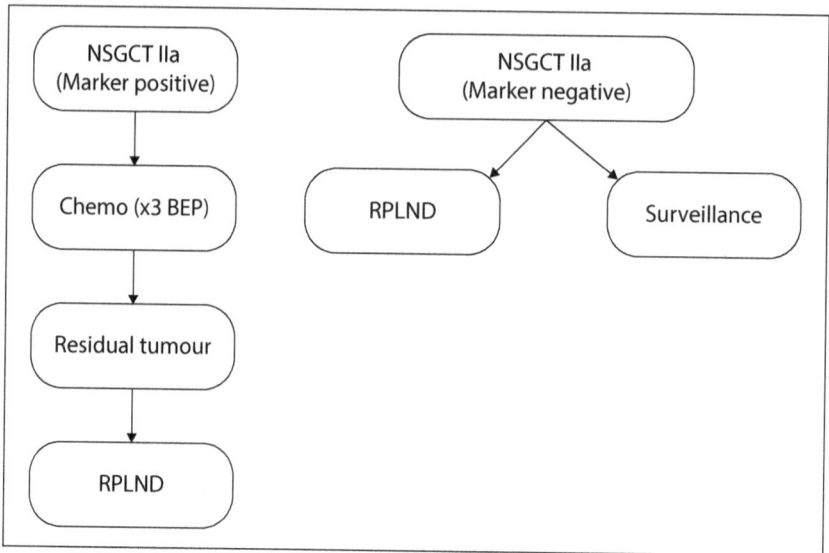

STAGE 2C/3 (METASTATIC) TREATMENT

SEMINOMAS

Good prognosis group

Patient should receive x3 cycles of BEP or x4 EP.

Intermediate prognosis group

Patient should receive x4 cycles of BEP.

There is no poor prognosis group.

NON-SEMINOMAS

Good prognosis group

Patient should receive x3 cycles of BEP.

Intermediate prognosis group and poor prognosis group

Patient should receive x4 cycles of BEP.

RESIDUAL TUMOUR RESECTION

Seminoma

Residual mass of seminoma should not be primarily resected irrespective of size but controlled by imaging and tumour markers.

This scenario rarely occurs and therefore tumour is not routinely expected within the mass.

PET is advised if residual volume > 3cm (4–6 weeks after chemotherapy) and if positive is a reliable predictor for viable tumour tissue in these patients.

A confirmatory biopsy is recommended.

If PET scan is positive and biopsy positive, consider RPLND.

Salvage therapy in the form of chemotherapy is given if indicated (or radiotherapy if they did not receive this initially). Surgical resection is challenging akin to retro-peritoneal fibrosis.

Non-seminoma

Following first-line BEP, < 10% of residual masses contain viable cancer (the vast majority harbour fibro-necrotic tissue) and salvage (second-line) chemotherapy must be considered.

This regime is PEI/TIP (cisplatin, ifosfamide and etoposide).

If residual mass is > 1cm, do not PET scan, rather refer for RPLND.

FOLLOW-UP REGIMENS

Table 16 – Recommended minimal follow-up for seminoma Stage I on active surveillance or after adjuvant treatment (carboplatin or RTx) [74]

Modality	Year 1	Year 2	Year 3	Year 4 and 5	After 5 years
Tumour markers	2 times	2 times	2 times	Once	Further management according to survivorship care plan
CXR	-	-	-	-	
Abdominopelvic CT/MRI	2 times	2 times	At 36 months	At 60 months	

Table 17 – Recommended minimal follow-up for NSGCT Stage I on active surveillance [74]

Modality	Year 1	Year 2	Year 3	Year 4 and 5	After 5 years
Tumour markers	4 times	4 times	2 times	1–2 times	Further management according to survivorship care plan
CXR	2 times	2 times	Once if LVI+	At 60 months if LVI+	
Abdominopelvic CT/MRI	2 times	At 24 months	At 36 months	At 60 months	

Table 18 – Recommended minimal follow-up after adjuvant treatment or complete remission for advanced disease (excluded poor prognosis and no remission) [74]

Modality	Year 1	Year 2	Year 3	Year 4 and 5	After 5 years
Tumour markers	4 times	4 times	2 times	2 times	
CXR	1–2 times	Once	Once	Once	Further management according to survivorship care plan
Abdominopelvic CT/MRI	1–2 times	At 24 months	At 36 months	At 60 months	
CT Thorax	1–2 times	At 24 months	At 60 months	At 60 months	

PROGNOSTIC TABLES

Table 19 – IGCCCG prognostic-based staging system for metastatic seminomatous GCT [75]

Good Prognosis Group	
(90% of cases)	*All* of the following criteria:
5-year PFS 89%	- any primary site - no non-pulmonary visceral metastases
5-year survival 95%	- normal AFP, any ßhCG, any LDH

Intermediate Prognosis Group	
(10% of cases)	*All* of the following criteria:
5-year PFS 79%	- any primary site - non-pulmonary visceral metastases
5-year survival 88%	- normal AFP, any ßhCG, any LDH

Poor Prognosis Group
No patients classified as poor prognosis group

Table 20 – IGCCCG prognostic-based staging system for metastatic NSGCT [76]

Good Prognosis Group	
(56% of cases)	*All* of the following criteria:
5-year PFS 90%	- Testis/retro-peritoneal primary tumour - No non-pulmonary visceral metastases
5-year survival 96%	- AFP < 1,000ng/mL, βhCG < 5,000 IU/L, LDH < 1.5 x ULN

Intermediate Prognosis Group	
(28% of cases)	*Any* of the following criteria:
5-year PFS 78%	- Testis/retro-peritoneal primary tumour - no non-pulmonary visceral metastases - 1,000ng/mL < AFP < 10,000ng/mL, or
5-year survival 89%	- 5,000 IU/L < βhCG < 50,000 IU/L, or - 1.5 x ULN < LDH < 10 x ULN

Poor Prognosis Group	
(16% of cases)	*Any* of the following criteria:
5-year PFS 54%	- Mediastinal primary tumour - non-pulmonary visceral metastases - AFP > 10,000ng/mL, or
5-year survival 67%	- βhCG > 50,000 IU/L, or - LDH > 10 x ULN

PENILE CANCER

EPIDEMIOLOGY

600+ new cases diagnosed in UK/year; < 1% of all new cancers in men; not in UK top-20 most common cancers; notable link with social deprivation.

Incidence rates are highest in males aged > 90 years and in areas with high prevalence of HPV.

Most cancers occur in the glans penis.

More common in developing countries where circumcision not a routine religious practice.

RISK FACTORS

Age   - Incidence increases as age rises.

Circumcision - Reduces risk as neonatal circumcision removes half the skin that could become cancerous in future (adult circumcision on healthy foreskin unlikely to change lifetime risk). [77]

HPV   - Main risk factor for penile cancer, types 16 and 18 (DNA found very commonly in intra-epithelial DNA). [78]

Phimosis   - Strongly associated with invasive penile cancer, due to underlying chronic infection.

Smoking   - Confers x5 increased risk. [79]

UV-A   - Therapeutic phototherapy for pathologies such as psoriasis.

HPV

Overall up to 50% cases of penile cancer show HPV infection (usually multiple strains), the most common being type 16 (~70%), 6 and 18.

Highest prevalence of HPV-associated carcinomas seen in basaloid (84%) and warty-basaloid (75%).

HPV infection has an inconsistent association with prognosis. [80]

HPV Vaccination

As part of the UK NHS vaccination schedule, it is currently offered to all children aged 12–13 years.

Gardasil® 9 is the HPV vaccine given in UK, in people < 25 years administered as single dose (2 doses for those aged 25–45 years, spaced 6–24 months apart).

All girls < 25 years and boys born after 1 September 2006 can receive it free on NHS (if missed in school), homosexual men < 45 years are also eligible.

Vaccine protects against HPV-related cancers (cervical, penile, oropharyngeal, genito-anal) and genital warts but not STI. More than 70% of unvaccinated people harbour HPV on skin. [81]

PATHOLOGY

SSCa accounts for > 95% of all penile malignancies.

Penile SSCa usually arises from epithelium of inner prepuce or glans penis.

The 2022 WHO classification sub-classifies precursor lesions and tumours into: [82]

- HPV-associated SCCa (e.g. basaloid, warty, warty-basaloid, clear cell)
- HPV-independent SCCa (e.g. usual, papillary, sarcomatoid, verrucous)
- Other (unclassified).

Rarely non-SCCa occur such as lymphomas, melanocytic (rare as penis seldom exposed to sunlight).

Secondary metastases to penis are rare and mostly prostatic/colorectal/bladder in origin.

Kaposi's sarcoma presents with a painful raised blue/violet papule, commonly associated with HIV infection. Reticulo-endothelial tumour of penis. (Associated with herpes-virus type 8.)

PRE-MALIGNANT LESIONS

Is it not known how often penile SCCa is preceded by pre-malignant lesions.

PeIN is considered the precursor lesion of penile SCCa.

PeIN classified into *HPV-independent* and *HPV-associated* as per scheme of their invasive counterparts.

Former terms such as *Erythroplasia of Queyrat, Bowen's disease* and *Bowenoid papulosis* are discouraged from use as per WHO 2022 classification. [83]

PeIN is effectively penile CIS (CIS implies lesions with all features of malignancy except invasion – not cross basement membrane and occurs in their normal place i.e. "in situ").

Benign Penile Lesions

Lichen sclerosus – (BXO) commonly presents as phimosis and histologically features epithelial atrophy/thinning, loss of rete pegs, hyper-keratinisation.

Found synchronously with penile cancer in 25% of cases; however, direct causal links not proven.

Zoon's balanitis – red shiny erythematous patches on the glans penis.

STAGING

Most commonly will start as an ulcerative/flat/papillary lesion on the glans penis (50%).

Spreads locally beneath foreskin and enters vertical phase where it will invade corpora cavernosa, urethra, perineum and pelvis.

Metastasis initially to superficial inguinal LN, then deep inguinal LN, then iliac and obturator LN.

Lymph node staging is the most important prognostic factor in penile cancer.

There is no tumour marker for penile cancer.

Imaging

Cancerous lesions of penis are usually evident on clinical examination, which can be reliably used to estimate tumour size and clinical T-stage.

MRI with/without artificial erection is helpful to assess in select circumstances such as evaluation of tumour invasion of the corpora, "skip lesions" or if organ-sparing treatment is being considered.

US can be used as alternative to evaluate corpora invasion, where MRI is not available.

Absence of palpable inguinal LN (cN0) still means chance of micro-metastatic disease is 25% (however, when palpable, points toward metastasis as cause rather than infection).

US, CT, MRI or 18FDG-PET are of limited value in cN0 patients as cannot reliably diagnose micro-metastatic disease – EAU 2023 does not recommend their routine use.

Clinically node-palpable patients (cN+) should be offered further CT TAP or 18FDG-PET for staging.

US along with FNA cytology will aid in confirming the diagnosis.

[More details of LN staging/assessment are covered in "Regional LN Management" section below.]

Penile Biopsy

Obtaining histology should address the penile lesion first, then focus on LN assessment.

In clinically evident lesions, certain penile cancer NHS Tertiary Referral Centres may prefer to receive referrals without prior biopsy to leave tumour untouched.

However, for purpose of FRCS (Urol) you should offer to perform an upfront penile biopsy under local anaesthesia for all suspicious lesions.

Incisional biopsy – removes only part of tumour (e.g. large tumour, clearly invasive) – and should be done only prior to more complex or invasive treatment.

Excisional biopsy – removes entire lesion (e.g. if flat/plaque) – this could effectively treat the cancer.

TNM Staging

T1 category is split into two prognostically different groups, depending on presence of lympho-vascular invasion, peri-neural invasion or poor differentiation (T1a and T1b).

Retro-peritoneal lymph node metastases are extra-regional and therefore classed as distant.

Table 21 – TNM classification for penile cancer [83]

T – Primary Tumour	
TX	Primary tumour cannot be assessed
T0	No evidence of primary tumour
Tis	Carcinoma in situ (PeIN)
Ta	Non-invasive verrucous carcinoma
T1	T1a – Invades sub-epithelial connective tissue without lympho-vascular invasion and not poorly differentiated T1b – Invades sub-epithelial connective tissue with lympho-vascular invasion and/or poorly differentiated
T2	Tumour invades corpus spongiosum with or without invasion of the urethra
T3	Tumour invades corpus cavernosum with or without invasion of the urethra
T4	Tumour invades other adjacent structures
N – Regional Lymph Nodes	
cNX	Regional lymph nodes cannot be assessed
cN0	No palpable or visibly enlarged inguinal lymph nodes
cN1	Palpable mobile unilateral inguinal lymph node
cN2	Palpable mobile multiple or bilateral inguinal lymph nodes
cN3	Fixed inguinal nodal mass or pelvic lymphadenopathy, unilateral or bilateral
M – Distant Metastasis	
cM0	No distant metastasis
cM1	Distant metastasis
G – Histological Grading	
GX	Grade of differentiation cannot be assessed
G1	Well differentiated
G2	Moderately differentiated
G3	Poorly differentiated
G4	Undifferentiated

pN – Regional Lymph Nodes on Pathology (on Biopsy or Surgical Excision)	
pNX	Regional lymph nodes cannot be assessed
pN0	No regional lymph nodes metastasis
pN1	Metastasis in 1–2 inguinal lymph nodes
pN2	Metastasis in > 2 unilateral inguinal lymph nodes or bilateral inguinal lymph nodes
pN3	Metastasis in pelvic lymph node(s), unilateral or bilateral extra-nodal extension of regional nodal metastasis
pM – Distant Metastasis	
pM1	Distant metastasis microscopically confirmed

TREATMENT

Treatment of penile cancer should focus on oncological outcomes as well as functional, sexual, psychological and voiding functions (i.e. consider penile preserving surgery).

Treatment of primary tumour and regional LN can either be simultaneous or staged.

SUPERFICIAL NON-INVASIVE DISEASE (PEIN, TA)

PeIN can progress to invasive disease, despite treatment, in up to 10% of patients – therefore successful eradication and minimum 5-year follow-up are essential.

Consider radical circumcision first – as most PeIN occurs on mucosal surface of glans or prepuce.

Topical Therapies

Topical treatments after circumcision include 5-FU or imiquimod – these should be undertaken with close surveillance and if unsuccessful at 6-week review, should not be repeated.

5-FU – anti-metabolite chemotherapy agent, acts at S-phase causing cell-cycle arrest + apoptosis: [83]

- No standard protocol exists
- Can apply 5% ointment over glans penis daily for 4 weeks
- High discontinuation rate (up to 25%) due to erythema/inflammation, erosion (use condom if continuing sexual intercourse).

Imiquimod – acts through several pathways, including activation of immune cells via TLR-7

- Can be used 3x/weekly for 12 weeks
- Also associated with adverse local side-effects e.g. erythema/erosion leading to discontinuation.

LASER Ablation

LASER ablation is an alternative treatment option:

- Energy-based therapies include Nd:YAG or CO2
- Response rates are high; however, the local recurrence rates after treatment are also high.

Surgery (Glans Resurfacing)

Surgical options can be considered for patients with:

- Extensive PeIN, or
- Recurrent disease after topical therapy.

Glans resurfacing involves complete abrasion of glandular epithelium followed by covering with split skin graft to cover the denuded glans (buccal mucosa if urethral reconstruction required).

Recurrence rates low, cosmetically acceptable and benefit of complete local histopathological staging which can occasionally lead to cancer upstaging.

Surgery involves single treatment session, as opposed to extended course needed in topical therapies.

TREATMENT OF INVASIVE DISEASE CONFINED TO GLANS (T1/T2)

Surgical

If opting for surgical management, EAU 2023 recommends undertaking organ-sparing operations to stage ≤ T2 penile cancers wherever possible, in compliant patients.

All patients should be circumcised before non-surgical treatments anyway (e.g. LASER, RTx).

There is no oncologically preferred penile preserving surgical technique.

Surgical options may include:

- *Circumcision* – a "radical" circumcision may be sufficient to treat a foreskin tumour alone
- *Wide local excision* – circumcision + excising margin of normal skin around tumour/erythema
- *Glans resurfacing* – as per PeIN/Ta; however, combined with deeper resection at site of invasion
- *Glansectomy* – can be *partial* or *total*, considering reconstructing neo-glans with split skin graft in appropriate patients (i.e. not if PVD, previous RTx, uncontrolled diabetics).

Partial penectomy/amputation offered to patients with more advanced disease, but may be considered in those unwilling to have organ-sparing surgery or to comply with strict follow-up.

Non-surgical (Radiotherapy or LASER)

RTx can be delivered as BTx alone +/- EBRT (60Gy) (patients must be circumcised prior to treatment).

RTx has a higher recurrence rate than surgical treatment; however, penile preservation rates are high and salvage surgery is always an option if RTx fails.

Complications of RTx – corpora cavernosa fibrosis, urethral stenosis, glans necrosis.

LASER (Nd:YAG or CO_2) can be considered as an option for smaller invasive lesions; however, recurrence rates are likely higher compared to surgical excision.

TREATMENT OF LOCALLY ADVANCED DISEASE (T3/4)

Disease may not be resectable, in which case (induction) chemotherapy can be offered:

- In responders, the disease may downstage and thus be amenable to surgery
- In combination with RTx as palliation for non-responders or those unkeen for surgery.

In resectable T3/4 disease, complex treatment planning is required in most cases if surgery considered.

Glansectomy + distal corporectomy can be undertaken in cases of minimal corporal involvement.

Partial penectomy may be performed if corporal involvement is obvious (penile length permitting); however, if penis is short than total penectomy may be necessary.

Total penectomy + perineal urethrostomy formation is offered if patient not amenable to partial amputation (neo-adjuvant platinum-based chemotherapy should be considered).

Hypercalcaemia is a common complication in patients with advanced metastatic penile cancer and is due to the tumour burden rather than bony involvement. (Often PTH secretion.)

| VIVA | You may be asked how to perform a partial penectomy, which many candidates may not have scrubbed in for during their training. Be aware of risks to consent for such as ED, penile shortening, urine spraying, cosmetic outcome. There are of course various techniques, but key steps include:

- Cover penile lesion with condom to exclude the lesion and apply tourniquet to base of penis
- Incise skin circumferentially around penis down to Buck's fascia
- Mobilise + divide urethra, leaving a distal redundancy > 1cm and spatulate it
- Divide/ligate NVBs, divide corpora (send frozen section) and close with 2'0 vicryl (glans can be reconstructed with split skin graft from thigh)
- Remove tourniquet and check for haemostasis
- Construct meatus by interrupted sutures between skin and spatulated urethra + insert catheter.

REGIONAL LN MANAGEMENT

Most important prognostic for survival of penile cancer is presence/extent of nodal metastases, thus detecting lymphatic spread as early as possible is crucial.

5-year CSS: N0 (95%), N1 (80%), N2 (65%), N3 (35%) [84]

The nodal spread of penile cancer follows a step-wise unilateral ascent – side cross-over is rare:

- Site of tumour -> superficial inguinal LN -> deep inguinal -> pelvic LN -> distant sites
- As inguinal LN are first involved, initial LN evaluation should focus on seeking metastases there.

Involvement of regional penile MDT is recommended.

Clinically Node Negative (cN0)

Even if LN are non-palpable, 25% of patients will have micro-metastases.

CT/US/MRI/PET cannot detect micro-metastases and are of limited value in cN0 patients and not recommended for routine use [84] where aim is to identify small sub-clinical metastatic LN.

As imaging accuracy is limited, invasive/surgical LN staging is key for detecting micro-metastases, although surgical staging over-treats most cN0 patients (only 25% have micro-metastases).

Therefore cN0 patients at highest risk of nodal metastases should be selected for invasive staging:

- T1 disease with LVI, peri-neural invasion or poorly differentiated
- T2–4 disease with any grade.

Low-risk patients (pTis, pTa, or G1pT1) – could be offered surveillance (in a compliant patient).

Intermediate-risk patients (G2pT1a) – consider invasive staging vs. surveillance on case-by-case basis.

The invasive diagnostic options which are available include:

1. *Modified superficial inguinal lymphadenectomy:*
   - Preserves the saphenous vein to reduce the degree of lymphoedema (20% incidence)

- Smaller incision and avoids transposition of sartorius muscles
- If intra-operative LN positive, then proceed to ipsilateral radical lymphadenectomy
- If multiple LN positive, or single LN with extra-capsular spread, then proceed to pelvic lymphadenectomy at a second operation [85]
- Furthermore if 2+ LN are found, contra-lateral staging LN assessment should be considered.

2. *DSNB*:
- Tc-99m injected peri-tumoral in morning, patient then goes to radiology for dynamic scanning to mark sentinel node on skin; in afternoon patient has peri-tumoral patent blue injection prior to GA, intra-operatively a gamma-ray probe detects sentinel node
- False negative 5% rate, as LN full of tumour will not uptake any radioisotope
- Intra-operative use of US can reduce this rate
- (Consider inguinal US before DSNB, as sonographic suspicious LN can have FNA as initial test which may obviate need for DSNB).

Both methods may still miss micro-metastatic disease.

DSNB was developed to try to minimise the morbidity of LND by avoiding resecting unnecessary LN.

EAU 2023 recommends DSNB should be offered, if available, when surgical staging is indicated.

Early lymphadenectomy is far more beneficial for long-term survival (> 90%) when compared to therapeutic lymphadenectomy when nodal disease becomes palpable (< 40%).

However, LND has considerable complication rates even in *modified* techniques and the patient should be evaluated and counselled carefully in terms of risks vs. benefits.

Clinically Node Positive (cN+)

Guiding principle – "palpable LN in context of significant penile cancer, need removing where possible".

Palpable LN (cN+) are presumed metastatic rather than infective (up to 80% of cN+ patients will harbour metastases) – do not prescribe antibiotics and reassess.

Offer full radiological staging (i.e. CT TAP or 18FDG-PET) to assess for distant spread.

Consider initial histological confirmation via CT/US guided biopsy (FNA).

If unilateral LN are palpable with confirmed diagnosis on FNA:

- Proceed to ipsilateral radical inguinal lymphadenectomy
- (If > 2 LN involved or pelvic LN or extra-capsular disease) proceed to ipsilateral pelvic lymphadenectomy with concomitant contra-lateral DSNB / modified groin dissection (if non-palpable contra-lateral LN).

Figure 7 – Schematic approach to evaluate lymph nodes in penile cancer

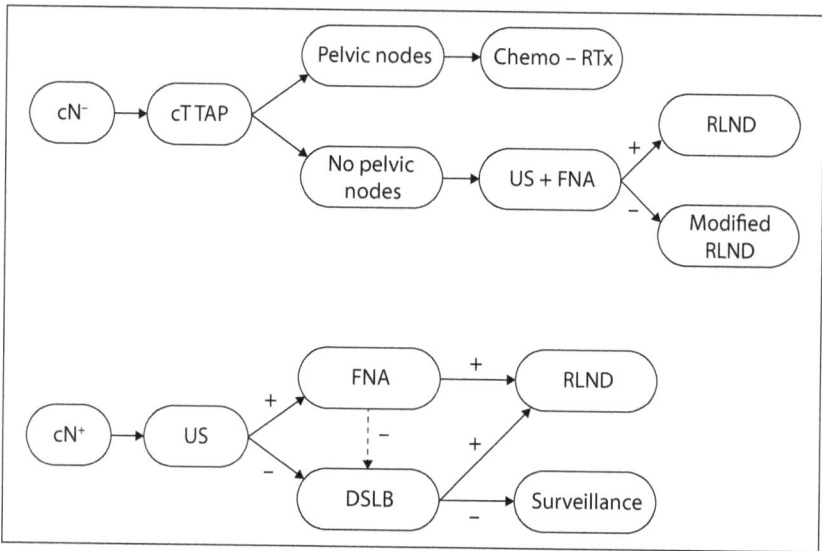

Radical Inguinal Lymphadenectomy

The boundaries of the dissection are those of the femoral triangle:

- Superiorly, the inguinal ligament
- Laterally, the lateral border of sartorius
- Medially, the lateral border adductor longus.

Morbidity is high (50%) – including wound infection, lymphoedema, lymphocoele. [12]

Pelvic Lymphadenectomy

Pelvic nodal disease does not occur without ipsilateral inguinal LN metastasis (side cross-over rare).

CSS with pelvic LN involvement is considerably lower (33%) vs. inguinal LN only (70%).

Prophylactic pelvic lymphadenectomy can be offered if:

- ≥ 3 nodes from radical inguinal lymphadenectomy are positive, and/or
- Extra-nodal extension is reported.

Boundaries of pelvic lymphadenectomy include:

- Proximal: iliac bifurcation
- Lateral: genito-femoral nerve
- Medial: bladder wall
- Inferior: Cloquet's node.

If LN recurrence occurs after surgery, there is no consensus on treatment and this should be multi-modal with chemotherapy.

cN3+ patients may be offered neo-adjuvant chemotherapy (cisplatin- and taxane- based) if fit, and considered for LND surgery if they have responded.

Disseminated disease or unfit patients may be offered palliative chemotherapy.

Post-operative Lymphoedema

Common complication after LDN surgery and patients should be warned pre-operatively.

Managed by mobilisation, compression stockings/underwear, +/- IR-guided drainage, consider involvement of *lymphoedema service* (clinical nurse specialist).

FOLLOW-UP REGIMEN

Most recurrences occur within 2 years post-operatively:

- Recommend follow-up every 3 months for first 2 years
- 6-monthly thereafter.

Follow-up should include examination of penis as well as inguinal LN assessment.

Psychological support should be offered due to impacts that penile cancer treatment can have on men.

Lymphoedema can be a chronic debilitating problem. This should be assessed at follow-up and referral to appropriate therapists considered early, when appropriate.

URETHRAL CANCER

EPIDEMIOLOGY

Rare cancer – estimated incidence 1.5/million in women and 4.3/million in men. [88]

Most commonly in age > 75 years.

More commonly will present with symptoms of locally advanced disease (blood discharge, bladder outlet obstruction, palpable mass, urethrocutaneous fistula).

RISK FACTORS

Exceedingly rare in those < 55 years; risk factors when TCC are similar to bladder cancer.

Infective   - HPV (type 16), chronic irritation from ISC, STI, recurrent UTI, local RTx treatment.

Gender   - More common in men (2.9:1 ratio vs. women).

PATHOLOGY

Occurs most commonly in bulbo-membranous urethra.

Anterior urethral carcinoma is more amenable to surgery and better prognosis than posterior urethral carcinoma.

Transitional cell carcinoma (TCC) is the most common (60%), followed by squamous cell carcinoma (20%) and rarely adenocarcinoma.

Lymphatic drainage in men will follow:

- Anterior urethra: superficial + deep inguinal LN -> pelvic LN (external, obturator, internal iliac)
- Posterior urethra: drain into pelvic LN.

Lymphatic drainage in women will follow:

- Proximal 1/3: pelvic LN chains
- Distal 2/3: superficial + deep inguinal nodes.

The WHO 1973 grading system has been replaced by the 2004 grading system, which differentiates urothelial carcinoma into papillary urothelial neoplasm of low malignant potential (PUNLMP) low-grade and high-grade.

Non-urothelial carcinoma is graded by a trinomial system (well, moderately and poorly differentiated tumours).

Table 22 – Pathological grading of urethral cancer

Urothelial carcinoma	
PUNLMP	Papillary urothelial neoplasm of low malignant potential
Low grade	Well differentiated
High grade	Poorly differentiated
Non-urothelial carcinoma	
GX	Tumour grade not assessed
G1	Well differentiated
G2	Moderately differentiated
G3	Poorly differentiated

INVESTIGATIONS

Examination of the external genitalia, inguinal lymphadenopathy.

Urgent cystoscopy and cold-cup biopsy of the lesion is investigation of choice (EAU 2023).

Cytology has a rather low sensitivity and should not be considered highly reliable.

Imaging – full staging CT should be requested; consider MRI with artificial erection for assessment of tumour depth/size and regional LN involvement.

Refer for urgent discussion at regional MDT for multi-modal approach due to rarity of tumour.

STAGING

Urothelial carcinoma is classified as per table below – note that there is a separate TNM staging system for prostatic urothelial carcinoma.

Table 23 – TNM eighth edition staging for urethral cancer [89]

T – Primary Tumour	
TX	Primary tumour cannot be assessed
T0	No evidence of primary tumour
Urethra (Male and Female)	
Tis	Carcinoma in situ
Ta	Non-invasive papillary, polypoid or verrucous carcinoma
T1	Tumour invades sub-epithelial connective tissue
T2	Tumour invades any of the following: corpus spongiosum, prostate, peri-urethral muscle
T3	Tumour invades any of the following: corpus cavernosum, EPE, anterior vagina, bladder neck
T4	Tumour invades other adjacent organs
Urothelial (TCC) of the Prostate	
Tis pu	Carcinoma in situ, involvement of prostatic urethra
Tis pd	Carcinoma in situ, involvement of prostatic ducts
T1	Tumour invades sub-epithelial connective tissue
T2	Tumour invades any of the following: prostatic stroma, corpus spongiosum, peri-urethral muscle
T3	Tumour invades any of the following: corpus cavernosum, beyond prostatic capsule, EPE
T4	Tumour invades other adjacent organs
N – Regional Lymph Nodes	
NX	Regional lymph nodes cannot be assessed
N0	No regional lymph node metastasis
N1	Metastasis in a single lymph node
N2	Metastasis in multiple lymph nodes
M – Distant Metastasis	
M0	No distant metastasis
M1	Distant metastasis

TREATMENT

Localised Primary Urethral Carcinoma

(Men)

Distal tumours have better prognosis than proximal. Aim for partial urethrectomy.

Wide local excision of urethra (along with tunica albuginea) and perineal urethostomy or hypospadiac opening if length adequate.

(Women)

Primary radical urethrectomy with bladder neck closure and appendico-vesicostomy.

Radiotherapy has high recurrence rates and complications.

Advanced Disease

Cisplatin-based chemotherapy – preferably neo-adjuvant before surgery rather than given alone.

REFERENCES

1. https://www.cancerresearchuk.org [last accessed 27 May 2020].
2. Kheirandish P, Chinegwundoh F (2011). Ethnic differences in prostate cancer. *British Journal of Cancer, 105*(4), 481.
3. Andriole G, Bostwick D, Brawley O, et al. (2004). Chemoprevention of prostate cancer in men at high risk: rationale and design of the reduction by dutasteride of prostate cancer events (REDUCE) trial. *Journal of Urology, 172*(4), 1,314–1,317.
4. Lippman SM, Klein EA, Goodman PJ, et al. (2009). Effect of selenium and vitamin E on risk of prostate cancer and other cancers: the Selenium and Vitamin E Cancer Prevention Trial (SELECT). *Jama, 301*(1), 39–51.
5. Brawer MK (2003). Androgen supplementation and prostate cancer risk: strategies for pretherapy assessment and monitoring. *Reviews in Urology, 5*(S1), S29.
6. Thompson IM, Ankerst DP, Chi C, et al. (2006). Assessing prostate cancer risk: results from the Prostate Cancer Prevention Trial. *Journal of the National Cancer Institute, 98*(8), 529–534.
7. Perner S, Demichelis F, Beroukhim R, et al. (2006). TMPRSS2: ERG fusion-associated deletions provide insight into the heterogeneity of prostate cancer. *Cancer Research, 66*(17), 8,337–8,341.
8. Andermann A, Blancquaert I, Beauchamp S, et al. (2008). Revisiting Wilson and Jungner in the genomic age: a review of screening criteria over the past 40 years. *Bulletin of the World Health Organization, 86*: 317–319.
9. Andriole GL, Crawford ED, Grubb III RL, et al. (2012). Prostate cancer screening in the randomized Prostate, Lung, Colorectal, and Ovarian Cancer Screening Trial: mortality results after 13 years of follow-up. *Journal of the National Cancer Institute, 104*(2), 125–132.
10. Hamdy FC, Donovan JL, Lane JA, et al. (2016). 10-year outcomes after monitoring, surgery, or radiotherapy for localized prostate cancer. *New England Journal of Medicine, 375*(15), 1,415–1,424.
11. Ilic D, Neuberger MM, Djulbegovic M, et al. (2013). Screening for prostate cancer. Cochrane database of systematic reviews.
12. http://www.aboutcancer.com/prostate_anatomy.htm [last accessed 9 April 2024].
13. Bostwick DG, Qian J (2004). High-grade prostatic intraepithelial neoplasia. *Modern Pathology, 17*(3), 360.
14. Mottet N, Bellmunt J, Bolla M, et al. (2017). EAU–ESTRO–ESUR–SIOG Guidelines on Prostate Cancer. *European Urology, 71*(4), 618–629.
15. Leone A, Rotker K, Butler C, et al. (2015). Atypical small acinar proliferation: repeat biopsy and detection of high grade prostate cancer. *Prostate Cancer.*

16. https://orchid-cancer.org.uk/prostate-cancer [last accessed 26 May 2020].

17. Humphrey PA (2004). Gleason grading and prognostic factors in carcinoma of the prostate. *Modern Pathology, 17*(3), 292.

18. Epstein JI, Egevad L, Amin MB, et al. (2016). The 2014 International Society of Urological Pathology (ISUP) consensus conference on Gleason grading of prostatic carcinoma. *American Journal of Surgical Pathology, 40*(2), 244–252.

19. Christensson A, Björk T, Nilsson O, et al. (1993). Serum prostate specific antigen complexed to α 1-antichymotrypsin as an indicator of prostate cancer. *Journal of Urology, 150*(1), 100–105.

20. Guess HA, Gormley GJ, Stoner E, et al. (1996). The effect of finasteride on prostate specific antigen: review of available data. *Journal of Urology, 155*(1), 3–9.

21. Oesterling JE, Jacobsen SJ, Chute CG, et al. (1993). Serum prostate-specific antigen in a community-based population of healthy men: establishment of age-specific reference ranges. *JAMA, 270*(7), 860–864.

22. D'Amico AV, Chen MH, Roehl KA, et al. (2004). Preoperative PSA velocity and the risk of death from prostate cancer after radical prostatectomy. *New England Journal of Medicine, 351*(2), 125–135.

23. Ng MK, Van As N, Thomas K, et al. (2009). Prostate-specific antigen (PSA) kinetics in untreated, localized prostate cancer: PSA velocity vs PSA doubling time. *BJU International, 103*(7), 872–876.

24. Catalona WJ, Southwick PC, Slawin KM, et al. (2000). Comparison of percent free PSA, PSA density, and age-specific PSA cutoffs for prostate cancer detection and staging. *Urology, 56*(2), 255–260.

25. Partin AW, Catalona WJ, Southwick PC, et al. (1996). Analysis of percent free prostate-specific antigen (PSA) for prostate cancer detection: influence of total PSA, prostate volume, and age. *Urology, 48*(6), 55–61.

26. Haese A, Huland E, Graefen M, et al. (1999). Supersensitive PSA-analysis after radical prostatectomy: a powerful tool to reduce the time gap between surgery and evidence of biochemical failure. *Anticancer Research, 19*(4A), 2,641–2,644.

27. Fradet Y, Saad F, Aprikian A, et al. (2004). uPM3, a new molecular urine test for the detection of prostate cancer. *Urology, 64*(2), 311–315.

28. Briganti A, Blute ML, Eastham JH, et al. (2009). Pelvic lymph node dissection in prostate cancer. *European Urology, 55*(6), 1,251–1,265.

29. Hövels A, Heesakkers RA, Adang EM, et al. (2008). The diagnostic accuracy of CT and MRI in the staging of pelvic lymph nodes in patients with prostate cancer: a meta-analysis. *Clinical Radiology, 63*(4), 387–395.

30. Husarik DB, Miralbell R, Dubs M, et al. (2008). Evaluation of [18F]-choline PET/CT for staging and restaging of prostate cancer. *European Journal of Nuclear Medicine and Molecular Imaging, 35*(2), 253–263.

31. Partin AW, Mangold LA, Lamm DM, et al. (2001). Contemporary update of prostate cancer staging nomograms (Partin Tables) for the new millennium. *Urology, 58*(6), 843–848.

32. Gleave ME, Coupland D, Drachenberg D, et al. (1996). Ability of serum prostate-specific antigen levels to predict normal bone scans in patients with newly diagnosed prostate cancer. *Urology, 47*(5), 708–712.

33. Turkbey B, Merino MJ, Gallardo EC, et al. (2014). Comparison of endorectal coil and nonendorectal coil T2W and diffusion-weighted MRI at 3 Tesla for localizing prostate cancer: correlation with whole-mount histopathology. *Journal of Magnetic Resonance Imaging, 39*(6), 1,443–1,448.

34. Ahmed HU, Bosaily AE, Brown LC, et al. (2017). Diagnostic accuracy of multi-parametric MRI and TRUS biopsy in prostate cancer (PROMIS): a paired validating confirmatory study. *Lancet, 389*(10,071), 815–822.

35. Hamoen EH, de Rooij M, Witjes JA, et al. (2015). Use of the Prostate Imaging Reporting and Data System (PI-RADS) for prostate cancer detection with multiparametric magnetic resonance imaging: a diagnostic meta-analysis. *European Urology, 67*(6), 1,112–1,121.

36. Nam RK, Saskin R, Lee Y, et al. (2010). Increasing hospital admission rates for urological complications after transrectal ultrasound guided prostate biopsy. *Journal of Urology, 183*(3), 963–969.

37. Remzi M, Fong YK, Dobrovits M, et al. (2005). The Vienna nomogram: validation of a novel biopsy strategy defining the optimal number of cores based on patient age and total prostate volume. *Journal of Urology, 174*(4), 1,256–1,261.

38. Pinkstaff DM, Igel TC, Petrou SP, et al. (2005). Systematic transperineal ultrasound-guided template biopsy of the prostate: three-year experience. *Urology, 65*(4), 735–739.

39. Bastacky SI, Walsh PC, Epstein JI (1993). Relationship between perineural tumor invasion on needle biopsy and radical prostatectomy capsular penetration in clinical stage B adenocarcinoma of the prostate. *American Journal of Surgical Pathology, 17*(4), 336–341.

40. https://www.nice.org.uk/guidance/ng131 [last accessed 9 April 2024].

41. Sundararajan V, Henderson T, Perry C, et al. (2004). New ICD-10 version of the Charlson comorbidity index predicted in-hospital mortality. *Journal of Clinical Epidemiology, 57*(12), 1,288–1,294.

42. van As NJ, Parker CC (2007). Active surveillance with selective radical treatment for localized prostate cancer. *Cancer Journal, 13*(5), 289–294.

43. Klotz L, Zhang L, Lam A, et al. (2009). Clinical results of long-term follow-up of a large, active surveillance cohort with localized prostate cancer. *Journal of Clinical Oncology, 28*(1), 126–131.

44. Wilt TJ, Brawer MK, Jones KM, et al. (2012). Radical prostatectomy versus observation for localised prostate cancer. *New England Journal of Medicine, 367,* 203–213.

45. Bill-Axelson A, Holmberg L, Garmo H, et al. (2014). Radical prostatectomy or watchful waiting in early prostate cancer. *New England Journal of Medicine, 370*(10), 932–942.

46. Gandaglia G, Martini A, Ploussard G, et al. (2020). External validation of the 2019 Briganti nomogram for the identification of prostate cancer patients who should be considered for an extended pelvic lymph node dissection. *European Urology, 78*(2), 138–142.

47. Gandaglia G, Ploussard G, Valerio M, et al. (2019). A novel nomogram to identify candidates for extended pelvic lymph node dissection among patients with clinically localised prostate cancer diagnosed with magnetic resonance imaging-targeted and systematic biopsies. *European Urology, 75*(3), 506–514.

48. Dearnaley D, Syndikus I, Mossop H, et al. (2016). Conventional versus hypofractionated high-dose intensity-modulated radiotherapy for prostate cancer: 5-year outcomes of the randomised, non-inferiority, phase 3 CHHiP trial. *Lancet Oncology, 17*(8), 1,047–1,060.

49. Bolla M, van Tienhoven G, Warde P, et al. (2010). External irradiation with or without long-term androgen suppression for prostate cancer with high metastatic risk: 10-year results of an EORTC randomised study. *Lancet Oncology, 11*(11), 1,066–1,073.

50. Ullah MI, Riche DM, Koch CA (2014). Transdermal testosterone replacement therapy in men. *Drug Design, Development and Therapy, 8:* 101–12.

51. Tannock IF, De Wit R, Berry WR, et al. (2004). Docetaxel plus prednisone or mitoxantrone plus prednisone for advanced prostate cancer. *New England Journal of Medicine, 351*(15), 1,502–1,512.

52. James ND, Sydes MR, Clarke NW, et al. (2016). Addition of docetaxel, zoledronic acid, or both to first-line long-term hormone therapy in prostate cancer (STAMPEDE): survival results from an adaptive, multiarm, multistage, platform randomised controlled trial. *Lancet, 387*(10,024), 1,163–1,177.

53. Sweeney CJ, Chen YH, Carducci M, et al. (2015). Chemohormonal Therapy in Metastatic Hormone-Sensitive Prostate Cancer. *New England Journal of Medicine, 373,* 737–746.

54. www.cancerresearchuk.org [last accessed 9 April 2024].

55. Schottenfeld D, Warshauer ME, Sherlock S, Zauber AG, Leder M, Payne R (1980). The epidemiology of testicular cancer in young adults. *American Journal of Epidemiology, 112*(2), 232–246.

56. Pettersson A, Richiardi L, Nordenskjold A, et al. (2007). Age at surgery for undescended testis and risk of testicular cancer. *New England Journal of Medicine, 356*(18), 1,835–1,841.

57. Frisch M, Biggar RJ, Engels EA, et al. (2001). AIDS-Cancer Match Registry Study Group. Association of cancer with AIDS-related immunosuppression in adults. *JAMA, 285*(13), 1,736–1,745.

58. Jacobsen R, Bostofte E, Engholm G, et al. (2000). Risk of testicular cancer in men with abnormal semen characteristics: cohort study. *BMJ, 321*(7,264), 789–792.

59. Bosl JG, Dmitrovsky E, Reuter VE, et al. (1989). Isochromosome of chromosome 12: clinically useful marker for male germ cell tumors. *Journal of the National Cancer Institute, 81*(24), 1,874–1,878.

60. Dogra VS, Gottlieb RH, Rubens DJ, et al. (2001). Testicular epidermoid cysts: sonographic features with histopathologic correlation. *Journal of Clinical Ultrasound, 29*(3), 192–196.

61. Heidenreich A, Engelmann UH, Vietsch HV, et al. (1995). Organ preserving surgery in testicular epidermoid cysts. *Journal of Urology, 153*(4), 1,147–1,150.

62. Moch H, Amin MB, Berney DM, et al. (2022). The 2022 World Health Organization Classification of Tumours of the Urinary System and Male Genital Organs – Part A: Renal, Penile, and Testicular Tumours. *European Urology, 82*, 458–468.

63. Al-Agha OM, Axiotis CA (2007). An in-depth look at Leydig cell tumor of the testis. *Archives of Pathology & Laboratory Medicine, 131*(2), 311–317.

64. Harland SJ, Cook PA, Fossa SD, et al. (1998). Intratubular germ cell neoplasia of the contralateral testis in testicular cancer: defining a high risk group. *Journal of Urology, 160*(4), 1,353–1,357.

65. Dieckmann KP, Kulejewski M, Pichlmeier U, et al. (2007). Diagnosis of contralateral testicular intraepithelial neoplasia (TIN) in patients with testicular germ cell cancer: systematic two-site biopsies are more sensitive than a single random biopsy. *European Urology, 51*(1), 175–185.

66. Mandybur TI (1977). Intracranial hemorrhage caused by metastatic tumors. *Neurology, 27*(7), 650.

67. Albers P, Albrecht W, Algaba F, et al. (2011). EAU guidelines on testicular cancer: 2011 update. *European Urology, 60*(2), 304–319.

68. DeCastro BJ, Peterson AC, Costabile RA (2008). A 5-year followup study of asymptomatic men with testicular microlithiasis. *Journal of Urology, 179*(4), 1,420–1,423.

69. Shukla AR, Woodard C, Carr MC, et al. (2004). Experience with testis sparing surgery for testicular teratoma. *Journal of Urology*, *171*(1), 161–163.

70. Robinson R, Tait CD, Clarke NW, et al. (2016). Is it safe to insert a testicular prosthesis at the time of radical orchidectomy for testis cancer: an audit of 904 men undergoing radical orchidectomy. *BJU International*, *117*(2), 249–252.

71. Warde P, Jewett MA (1998). Surveillance for stage I testicular seminoma: is it a good option? *Urologic Clinics of North America*, *25*(3), 425–433.

72. Warde P, Specht L, Horwich A, et al. (2002). Prognostic factors for relapse in stage I seminoma managed by surveillance: a pooled analysis. *Journal of Clinical Oncology*, *20*(22), 4,448–4,452.

73. Cornelison TL, Reed E (1993). Nephrotoxicity and hydration management for cisplatin, carboplatin, and ormaplatin. *Gynecologic Oncology*, *50*(2), 147–158.

74. Patrikidou A, Cazzaniga W, Berney D, et al. (2023). EAU Guidelines on Testicular Cancer: 2023 Update. *European Urology*, *84*(3), 289–301.

75. Beyer J, Collette L, Sauve N, et al. (2021). Survival and new prognosticators in metastatic seminoma: results from the IGCCCG – Update Consortium. *Journal of Clinical Oncology*, *39*(14), 1,553–1,562.

76. Gillessen S, Sauve N, Collette L, et al. (2021). Predicting outcomes in men with metastatic nonseminomatous germ cell tumors (NSGCT): results from the IGCCCG Update Consortium. *Journal of Clinical Oncology*, *39*(14), 1,563–1,574.

77. Maden C, Sherman KJ, Beckmann AM, et al. (1993). History of circumcision, medical conditions, and sexual activity and risk of penile cancer. *JNCI: Journal of the National Cancer Institute*, *85*(1), 19–24.

78. Lebelo RL, Boulet G, Nkosi CM, et al. (2014). Diversity of HPV types in cancerous and pre-cancerous lesions of South African men: implications for future HPV vaccination strategies. *Journal of Medical Virology*, *86*(2), 257–265.

79. Pow-Sang MR, Ferreira U, Pow-Sang JM, et al. (2010). Epidemiology and natural history of penile cancer. *Urology*, *76*(2), S2–6.

80. Bandini M, Ross JS, Zhu Y, et al. (2021). Association between human papillomavirus infection and outcome of perioperative nodal radiotherapy for penile carcinoma. *European Urology Oncology*, *4*(5), 802–810.

81. https://www.gov.uk/government/publications/hpv-vaccine-vaccination-guide-leaflet/information-on-the-hpv-vaccination-from-september-2023 [last accessed 9 April 2024].

82. Menon S, Moch H, Berney DM, et al. (2022). WHO 2022 classification of penile and scrotal cancers: updates and evolution. *Histopathology*, *82*(4), 508–520.

83. Hakenburg OW, Comperat E, Minhas S, et al. (2017). EAU Guidelines on Penile Cancer. *European Urology, 71*(4), 1–29.

84. Horenblas S, van Tinteren H (1994). Squamous cell carcinoma of the penis. IV. Prognostic factors of survival: analysis of tumor, nodes and metastatis classification system. *Journal of Urology, 151*(5), 1,239–1,243.

85. Heyns CF, Fleshner N, Sangar V, et al. (2010). Management of the lymph nodes in penile cancer. *Urology, 76*(2), S43–57.

86. Lont AP, Kroon BK, Gallee MP, et al. (2007). Pelvic lymph node dissection for penile carcinoma: extent of inguinal lymph node involvement as an indicator for pelvic lymph node involvement and survival. *Journal of Urology, 177*(3), 947–952.

87. Bouchot O, Rigaud J, Maillet F, et al. (2004). Morbidity of inguinal lymphadenectomy for invasive penile carcinoma. *European Urology*, 45(6), 761–766.

88. Wenzel M, Nocera L, Ruvolo CC, et al. (2021). Incidence rates and contemporary trends in primary urethral cancer. *Cancer Causes Control, 32*(6), 627–634.

89. Gakis G, Witjes JA, Bruins M, et al. (2023). EAU Guidelines on Primary Urethral Carcinoma, European Urology. Available at: https://d56bochluxqnz.cloudfront.net/documents/full-guideline/EAU-Guidelines-on-Primary-Urethral-Carcinoma-2023.pdf [last accessed 24 May 2024].

UROLOGICAL ONCOLOGY 2 MCQS

1. Which of the following has not been associated with an increased incidence of prostate cancer and/or ISUP grade at diagnosis and/or prostate cancer death?

    A) Inflammatory bowel disease
    B) UV radiation exposure
    C) Gonorrhoea
    D) Balding
    E) Occupational exposure to cadmium

2. With regard to genetics of prostate cancer, which of the following genes is a tumour suppressor gene?

    A) CyclinD2
    B) GPX3
    C) ERαA
    D) DKK3
    E) RAR-β

3. Which of the following statements about intraductal prostatic carcinoma is true?

    A) It is associated with favourable prognosis of prostate cancer
    B) It does not share morphological features of HGPIN
    C) Basal cells are damaged/destroyed
    D) Prostatic ducts are distended
    E) Incidence of this type of prostate cancer is unchanged in patients with BRCA gene mutations

4. On which chromosome number is PSA encoded?

    A) 11
    B) 13
    C) 15
    D) 17
    E) 19

5. The Briganti 2019 nomogram for calculating risk of lymph nodal involvement during radical prostatectomy proposes which cut-off percentage risk, above which pelvic node dissection should be offered?

   A) 6%
   B) 7%
   C) 8%
   D) 9%
   E) 10%

6. Which of the following is not a sequence on a multi-parametic MRI for prostate cancer?

   A) T2
   B) DWI
   C) FLAIR
   D) DCE
   E) ADC

7. Which one of the following conditions is not used in the Charlson Comorbidity Index calculation?

   A) Hypertension
   B) AIDS
   C) Peptic ulcer disease
   D) Dementia
   E) Diabetes

8. Regarding radical prostatectomy surgery, which of the following statements is false?

   A) Bladder neck preservation does not benefit post-operative urinary continence rates
   B) Neo-adjuvant hormones decrease positive margin rates
   C) Prophylatic antibiotics are recommended by EAU 2023
   D) Surgical volume is inversely proportional to positive margin rates
   E) Ligation of dorsal venous complex can be performed before or after its transection

9. What is the most appropriate level of testosterone which defines castration?

   A) 10ng/dL
   B) 20ng/dL
   C) 30ng/dL
   D) 40ng/dL
   E) 50ng/dL

10. *How many freeze–thaw cycles are routinely used in cryotherapy to treat PCa?*

   A) 2
   B) 3
   C) 4
   D) 5
   E) 6

11. *Which of the following is the correct dosage of degarelix?*

   A) 120mg stat, then 40mg monthly
   B) 120mg stat, then 80mg monthly
   C) 120mg stat, then 120mg monthly
   D) 240mg stat, then 80mg monthly
   E) 240mg stat, then 120mg monthly

12. *What is the correct dose of docetaxel chemotherapy for mPCa?*

   A) 25mg/m2 once every 3 weeks
   B) 50mg/m2 once every 3 weeks
   C) 75mg/m2 once every 3 weeks
   D) 100mg/m2 once every 3 weeks
   E) 125mg/m2 once every 3 weeks

13. *In patients with mCRPC and progression following docetaxel chemotherapy, as per EAU 2023, which of the following would not be a suitable option of treatment?*

   A) Abiraterone
   B) Cabazitaxel
   C) Radium-223
   D) Olaparib
   E) Paclitaxel

14. *Which of the following statements regarding the incidence of testicular cancer is false?*

   A) In females and males combined, testicular cancer is not among the 20 most common cancers in the UK
   B) Testicular cancer accounts for 1% of all new cancer cases in males in the UK
   C) Incidence rates are higher in Scotland than other UK constituent countries
   D) Less than 100 people die per year of testicular cancer in the UK every year
   E) 85–90% of men diagnosed with testicular cancer in England survive their disease for 10 years or more

15. *A 32-year-old male has testicular cancer. Histology after radical orchidectomy reveals classical seminoma, with vascular invasion and invasion of tunica albuginea, Staging CT scan reveals retro-peritoneal lymph node mass of 3cm, no further distant metastasis. Tumour markers were not performed. What is the correct staging for the patient?*

A) pT1pN1M0SX
B) pT1pN2M0SX
C) pT2pN1M0SX
D) pT2pN2M0SX
E) None of the above

16. *A 35-year-old male has testicular cancer. Histology after radical orchidectomy reveals non-seminomatous GCT (mature teratoma) with vascular invasion and involvement of tunica vaginalis. Staging CT scan + RPLND reveals 5 regional lymph nodes involved measuring 1.5cm, no further distant metastasis. Tumour markers taken prior to surgery: LDH < 1.5 x N, hCG 1,500, AFP 5,000. What is the correct staging for the patient?*

A) pT2pN1M0S1
B) pT3pN1M0S1
C) pT2pN1M0S2
D) pT3pN2M0S2
E) pT2pN2M0S1

17. *What is the correct serum half-life for the testicular tumour marker AFP?*

A) 24 hours
B) 36 hours
C) 3 days
D) 5 days
E) 7 days

18. *What is the correct serum half-life for the testicular tumour marker þhCG?*

A) 24 hours
B) 36 hours
C) 3 days
D) 5 days
E) 7 days

19. Which of the following statements regarding sperm banking in testicular cancer is false?

   A) HFEA code of practice says clinics should provide a cost plan to the patient prior to banking
   B) Correct storage temperature is -196°C
   C) The sperm cannot be used after the patient dies
   D) Recent COVID-19 infection prior to banking can adversely affect sample quality
   E) Up to a quarter of testicular patients are azoospermic before treatment

20. As per the IGCCCG prognostic system for metastatic NSGCT, which of the following factors would enter a patient in the "intermediate risk" group?

   A) AFP 5,000ng/mL
   B) ßHCG 1,000IU/L
   C) LDH 15x ULN
   D) Non-pulmonary visceral metastases
   E) Mediastinal primary tumour

21. Regarding HPV in penile cancer, which of the following statements is false?

   A) HPV vaccine in healthy teenagers is usually administered in 2 doses spaced in time
   B) Among HPV-associated penile carcinomas, basaloid has the highest prevalence of the infection
   C) HPV is prevalent in approximately 1 in 5 HPV-independent penile carcinomas
   D) Presence of HPV is not clearly associated with adverse prognosis
   E) In the UK, the HPV vaccine is offered routinely to boys in year 8

22. Which HPV vaccine is used in the NHS vaccination schedule?

   A) Cervarix
   B) Gardasil 9
   C) Revaxis
   D) Priorix
   E) Repevax

23. Which of the following is an HPV-related penile SCCa?

   A) Pseudohyperplastic carcinoma
   B) Verrucous carcinoma
   C) Adenosquamous carcinoma
   D) Papillary carcinoma
   E) Clear-cell carcinoma

24. Which of the following best describes the mechanism of action of 5-FU used to treat PeIN?

   A) Activation of TLR-7 which secretes inflammatory cytokines and activates Langerhans cells
   B) Anti-metabolite chemotherapy drug, works at S-phase causing cell-cycle arrest + apoptosis
   C) Cytotoxic activity via promoting and stabilising microtubule assembly
   D) Interferes with DNA replication and undergoes aquation, then involved in DNA cross-linking
   E) Inhibits DNA replication by forming a complex with DNA by intercalation of its planar rings

25. Regarding non-surgical options of treatment of stage ≤ T2 penile cancers, which of the following statements is true?

   A) Minimum dose of 70Gy should be delivered if RTx is selected treatment option
   B) Significantly higher power is required for CO2 LASER compared to Nd:YAG
   C) Nd:YAG LASER treatment healing time is faster than CO2 LASER, due to reduced depth of tissue coagulation
   D) CO2 LASER wavelength for treatment is $10.6\mu m$
   E) Brachytherapy should not be offered for lesions > 2cm in size

STATION 3
PAEDIATRIC
UROLOGY

ANTENATAL HYDRONEPHROSIS

EPIDEMIOLOGY

Widespread use of US during pregnancy has increased detection rates of antenatal hydronephrosis.

Incidence is 0.6% on second trimester (20 weeks gestation). [1]

65% of cases will resolve without treatment and < 5% require surgical intervention.

Standard minimum antenatal scans offered in the NHS are at 12 and 20 weeks gestation.

AETIOLOGY

Potential causes of antenatal hydronephrosis include PUJO (40% of cases i.e. most common), VUR, megaureter, PUV, ureterocoele, renal cysts, MCDK, physiological hydronephrosis. [2]

Each of these conditions will be covered separately in their appropriate sections below.

MANAGEMENT

The key challenge in managing the child with dilated upper urinary tract is deciding which patient should be observed, which managed medically and which requires surgical intervention.

Antenatal

Kidneys can be visualised clearly at the 20-week gestation (NHS anomaly scan), when almost all the amniotic fluid is urine.

The most sensitive time for foetal urinary tract assessment is at 28 weeks gestation (i.e. repeat US may be planned at this point if an anomaly was detected at 20-week scan).

If antenatal hydronephrosis is found, the following additional findings should be checked for on US:

- Degree of hydronephrosis (APD renal pelvis > 5mm)
- Cortical thinning and echogenicity of renal parenchyma
- Ureteric assessment for dilatation

- Bladder assessment for thickness, emptying or not seen (bladder exstrophy)
- Visible penis to determine male gender
- Amniotic fluid volume (oligo- or an-hydramnios is a marker of poor outcome)
- Health of contra-lateral kidney.

US should be repeated later in third trimester of pregnancy to review progression of hydronephrosis.

Parental counselling – important for expectations particularly for severe cases with massive progressive bilateral dilatation, oligo-/an-hydramnios and pulmonary hypoplasia.

Delivery – high-risk cases should be delivered in appropriate tertiary centre with NICU available

Intra-uterine intervention is rarely indicated.

Postnatal

Postnatal investigation/management of antenatal hydronephrosis will depend on underlying diagnosis and severity. These are described in the appropriate sections for each condition.

Initial assessment should follow systematic A-to-E APLS protocol. Further consider:

- Blood-pressure monitoring and follow-up
- Blood tests, including UE, FBC, gas sampling
- Continuous antibiotic prophylaxis (e.g. trimethoprim 2mg/kg OD) in higher-risk cases (e.g. uncircumcised males and/or high-grade hydronephrosis).

Postnatal imaging will always be required.

Transitory neonatal dehydration lasts 48 hours after birth; therefore if safe, postnatal US should be deferred following this period of neonatal oliguria (i.e. consider 1–2 weeks post-partum).

Urgent postnatal US warranted in severe cases (oligo-hydramnios, single kidney, bilateral obstruction).

MCUG can be deferred until the child is older in non-urgent clinical scenarios (e.g. VUR).

In urgent cases, MCUG should be performed urgently after birth (e.g. suspected PUV with bilateral hydro-ureteronephrosis and thick-walled bladder).

DMSA/MAG3 renogram are otherwise usually deferred until child is > 6 weeks of age.

Figure 1 – Algorithm for antenatal hydronephrosis

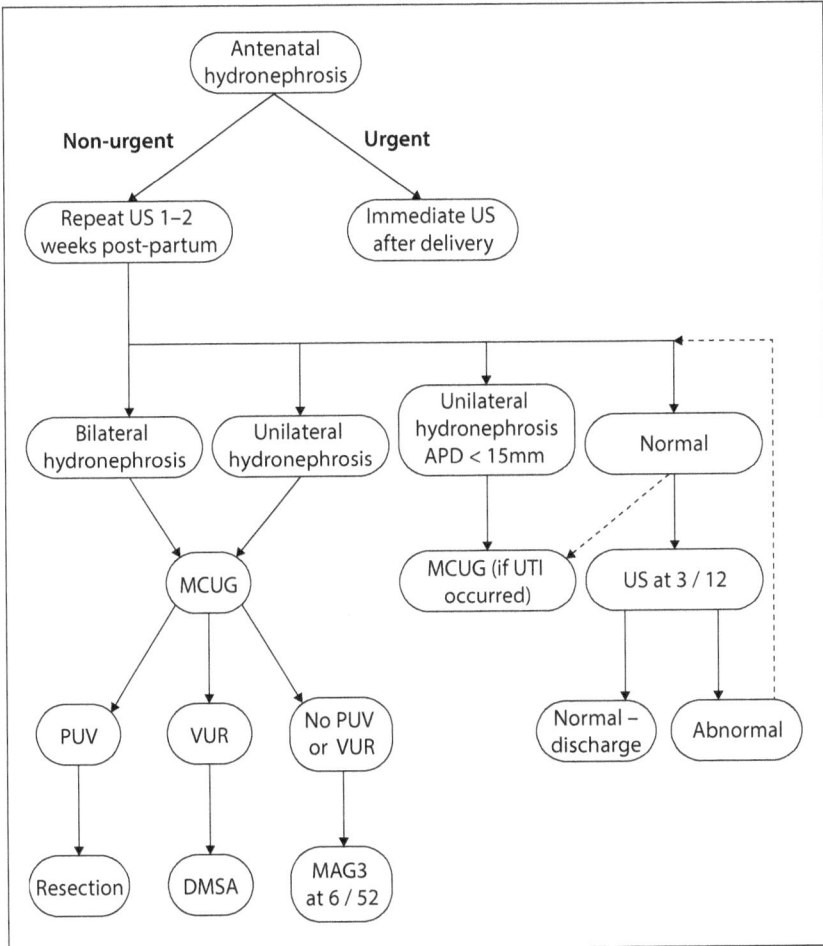

VESICO-URETERIC REFLUX

VUR is an anatomical and/or functional disorder arising from abnormal retrograde urinary flow from the bladder to the upper tracts, which may cause renal scarring, hypertension and renal failure.

Lack of strong RCTs limits ability to establish definitive guidelines for the management of VUR.

EPIDEMIOLOGY

Overall incidence in children is 1% – significant proportion will not require intervention.

Offspring of affected parent have 40% incidence of VUR, siblings of affected child have 30% risk; however, screening remains controversial (e.g. US as screening tool). [3]

Sibling screening is challenging due to lack of non-invasive tests (MCUG requires catheterisation).

Female to male ratio is 5:1.

VUR in males tends to be diagnosed at younger age (0–2 years) and be of a higher grade but has a greater chance of spontaneous resolution. [4]

VUR in females tends to be diagnosed later (2–7 years) but be of lower grade.

Incidence of VUR in children with UTIs is 30% and in antenatal hydronephrosis is 15%.

There is a clear co-prevalence of LUTD and VUR implying functional element to the condition.

Reflux nephropathy is one of the commonest causes of hypertension in children.

PATHOGENESIS

Anti-reflux mechanisms include the oblique entry of ureter through bladder wall (1–2cm) and muscular attachments which prevent reflux during bladder filling and voiding.

VUR arises from deficiency of valvular mechanism of longitudinal muscle of intra-vesical ureter

The normal ratio of intra-mural ureteric length to ureteric diameter is 5:1.

Paquin's law, where reflux occurs due to short intra-mural length (ratio < 5:1).

CLASSIFICATION

Primary

Results from congenital abnormality of the VUJ (e.g. Paquin's law).

In duplication, the *Weigert–Meyer rule* states the lower moiety ureter enters the bladder proximally and laterally, resulting in shorter intra-mural length and thus higher risk of reflux.

Genetically recognised cause with autosomal dominant inheritance.

Secondary

Results from LUTD associated with raised intra-vesical pressures – VUR tends to resolve once bladder pressures brought down to normal by treating the LUTD.

Reflux of sterile urine at physiological voiding pressures does not cause renal scarring.

The most common anatomic bladder obstruction causing VUR in boys is PUV, and VUR is present in the majority of patients with this condition.

In females the most common anatomical cause is ureterocoele.

Neuropathic bladders with intra-vesical pressures > 40cm H20 have strong association with VUR.

Other causes include PUV, DSD, urethral stenosis.

Treatment for secondary reflux is to target the underlying cause.

GRADING

Grading of VUR is based on the extent of retrograde filling and dilatation of the ureter, renal pelvis and calyces on MCUG. (Accurately grading VUR is impossible with co-existent ipsilateral obstruction.)

Table 1 – Grading system for VUR on MCUG according to International Reflux Study Committee [2]

VUR Grade	Characteristics	Rate of Spontaneous Resolution (%)	Distribution of Grades (%)
1	Reflux does not reach renal pelvis with varying degrees of ureteral dilatation	90	7
2	Reflux reaches renal pelvis, no dilatation of collecting system, normal fornices	80	53
3	Mild/moderate ureteric dilatation +/- tortuosity, moderate dilatation of collecting system, normal or minimally deformed fornices	50	32
4	Moderate ureteric dilatation +/- tortuosity, moderate dilatation of collecting system, blunt fornices, papillae impressions still visible	20	6
5	Gross ureteric dilatation and tortuosity, marked dilatation of collecting system, papillary impressions not visible, intra-parenchymal reflux	< 10	2

PRESENTATION

VUR presents with varying degrees of severity; however, most do not result in renal scarring and do not require any surgical intervention.

Asymptomatic bacteriuria is not associated with renal scarring.

VUR may present acutely with UTI, failure to thrive or even chronic vomiting and diarrhoea.

Pyelonephritis in children may result in renal scarring (however, rarely resulting in renal impairment) which does carry a long-term risk of hypertension (10% if unilateral, 20% if bilateral).

Greatest risk of renal scarring is < 4 years of age (as intra-mural ureter elongates with growth), scarring occurs maximally after first episode of pyelonephritis.

Having VUR that is symptomatic (i.e. UTI) increases risk of scarring. [5]

Acute pyelonephritis in children has 20% risk of recurrence within 12 months.

VUR may also present with LUT dysfunction (LUTD), including urge +/- incontinence, frequency, prolonged voiding or even bowel dysfunction.

VUR is the most common cause of severe hypertension in children and young adults.

DIAGNOSTIC EVALUATION

History from the parent and/or child should enquire regarding:

- Overall health and development of child
- Presence of LUTD, UTI, constipation
- Parental and sibling history of VUR.

Examination of the child (with the parent/guardian present) should cover:

- General examination of height, weight (growth chart)
- Urological assessment for palpable bladder or kidneys, external genitalia
- Blood pressure, urinalysis and MSU.

Blood tests may include UE and FBC if bilateral renal cortical abnormalities.

IMAGING

MCUG is gold-standard investigation to diagnose VUR, assess grade and reversible causes. [6]

- Patient is catheterised and iodine-based contrast injected into bladder.
- X-rays are taken and catheter is then removed.
- Patient voids and x-rays taken again.
- It is, however, an invasive test and child/parents need counselling appropriately.

DMSA renogram is useful in assessment of VUR for:

- Detecting and monitoring renal cortical scarring (photo-deficient lesions)
- Providing baseline at diagnosis which can be used for comparison with successive scans

- Split kidney function
- Diagnostic tool during suspected acute pyelonephritis (dimercaptosuccinic acid uptake is poor in areas of inflammation and will appear as cold-spots).

VUDS not routinely used unless underlying secondary reflux is suspected e.g. spina bifida, PUV.

US can be used as first evaluation tool for antenatal hydronephrosis, repeated > 7 days after birth.

US can reliably assess kidney size, collecting system dilatation and parenchymal thickness.

US is not sensitive for VUR – absence of hydronephrosis does not exclude VUR; however, two sequentially normal US scans make the chance of significant VUR unlikely.

The presence of cortical scarring on US warrants further assessment with MCUG.

MANAGEMENT

Main aim of management is kidney function preservation by minimising risk of pyelonephritis episodes.

Risk factors for each patient (age, sex, grade of reflux, associated LUTD, abnormal anatomy and kidney appearance) should be evaluated to identify those at highest risk of renal scarring.

The majority of primary VUR grades I–II will resolve spontaneously (≤ 80%).

Overall ≤ 50% resolution seen in grades III–V as child's growth elongates the intra-mural segment of ureter, within 4–5 years follow-up.

Postnatal renal damage is very unlikely provided child does not have UTIs or any associated LUTD.

CONSERVATIVE THERAPY

General advice, including fluid intake, treatment of any constipation, regular voiding.

Education, including informing parents that UTI or febrile presentations need urgent treatment.

LUTD management is key if present.

Whilst on conservative treatment, child's growth, blood pressure, urinalysis, UTI events should be monitored regularly, follow-up imaging depends on each case (consider annual US as minimum).

Continuous Antibiotic Prophylaxis

CAP is not required in asymptomatic children with low-grade VUR (EAU 2024).

CAP can prevent UTIs in children with higher-grade VUR, but reduction in renal scarring is not proven.

Challenging to determine which high-grade should receive CAP – factors such as gender, circumcision status, age all play a part. Safe approach likely to consider CAP in all patients.

No standard recommended age when to discontinue CAP; however, cessation could be considered once child is suitably toilet trained, not suffering with LUTD and no UTI > 1 year.

| **VIVA** | The topic of CAP in VUR is a FRCS (Urol) viva favourite, as it allows the candidate to discuss the available evidence (see key papers below) as well as recognise that its use should not be dogmatic but relies on sound clinician background knowledge to apply on a case-by-case basis.

KEY PAPER | RIVUR Trial (2014) [7]

Randomised, placebo-controlled trial published in *NEJM* regarding CAP for children with VUR.

600+ children with VUR randomised to receive CAP vs. placebo.

Found reduced risk of recurrent UTI by 50% but not renal scarring and its consequences (hypertension, ESRF) and no significant increased antimicrobial resistance.

KEY PAPER | Swedish Reflux Study (2010) [8]

Evaluated > 200 children with grade 3–4 VUR randomised equally to:

• CAP vs. endoscopic injection vs. surveillance.

MCUG and DMSA performed before randomisation and after 2 years.

Findings: Girls – prophylactic antibiotics reduced scarring and UTI, injections reduced UTI

Boys – no benefit from any active treatment

SURGICAL TREATMENT

The indications for surgical treatment for VUR may include:

- Failure of conservative therapy (breakthrough UTI, non-compliance, new renal scarring)
- Persistent high-grade VUR (IV or V).

There is no consensus regarding the optimum timing of surgical correction.

Circumcision is beneficial in males with VUR and anatomical abnormalities and should be offered.

Surgical options involve either endoscopic injection of bulking agents or ureteric reimplantation.

Endoscopic Options

Endoscopic options are preferable for lower grades of reflux.

Day-case cystoscopy and injection of bulking agent Deflux around the ureteric orifice with success rates of 80% (can be repeated). [9]

Injected bulking agent elevates ureteric orifice which lengthens the submucosal tunnel, narrowing the lumen but still allowing antegrade flow of urine.

Sub-ureteric Teflon injection (STING) fallen out of favour due to Teflon migration to distant organs.

Reimplantation Options

Major reconstruction should be considered for persisting higher-grade reflux as outcomes are better compared to endoscopic injection.

There are various surgical options involving reimplantation of the ureter (open/robotic): [9]

- *Intra-vesical*, by opening the bladder, mobilising the ureter and advancing it across the trigone (*Cohen's* repair) or implanting it higher and more medially (*Leadbetter–Politano* repair), always respecting the 5:1 Paquin's rule
- *Extra-vesical*, by suturing the distal ureter onto the bladder and constructing a tunnel of detrusor muscle around it (*Lich–Gregoir* procedure).

POSTERIOR URETHRAL VALVES

EPIDEMIOLOGY

PUV are one of the few life-threatening congenital abnormalities of the urinary tract found during the neonatal period.

Alternative term is congenital obstructive posterior urethral membrane (COPUM).

Incidence is 1 in 5,000 males. [10]

50% will have day- and night-time incontinence at age 5 years.

Risk of long-term CKD ≤ 32% and ESRF ≤ 20%. [11]

PATHOLOGY

PUV arise through abnormal Wolffian duct insertion in urogenital sinus during foetal development (does not occur in females).

Outflow obstruction leads to abnormalities in bladder wall components (increased collagen content, aberrations in nerve supply and renal dysplasia).

A secondary reflux is noted in ≥ 50% of children with PUV.

CLASSIFICATION

PUV were originally described by H.H. Young using three categories: [12]

- *Type 1* – bicuspid valves from verumontanum through to membranous urethra, fusing with anterior wall of urethra
- *Type 2* – this is a fold and non-obstructive and therefore not associated with PUV
- *Type 3* – sheet membrane attached to entire urethral circumference with a central aperture (iris-shaped); this will be converted to Type 1 when a catheter is passed.

PRESENTATION

Majority diagnosed antenatally – 60% identified on US at 20 weeks gestation (accounting for 1% of all cases of antenatally detected hydronephrosis).

Antenatal US findings may include:

- Bilateral hydro-ureteronephrosis
- Thick-walled bladder
- Dilated posterior urethra (keyhole sign)
- Renal dysplasia
- Oligo-hydramnios.

Newborns/infants may present with urinary sepsis, palpable bladder, signs of renal failure and respiratory distress secondary to pulmonary hypoplasia (most common cause of early mortality).

Potter's facies (due to oligo-hydramnios) include flattened nose, epicanthal folds, low-set ears.

Older children may present with rUTI, weak stream, incontinence, failure to thrive, renal impairment.

Pop-off pressure valve, self-defence mechanisms to reduce urinary tract pressures, including:

- Bladder diverticula
- Reflux in renal units to protect contra-lateral kidney
- Bladder or renal pelvis rupture (seen as extravasation on MCUG) with or without urinary ascites.

This, however, has not been proven to preserve overall long-term renal function. [13]

MANAGEMENT

ANTENATAL MANAGEMENT

Most cases are detected antenatally and note oligo- or an-hydramnios. Amniotic fluid is necessary for healthy lung development and its absence may lead to pulmonary hypoplasia.

Vesico-amniotic shunt insertion does not make a difference to long-term outcomes.

LASER ablation of foetal PUV currently has no proven benefit.

Repeat antenatal US to review progression in third trimester – if bilateral/severe hydronephrosis, plan for delivery in specialist centre with NICU and paediatric nephrology; counsel parents carefully.

POSTNATAL MANAGEMENT

Resuscitate in a systematic fashion following Airway-to-Exposure protocol, with paediatric support at hand and access to neonatal ITU.

The following aspects of management must be addressed:

- *Catheter insertion*, using 6F feeding tube (although the risk of this is that it may fall out) or an SPC (risk of urethral catheter is balloon inflation may occlude ureteric orifices)
- *Treat diuresis*, by replacing fluids, monitoring urine output and UEs, liaise with nephrology
- *Prophylactic antibiotics*, e.g. trimethoprim 2mg/kg daily
- Urgent imaging to include repeat USS and proceeding to MCUG.

Once emergency management is in place, proceed to establish a diagnosis.

The investigation of choice is the MCUG. [2]

On the MCUG in PUV a secondary reflux is observed in > 50% (associated with renal dysplasia) and it is important to check catheter is in bladder and not posterior urethra. [14]

MCUG may show dilated ureter, trabeculated bladder, narrowed junction between dilated posterior urethra and narrower anterior urethra (site of PUV).

Valve Ablation

Definitive treatment is cystoscopy and ablation/resection of valves under general anaesthesia.

Main complication is urethral stricture (i.e. limit electrocoagulation and use cold knife). [15]

If the urethra is too small to allow cystoscope, a temporary vesicostomy is performed (unless SPC already in situ which can be left up to 12 weeks).

FOLLOW-UP

Following valve resection, a follow-up cystoscopy or MCUG should be repeated at 3 months, to assess for any residual valve tissue.

DMSA should be performed to assess split kidney function. [2]

VUDS should be considered to assess any voiding dysfunction in childhood.

Despite early intervention, bladder function is abnormal in 70% of boys in the long term (consider stating in the FRCS (Urol) viva that you would never discharge a boy with PUV).

Long-term follow-up is warranted due to implications of PUV – renal function monitoring, assessments of LUTS conditions, recurrent UTI and overall development.

Poor prognosis associated with oligo-hydramnios, high levels B2 micro globulin in foetal urine (antenatally) and low GFR, day-time incontinence, urodynamic detrusor failure (postnatally).

PELVIURETERIC JUNCTION OBSTRUCTION AND MEGAURETER

EPIDEMIOLOGY

Most common pathological cause of neonatal hydronephrosis

Childhood incidence is 1 in 1,500.

Male-to-female ratio is 2:1, left-to-right ratio is 2:1, bilateral in 10%. [16]

AETIOLOGY

In most children the PUJO is congenital.

Extrinsic – due to compression of PUJ by aberrant crossing vessels.

Intrinsic – due to abnormal insertion of ureter into renal pelvis, ureteric folds or PUJ muscle which is hypo-plastic or aperistaltic.

PRESENTATION

Most commonly diagnosed via antenatal US with unilateral hydronephrosis (PUJO is most common cause of hydronephrosis without ureteric dilatation).

UTI, haematuria, loin pain or palpable mass.

Deitl's crisis – pain exacerbated by drinking large fluid volumes where subsequent diuresis exacerbates stretching of the upper tract. [17]

INVESTIGATION

US assesses degree of hydronephrosis, calyceal dilatation and cortical thinning.

US should be repeated urgently after birth (if severe bilateral hydronephrosis); for less urgent cases defer > 7 days to allow for physiological diuresis, which may resolve hydronephrosis.

If US excludes ureteric dilatation then there is no need for MCUG (i.e. VUR highly unlikely).

MAG3 renogram performed at 6–12 weeks of age to confirm the diagnosis of PUJO.

MANAGEMENT

Consider covering child with CAP until diagnosis is made, particularly if uncircumcised, or if hydronephrosis is severe.

Asymptomatic cases should initially be managed conservatively.

Symptomatic obstruction (e.g. UTI, pain, pyelonephritis) will require surgical correction.

Pyeloplasty can be performed open/laparoscopic/robotically with comparable long-term success rates, minimally invasive benefits cosmesis, length of in-patient stay and complication rates.

Standard technique is Anderson–Hynes dismembered pyeloplasty.

The following are indications for surgery: [2]

- Symptomatic children
- Impaired split function of kidney (< 40% on affected side is significant)
- Sequential deterioration of affected kidney function (decrease in > 10% differential function or increasing hydronephrosis on USS
- Hydronephrosis > 50 mm of renal AP pelvic diameter.

If the kidney is confirmed non-functioning, then simple nephrectomy is recommended.

Most children with an APD renal pelvis > 40mm will require surgery; however, only 1–3% of those with APD < 20mm require this (20% of those 20–30mm). [9]

MEGAURETER

Megaureter is the term that describes a dilated ureter (> 7mm).

Megaureter most commonly arises due to obstruction at the level where the distal ureter enters the bladder (VUJ), also called *primary obstructive megaureter*.

Megaureter can also be secondary to any other condition which may dilate/obstruct the ureter, such as urolithiasis, stricture, tumour or BOO (if bilateral).

CLASSIFICATION

Megaureter can be divided into 4 groups:

- Obstructed
- Refluxing
- Non-refluxing, non-obstructed
- Refluxing and obstructed.

EPIDEMIOLOGY

Affects 1 in 200 children, boys more frequently than girls, left more than right.

4% of cases of antenatally detected hydronephrosis.

The most common presenting symptom is UTI.

AETIOLOGY

Refluxing megaureter is due to VUR (discussed in "Vesico-ureteric Reflux" section above)

Obstructive megaureter is associated with a stenotic or aperistaltic segment of distal ureter.

INVESTIGATION

US – repeat > 7 days after birth to reassess persistence of ureteric dilatation after physiological diuresis.

MCUG can help distinguish between obstructive and refluxing cause.

MAG3 may be performed 6–12 weeks after delivery (ipsilateral PUJO is found in 13% of cases) and can help distinguish obstructed vs. non-obstructed.

MANAGEMENT

Principles of management are similar as per strategic approach to PUJO.

Conservative treatment is warranted with CAP, providing child is symptom-free, split function > 40% and no sequential deterioration in sonographic/ renogram results.

Surgery < 12 months of age is usually limited to stent insertion.

Most primary obstructive megaureters will resolve spontaneously – therefore, any corrective surgery should be deferred for as long as possible provided child is well.

Definitive surgery includes ureteric reimplantation +/- excision of stenotic segment of ureter.

ECTOPIC URETER, URETEROCOELE AND RENAL DYSPLASIA

ECTOPIC URETER

EPIDEMIOLOGY

Ectopic ureter is caused by the ureteric bud which arises from an abnormally high or low position on the mesonephric duct during embryological development.

80% are associated with a duplicated collection system.

5x more common in females than males (incidence difficult to determine as many are asymptomatic).

Most ectopic ureters in females are associated with a duplex kidney.

In girls the ectopic ureter orifice may be located in vagina, urethra, uterus, fallopian tube.

Most common site for ectopic ureter orifice drainage in boys is the posterior urethra, and it is never sited below the external sphincter.

CLASSIFICATION

Two ureters may join to form a single ureter, or they may both pass down individually into the bladder (complete duplication).

Weigert–Meyer rule – in complete duplication, the upper renal moiety always opens onto bladder below and medial to the lower moiety ureter (i.e. the upper moiety obstructs, the lower moiety refluxes).

PRESENTATION

Antenatally – may be detected by antenatal US revealing hydronephrosis of affected side.

Postnatally – with acute or rUTI, dribbling of urine, epididymitis (in pre-adolescent boys).

Females – if the ureteric opening is below the urethral sphincter, girl may present with persistent incontinence/leakage (this does not occur in males as never below external sphincter).

INVESTIGATION

US for initial assessment, MCUG evaluates for reflux.

DMSA assesses split function and differential function between upper and lower pole moieties of a duplex kidney to help plan surgery.

MANAGEMENT

Conservative with CAP cover is an option in the well child.

An ectopic ureter associated with dilated poorly functioning upper moiety of kidney is an indication for hemi-nephrectomy.

URETEROCOELE

EPIDEMIOLOGY

A ureterocoele is a cystic dilatation of the distal intra-vesical ureter as it drains into the bladder.

Ureterocoele is 4–7x more common in females vs. males.

80% associated with upper pole ureter in duplicated systems, 20% in single systems, 10% are bilateral.

CLASSIFICATION

Intra-vesical/Orthotopic (20%) [2]

Ureterocoele completely confined within the bladder, more common in males and single system:

- Stenotic, small stenotic ureteric orifice associated with obstruction
- Non-obstructed, large ureteric orifice.

Extra-vesical/Ectopic (80%) [2]

Ureterocoele extends to bladder neck or urethra, more common in females and duplex systems:

- Sphincteric (extends into bladder neck and urethra)
- Sphinctero-stenotic (ureteric orifice stenosed)
- Caeco-ureterocoele
- Blind ectopic.

PRESENTATION

Antenatally – with US detected hydronephrosis, postnatally – with UTI, pain, vaginal mass in girls (if prolapsing ureterocoele).

Ureterocoeles usually cause obstruction of the upper pole.

INVESTIGATION

US shows a thin-walled cyst-like appearance in the bladder; may reveal dilated ureter behind bladder.

MCUG identifies ureterocoele location, size, evaluates for associated VUR which is common.

DMSA for split renal moiety function and cortical abnormalities in the presence of VUR.

MANAGEMENT

Commence treatment with CAP at birth.

The choice of treatment modality depends on the following criteria:

- Clinical status of patient
- Age of child
- Presence of reflux or obstruction
- Function of upper pole
- Intra-vesical vs. ectopic ureterocoele.

Management is controversial with a choice between conservative, endoscopic decompression, ureteral reimplantation, partial nephroureterectomy or complete reconstruction.

Early treatment – antibiotics, immediate endoscopic incision of ureterocoele if septic or if featuring bladder neck obstruction.

Re-evaluation – appropriate if child is asymptomatic, no severe hydro-ureteronephrosis and no evidence of bladder outlet obstruction.

Surgery may vary from upper pole nephrectomy to complete ipsilateral LUT reconstruction.

RENAL DYSPLASIA

HORSESHOE KIDNEY

Horseshoe kidney is the most common example of renal fusion – prevalence 1 in 400. [18]

The kidneys lie vertically rather than obliquely and are joined by an isthmus (located anterior to L3–L4) which in 95% of cases joins the lower poles.

Ascent of the kidney is obstructed by the inferior mesenteric artery; hence it lies lower in the abdomen.

Normal rotation is prevented, therefore renal pelvis lies anteriorly and ureters pass anteriorly over the kidneys and isthmus.

Most patients are asymptomatic with a normal renal function.

Horseshoe kidney in presence of coarctation of aorta may suggest Turner's syndrome. [19]

ECTOPIC KIDNEY

Kidneys fail to achieve normal position, and can be thoracic, abdominal, pelvic or lumbar.

The affected kidney is usually smaller.

Left is more common than right, bilateral in < 10%.

Pelvic location is most common (60%) and most frequent cause of hydronephrosis in this scenario is due to PUJO – as a result of incomplete rotation of kidney.

Pelvic kidneys lie opposite the sacrum and below the bifurcation of the aorta.

RENAL AGENESIS

Unilateral renal agenesis is the absence of one kidney due to embryological abnormality or absence of the ureteric bud (failed induction of nephrogenesis).

Incidence of unilateral renal agenesis is 1:1,000 (left more than right, males more than females).

Many patients are asymptomatic.

Associated with absent ipsilateral ureter, uterine abnormalities (uni-cornuate, where one side failed to develop; didelphys, double uterus), absence of vas deferens.

Bilateral renal agenesis is incompatible with life.

DUPLEX KIDNEY

Duplex kidneys arise from two separate ureteric buds which induce separate segments of the metanephric blastema.

PUJO and VUR most commonly occur in the duplex lower pole/moiety.

Ectopic ureter is almost always associated with the duplex upper pole/moiety.

PHIMOSIS AND CIRCUMCISION

EPIDEMIOLOGY

By 12 months of age, foreskin retraction behind glandular sulcus is achieved in 50%, therefore in those where this is not possible it is termed "physiological".

Phimosis is present in 8% of 6 year olds and 1% of 16 year olds (i.e. most cases will resolve). [20]

PHYSIOLOGICAL PHIMOSIS

Physiological phimosis can be also termed primary phimosis.

This arises due to adhesions between the glans epithelium with the inner epithelium lining layer.

Physiological phimosis should resolve naturally by processes which separate these layers of skin:

- Spontaneous erections
- Penile growth
- Epithelial desquamation.

Non-surgical treatment includes 4–6 weeks of topical corticosteroid cream (e.g. 0.05% betamethasone) applied twice daily directly onto the narrow ring under gentle retraction.

This treatment strategy has no long-term demonstrable risks or side-effects; success rates ≤ 90% and therefore indicated as first-line treatment. [2]

BALANITIS XEROTICA OBLITERANS

BXO (also known as lichen sclerosus) can affect any part of the skin, but has a predilection for genitalia.

Cardinal signs on histology:

- Loss of rete pegs
- Hyper-keratosis
- Thinned epithelium.

BXO is not contagious. The pathophysiology remains unknown; however, auto-immune mechanism has been suggested as well as a sequalae of chronic infections.

Can affect glans, foreskin, external urethral meatus and urethra.

Examination when retracting the foreskin will reveal a white thickened ring of tissue, rather than the pink inner mucosa of foreskin which should appear as a carnation flower.

BXO should not be treated with topical steroids or preputioplasty, but requires a circumcision.

CIRCUMCISION

The medical indications for circumcision in children include:

- Treatment of BXO [2]
- Recurrent symptomatic balanoposthitis
- Symptomatic phimosis
- Recurrent paraphimosis.

Circumcision can contribute to management of children with VUR (NNN = 4 to prevent 1 UTI) and rUTI (NNT = 11). [9]

Routine neonatal circumcision is not recommended to prevent penile carcinoma. [21]

Circumcision contraindicated in:

- Presence of hypospadias (foreskin required for reconstructive surgery)
- Active balanitis
- Buried penis megaprepuce
- Uncorrected coagulopathy.

Risks include infection requiring antibiotics (2%), bleeding and return to theatre, cosmetic dissatisfaction, meatal stenosis, urethro-cutaneous fistula.

PREPUTIOPLASTY

Longitudinal preputial incision sutured transversely in the aim of widening the preputial opening.

Not a treatment for BXO.

Requires child co-operation to regularly retract foreskin after surgery and maintain hygiene.

BURIED PENIS MEGAPREPUCE

Also known as congenital megaprepuce.

Patients will present with buried penis; whereby outer preputial skin appears to meet directly with abdominal wall skin dorsally and scrotum ventrally. [22]

It is not a true phimosis.

Urine collects in foreskin and has to be milked out.

Surgical correction involves removing the inner preputial skin and using the outer preputial skin to substitute penile shaft.

Megameatus is congenital appearance of a large meatus; patient can be discharged.

UNDESCENDED TESTIS

EPIDEMIOLOGY

Cryptorchidism (UDT) is one of the most common congenital malformations of male neonates.

Incidence depends on gestational age: ≤ 4% of full-term and ≤ 40% of pre-term infants.

Many will spontaneously descend, hence incidence at 1 year in full-term infants reduces to 1% (most will have descended by 3 months of age due to neonatal LH surge).

If testis has not descended by 3 months of age, it is unlikely to happen spontaneously.

If bilateral UDT is noted (≤ 30% of cases) and/or concomitant hypospadias, undertake thorough examination to assess for DSD.

Only 1–3% of boys with UDT will develop TC (however, 10% of patients with testicular cancer have a history of UDT).

AETIOLOGY

Until 6 weeks gestation the gonads remain undifferentiated (until SRY gene influence occurs).

SRY is the master gene responsible for male sexual differentiation. [9]

First Phase (7–8 weeks) – testicular descent from genital ridge to internal inguinal ring, occurs under influence of MIS.

Second Phase (25–30 weeks) – testicular descent through inguinal canal into scrotum, occurs under the influence of testosterone.

Endocrine abnormalities – low levels of androgens, HCG, LH, MIS

Decreased intra-abdominal pressure – prune belly syndrome, gastroschisis

RISK FACTORS

Premature birth is the most significant risk factor.

Twins or family history (14% of boys with UDT have positive family history).

Low birth weight.

CLASSIFICATION

The most useful classification for UDT is palpable (80%) vs. non-palpable.

Possible locations of a non-palpable testis include intra-abdominal and inguinal (50%), absent (20%), atrophic (30%) and ectopic.

Most intra-abdominal testes are close to internal inguinal ring opening.

Palpable includes true UDT and ectopic.

Ectopic Testis (< 5%)

Abnormal testis migration below external ring of the inguinal canal (perineum, base of penis, femoral).

The most common aberrant position is in the superficial inguinal pouch.

It is not usually possible for an ectopic testis to descend into its normal position into the scrotum, therefore surgical intervention is warranted.

Retractile Testis

An intermittent overactive cremasteric reflex causing testis to retract up and out of scrotum, which however can be manipulated down into scrotum (and stays there). [23]

Testis itself is usually normal in size and consistency.

1/3 can ascend and become undescended; therefore patients should be monitored in clinic as they may require future orchidopexy.

Gliding Testis

Differs from retractile testis in that manipulation down into scrotum is possible but painful, and the testis will migrate upwards again on release.

Gliding testis will therefore only enter the scrotum under tension.

Surgical intervention is required (unlike retractile testis, which can be observed).

Absent Testis

Monorchidism (absent testis) noted in ≤ 4% of boys with UDT (bilateral monorchidism < 1%).

An intra-uterine gonadal vessel torsion may have led to infarction of a normal testis, a condition termed *vanishing testis syndrome*. [24]

In most cases the PPV is closed. If bilateral then patient may have raised FSH or micropenis.

DIAGNOSTIC EVALUATION

Enquire regarding risk factors such as prematurity, low birth weight, family history and maternal exposure to hormones.

Previous palpable testicle suggests testicular ascent.

Clinical examination should evaluate:

Infant's overall health:	- Presence of other genital or constitutional abnormalities
For palpable testis:	- Define the location - Can it be brought down into scrotum? (Painful or pain-free?)
For non-palpable:	- Is contra-lateral testis palpable? (If not, consider DSD) - Compensatory hypertrophy suggests UDT absence or atrophy.

Imaging cannot determine with certainty that a testis is present or not (US high false negative) and MRI is likely to require a GA anyway.

Imaging is therefore not routinely recommended in further assessment of UDT.

Repeat examination should be deferred until child reaches > 3 months of age.

The first step in further evaluation should include EUA, to then proceed to surgical intervention based on examination findings.

> **VIVA** In any paediatric station, consider mentioning that you would review the child's *"Personal Child Health Record"* (also termed "red book"), as this is where all the baby checks will be documented, immunisation records, etc. In particular to UDT you would be keen to know if the testes were found on the newborn first health check.

MANAGEMENT

Most testes will have descended by 3 months of age – it is unlikely they will descend after.

BAPU suggests orchidopexy should be performed at 3–6 months of age (although 6–12 months is considered acceptable).

Any treatment leading to scrotally positioned testis should be completed by 12 months of age.

Histological examination after this age has revealed:

- Leydig cell hypoplasia
- Delayed disappearance of gonocytes
- Reduced number of adult dark (Ad) spermatogonia
- Reduced total numbers of germ cells per testicular tubule.

Earlier orchidopexy is more technically challenging (delicate vas and testicular vessels) and higher anaesthetic risk must be taken into consideration.

Reasons for correcting an UDT include:

- 10x risk of TC, therefore correction allows patient to self-examine later in life (cancer risk is related to degree of UDT descent; significantly higher risk in intra-abdominal testis)
- Preserve fertility (paternity rates match controls if orchidopexy performed < 2 years)
- Cosmetic
- Reduce the risk of testicular torsion (UDT carries a higher risk of torsion)
- Abolish risk of hernia arising from PPV.

Medical therapy (e.g. endocrine therapy) to promote testicular descent is not recommended.

INGUINAL ORCHIDOPEXY

Widely used technique with a high success rate.

The key surgical steps for performing standard inguinal orchidopexy:

- WHO checklist completed, supine position, patient suitably prepped, draped and marked
- EUA to confirm palpable testis in groin

- Skin crease incision superior and lateral to pubic tubercle
- Open the external oblique to enter the inguinal canal and identify testis
- Divide gubernaculum
- Mobilise vas and vessels away from processus vaginalis (which is transfixed and divided at internal ring) and gain length by mobilisation
- Create dartos pouch in scrotum and pass the testis into this
- Close both wounds and instil local anaesthetic.

Parental consent must include discussing potential failure to bring testicle down into scrotum, orchidectomy or subsequent testicular atrophy, further surgery.

NON-PALPABLE TESTIS MANAGEMENT

Requires treatment decisions that will be made in theatre depending on findings of EUA.

If the testis is now palpable in groin on EUA, patient proceeds to inguinal orchidopexy.

If testis is not palpable, immediate laparoscopy performed to assess for intra-abdominal testis.

If testis is located within the abdominal cavity:

- If close to inguinal ring, may be possible to achieve single-stage orchidopexy
- Higher testis requires two-stage Fowler–Stephens (first stage divides testicular artery allowing growth of artery to vas from inferior vesical artery; second stage brings testis into scrotum) with ≤ 20% risk of loss of testicle [25]
- If vessels are blind ending or end in poor nubbin of tissue, orchidectomy recommended with contra-lateral testicular fixation (risk of future torsion).

To check whether adequate length has been achieved, draw the testis and cord to the contra-lateral deep inguinal ring.

Note laparoscopy is not used to repair ipsilateral inguinal hernia or PPV if found intra-operatively.

Figure 2 – EAU 2024 algorithm for unilateral non-palpable UDT [2]

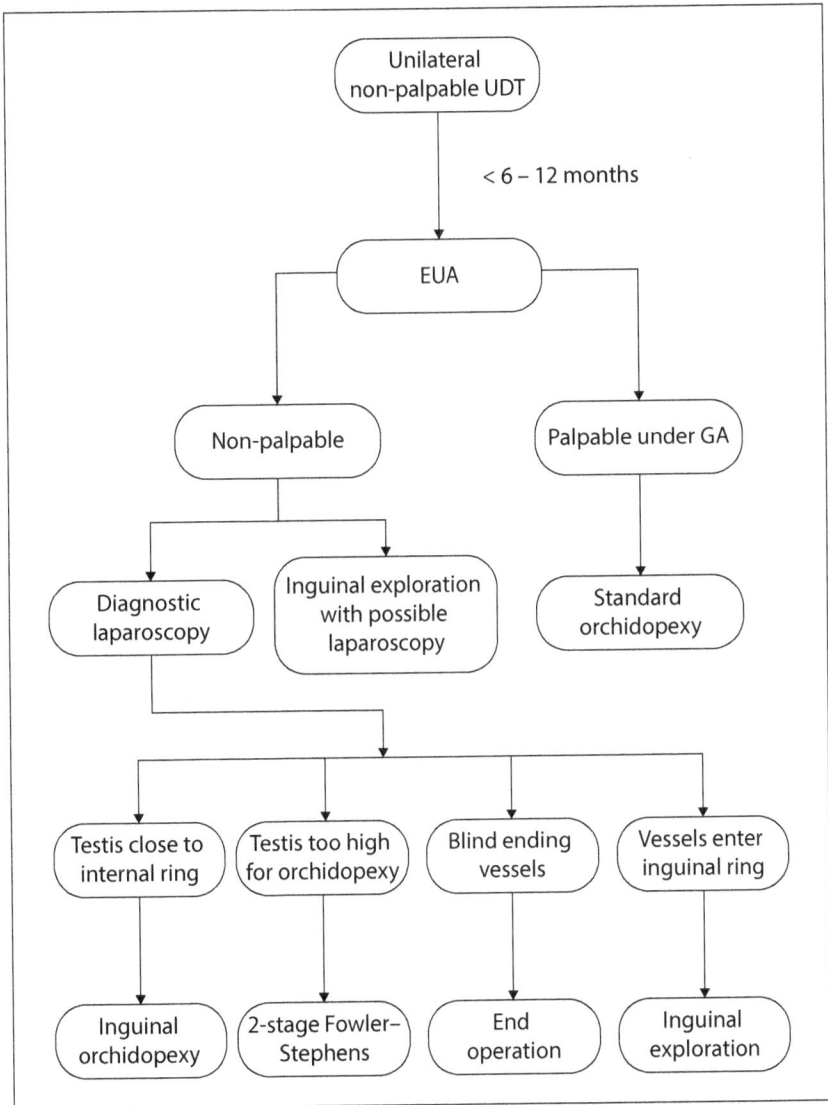

MANAGEMENT OF OLDER PATIENTS

Patients with UDT occasionally present later in life. Consider the following guide for treatment options:

Pre-pubertal management:

- < 10 years and/or bilateral UDT – proceed to bilateral orchidopexy
- > 10 years and normal contra-lateral testis – proceed to orchidectomy

Post-pubertal management:

- < 32 years and normal contra-lateral testis – proceed to orchidectomy
- > 32 years and unilateral UDT – observe and self-examine (offer orchidectomy if self-examination is difficult)

HYPOSPADIAS

EPIDEMIOLOGY

Congenital abnormality found in 1/250 live male births (second most common congenital birth defect in the male reproductive system).

7% risk of hypospadias in offspring of affected male, 14% risk in male siblings. [26]

Higher risk in babies with low birth weight.

Often associated with hooded foreskin and chordee.

CLASSIFICATION

Typically described in relation to the degree of proximal displacement of the urethral meatus: [27]

- *Distal* – (anterior) meatus situated on glans or corona (most common 80%)
- *Intermediate* – meatus on distal- or mid-penile shaft (10%)
- *Proximal* – (posterior) meatus on proximal shaft, scrotum or perineum (10%).

This classification, however, has limited use in characterising condition's severity and indeed predicting which patients will benefit from surgery.

Other relevant factors in classification include concomitant chordee, penile length, urethral plate quality.

AETIOLOGY

Hypospadias is a congenital deformity whereby the urethral meatus opening is abnormally sited on the ventral side of the penis.

Results from incomplete closure of urethral folds on the underside of the penis during development.

Defect in production/metabolism of foetal androgens or abnormality in tissue androgen receptors.

Chordee arises due to abnormal urethral plate development or intrinsic corpora cavernosa abnormality.

Hooded foreskin results from failed fusion of preputial folds.

ASSOCIATED ABNORMALITIES

Diagnostic evaluation also includes assessment of associated abnormalities, including: [2]

- Undescended testis/cryptorchidism (≤ 10%)
- PPV or inguinal hernia (≤ 10%).

Severe hypospadias with associated uni- or bilaterally impalpable testis, warrants assessment for DSD (i.e. chromosomal karyotyping).

Incidence of upper-tract abnormalities is comparable to that of general population.

DIAGNOSTIC EVALUATION

The descriptive evaluation of hypospadias should include the following factors:

- Presence of hooded foreskin
- Curvature of penis on erection
- Size and length of the penis
- Position, shape and width of urethral opening
- Presence of bilateral palpable testes.

MANAGEMENT

Presence of hypospadias does not mandate surgical intervention.

The considerations/aims of surgery focus on voiding, future sexual function and cosmetic factors.

Cornerstone principles of surgery include:

1. Correcting any curvature (orthoplasty)
2. Dealing with hooded foreskin
3. Re-siting urethral meatus.

Preferred age for primary hypospadias repair is 6–18 months, balancing anaesthetic risk, size of penis and compliance with post-operative catheter and dressings.

Haemostasis should be meticulous and achieved by bipolar diathermy.

Sutures should be fine (6'0 or 7'0) and hence magnification lenses recommended.

Difficulty of catheter placement is most commonly due to enlargement of the utricle.

There are many different types of hypospadias repair – choice will depend on surgeon experience; outcomes, however, strongly correlated with surgeon case volume.

Pre-operative Hormones

Local or parenteral administration of testosterone, DHT or β-HCG is an option to enlarge glans and shaft of penis, to allow better tubularisation of urethral plate.

This may be indicated in proximal hypospadias, small penis and reduced glans circumference. [28]

Limited evidence supporting its use such that its use is only *weak* recommendation by EAU 2024.

CORRECTION OF CURVATURE

Functionally, probably the most important aspect of the operation.

Often due to the ventral skin being too short, which is corrected by de-gloving the penis and excising tissue on ventral aspect (first step in most cases which may be sufficient).

Residual curvature is due to corporeal disproportion and requires straightening by dorsal plication (similar to Nesbit procedure).

Curvatures < 30° can be straightened by single dorsal plication without apparent penile shortening.

Urethral plate transection and/or ventral corporal grafting surgery are reserved for patients with curvature > 30° after de-gloving.

DEALING WITH HOODED FORESKIN

Hooded foreskin may be used as a source of dartos layer, free graft or correcting skin layer curvature.

Residual foreskin is excised to achieve circumcised appearance, although it can be preserved for foreskin reconstruction if this is the parental preference.

RE-SITING URETHRAL MEATUS

For distal forms of hypospadias, a range of surgical techniques exist, and none is demonstrably superior in outcome.

Examples of distal hypospadias repair techniques include:

- *Mathieu* – meatal-based flap technique
- *MAGPI* – meatal advancement and glanuloplasty incorporated
- *TIP (Snodgrass)* – narrow urethral plate can be incised and then tubularised
- *Thiersch–Duplay* – tubularising a wide urethral plate.

Key principle of hypospadias repair is preservation of well-vascularised urethral plate for its use in urethral reconstruction.

Two-stage repair may be required for proximal cases, using buccal or preputial mucosa over a catheter (in situ for 7 days). Second-stage tubularisation of neo-urethra is delayed for 6 months.

> | VIVA | Hypospadias repair surgery is a vast topic and intimate knowledge of it and all its techniques is beyond the scope of the FRCS (Urol) exam. I recommend however reading up to understand the key principles and being able to name and very briefly describe several techniques as detailed above.

COMPLICATIONS

Early – bleeding, infection, dehiscence

Late – fistula (most common), meatal stenosis, urethral stricture or diverticulum, psychological [29]

Complication rates are inversely proportional to surgeon case volume.

Re-do repairs are associated with higher complication rates (> 20%).

For fistulas, management includes initially replacement of catheter and referral to tertiary centre for further management and consideration of re-do surgery (≤ 50% recurrence).

PAEDIATRIC HYDROCOELE

Hydrocoele is defined as collection of fluid between parietal and visceral layers of tunica vaginalis.

- *Primary* hydrocoele (communicating) – based on patency of processus vaginalis
- *Secondary* hydrocoele (non-communicating) – reactive fluid due to infection/trauma/tumour

PRIMARY HYDROCOELE

An open processus vaginalis will allow communication with the peritoneal cavity and thus fluid transmission, as well as the possibility of an inguinal hernia.

Size/presence of hydrocoele may depend on the patient's position, or indeed be intermittent.

The exact time of spontaneous PPV closure is not known.

90% of these hydrocoeles will resolve by 12 months of age and do not require surgery.

SECONDARY HYDROCOELE

Non-communicating hydrocoeles are based on an imbalance between secretion and reabsorption of fluid, secondary to trauma, torsion or infection.

Hydrocoele of the Cord

If PPV obliterates with patency of mid-portion, a hydrocoele of the cord occurs. This is fixed in line with the cord, the testis is separate (you can get above testis on examination).

Idiopathic Scrotal Oedema

Presents as painless hemi-scrotal swelling often extending into perineum and inguinal area.

Peak incidence age 6–7 years.

Warrants sonographic evaluation to rule out hydrocoele. Treated conservatively +/- NSAIDs.

DIAGNOSTIC EVALUATION

History of the swelling to include:

- Age of onset
- Related symptoms such as pain, inflammation, change in nappies
- Variation with position/ambulation.

Examination of the abdomen and scrotum:

- If unable to get above swelling – consider inguinal hernia, communicating hydrocoele
- If able to get above swelling – consider hydrocoele of cord, testicular tumour
- Transillumination – suggests hydrocoele (although intestines and tumours can transilluminate).

US +/- Doppler is best imaging with almost 100% sensitivity.

MANAGEMENT

In most infants surgical treatment of hydrocoele is not indicated within the first 12 months of life, as most will resolve by this age. [30]

There is little risk with conservative management as progression to herniation is rare and does not result in incarceration (i.e. safe to wait until > 2 years of age).

If concurrent inguinal hernia is identified at presentation then surgical fixation is warranted. [31]

If herniotomy/PPV ligation is required:

- Identify PPV in inguinal canal and mobilise vas and testicular vessels away from this
- Ligate and divide processus vaginalis close to internal inguinal ring.

DAY-TIME LOWER URINARY TRACT CONDITIONS

LUTS in children may be caused by congenital/neurological abnormalities.

When there is no such obvious cause, children are deemed to have functional bladder problems.

The term *"day-time LUT conditions"* is proposed by the ICCS as a term to group together all functional bladder problems in children. [32]

Uropathy and/or neuropathy must be ruled out prior to labelling a child as having LUT condition.

Night-time bedwetting is known as "enuresis" – if this is the only symptom present in the child, this is termed *"mono-symptomatic nocturnal enuresis"*.

Normal day-time control of bladder function matures 2–3 years, night-time control 3–7 years.

Frequency of voiding is ≤ 20/day at 0–12 months, decreasing to 10x/day over ensuing years and at age 7 years it is approximately 7/day.

CLASSIFICATION

LUT conditions arise from incomplete or delayed maturation of bladder sphincter complex.

The two main groups of LUTD are:

1. *Filling-phase* dysfunctions

   - Detrusor can be overactive (more common) or underactive
   - Urgency, frequency, UUI
   - Habitual postponement of micturition (e.g. leg-crossing, squatting) which may be associated with behavioural/psychological problems.

2. *Voiding-phase* dysfunctions

   - E.g. incomplete relaxation of sphincter/pelvic floor during voiding (*staccato voiding*) [33]
   - E.g. unsustained detrusor contractions resulting in infrequent/incomplete micturition (*interrupted voiding pattern*)
   - High bladder pressures against contracted sphincter jeopardises upper tract/VUR

- General term for this condition is *dysfunctional voiding*
- Treatment relies on pelvic-floor relaxation and biofeedback.

Incontinence in children can be broadly categorised as:

1. *Functional* – e.g. overactive bladder, dysfunctional voiding, vaginal reflux, giggle incontinence
2. *Structural* – relating to an anatomical cause or bladder outflow obstruction, e.g. labial adhesions or masses, meatal stenosis, phimosis, posterior urethral valves, duplex kidney with abnormal moiety may suggest ectopic ureter
3. *Neurogenic* – suggested if patient exhibits spinal abnormalities, peripheral neurology, severe bowel symptoms, background of known underlying neurological conditions.

Vaginal Reflux

Urine enters the vagina during voiding and then leaks out a short time after when standing, characterised by incontinence following normal voiding in absence of other LUTS. [34]

Treated by getting the girl to void with widely abducted legs.

If labial adhesions are present, these can be treated with topical oestrogen or surgical division.

Giggle Incontinence

Incontinence triggered by laughing; this mainly affects girls who typically leak large amounts of urine (entire bladder content); however, the bladder is normal between episodes.

Managed with biofeedback or in select cases with methylphenidate or oxybutynin. [35]

Pollakiuria

Disorder characterised by very high frequency of day-time micturition (up to 50x); however, differentiated from OAB in that there are no night-time symptoms. [36]

Often due to significant life-event stressor, condition should resolve within 6 months.

DIAGNOSTIC EVALUATION

HISTORY

History is often the most important component of the patient evaluation and may be obtained from the parents and/or child.

The following points should be clarified in the patient history:

- *Drinking habits* – enquire regarding caffeinated or stimulant energy drinks
- *Bowel habits* – enquire about constipation (if treated can resolve LUTS) and co-existence of bowel problems which may suggest neuropathic aetiology
- *UTIs* – enquire about antibiotic use, fevers and review any available MSU results
- *Voiding frequency* – (via FVC) enquire about withholding behaviour; does child use toilet at school?
- *Night-time symptoms*
- *General wellbeing assessment* – screening for other medical conditions, developmental progress, social/domestic stressors.

In particular for children presenting with incontinence, the following should be defined:

- *Primary vs. secondary* – was incontinence present since birth (*primary*) or did child previously achieve a period of > 6 months of continence?
- *Incontinence pattern* – such as associated urgency (UUI), continuous (ectopic ureter), after laughing (giggle incontinence), shortly after voiding (vaginal reflux in girls)
- *Severity* – both in terms of frequency of episodes and amount of urine leaked.

Frequency–volume Chart

Accurate completion of FVC is mandatory for determining child's voiding frequency and volumes, and should be completed on at least two days (most sensibly for age > 5 years).

FVC records time/volume of each void, wetting episodes, and time/volume/type of fluid intake.

ICCS defines normal voiding frequency as 4–7/day.

Formula to calculate bladder capacity in children < 12 years (mL) = 30 x (age in years + 1).

EXAMINATION

Thorough examination of the child should cover the following regions:

- *Abdomen* – for palpable bladder, masses, loaded bowel
- *Male genitalia* – meatal opening (hypospadias) and stenosis, foreskin pathology (e.g. phimosis)
- *Female genitalia* – split or bifid clitoris (epispadias), perineal excoriation due to severe wetting or vaginal reflux
- *Spine* – hair patch/lipoma/pigmented lesions over midline may suggest spinal dysraphism which warrants peripheral neurological examination.

Perform urine dipstick testing and blood pressure recording.

Uroflowmetry (ideally repeated more than once) with PVR should be undertaken if child can comply.

VUDS may be warranted if concomitant VUR is suspected, but as it is an invasive test it should not be routinely used to assess LUTS in children.

IMAGING

US urinary tract may be indicated evaluating for:

- Thickened bladder with upper-tract dilation, suggesting BOO
- Post-void residual > 20mL is significant
- Duplex kidney with abnormal upper moiety, may suggest ectopic ureter.

MANAGEMENT

The mainstay of LUT conditions treatment in children involves "urotherapy", which is a broad field of non-medical/non-surgical strategies. [2]

Address constipation first since bowel problems will perpetuate bladder symptoms.

Urotherapy can be divided into "standard therapy" and "specific interventions".

Standard Therapy

Non-surgical, non-pharmacological treatment for LUT conditions.

Large part of this involves education of parent and child:

- Information about normal bladder function
- Ensure correct voiding posture, avoid withholding urination, pelvic-floor relaxation
- Advice regarding fluid intake, limiting evening fluids, emptying before bedtime.

Specific Interventions

Additional management options should address specific components of the day-time LUTS condition:

- Oxybutynin 2.5–5mg BD for OAB or giggle incontinence
- ISC for large PVR
- Biofeedback sessions for pelvic-floor muscle awareness.

UDS considered if neuropathic pathology suspected, or all treatment strategies have failed. [37]

Bladder pressures consistently > 40cm H2O may jeopardise the upper urinary tract.

MONOSYMPTOMATIC NOCTURNAL ENURESIS

MNE is night-time urinary incontinence in children without other LUTS or history of bladder dysfunction.

Primary MNE refers to children who have never been dry at night for more than 6-month period.

Secondary MNE refers to the emergence of bed-wetting after a period > 6 months of being dry.

Non-MNE is the condition of enuresis in association with concurrent day-time LUTS.

EPIDEMIOLOGY

One of the most prevalent conditions in childhood.

5–10% of 7-year-old children have MNE. [38]

Expect a yearly resolution rate of 15%; however, 7% of children wetting the bed at age 7 years will continue to have enuresis into adulthood. [39]

More common in boys than girls (2:1 ratio at any age).

PATHOPHYSIOLOGY

Three main factors contribute to nocturnal enuresis:

1. *Kidneys* – high night-time urine output occurs if ADH secretion is reduced (nocturnal polyuria), the normal circadian reduction in urine output during sleep is diminished

2. *Brain* – altered sleep/arousal mechanism in response to full bladder (parents report difficulty in waking child at the time of bedwetting)

3. *Bladder* – reduced functional bladder capacity +/- DO.

Other potential contributing factors may include:

- *Family history* – significantly higher risk of MNE if one or both parents suffered from the condition
- *Psychological* – such as ADHD, trauma, neglect, abuse
- *Genetic* – with loci described on chromosomes 12, 13 and 22.

DIAGNOSTIC EVALUATION

HISTORY

Diagnosis mainly via careful history-taking, as clinical examination in MNE is often unremarkable.

The following aspects should be covered during the history:

- Distinguishing between primary or secondary MNE
- Presence of day-time LUTS including day-time incontinence
- Frequency, character and impact of the episodes on child and parents
- Family history of enuresis and potential psychological contributors.

EXAMINATION

Physical examination of a child with MNE is usually normal – assess the abdomen, genitalia, spine and peripheral neurology.

FVC is essential – allows evaluation of nocturnal polyuria and functional bladder capacity.

Urinalysis, assessing for UTI and presence of glucose.

Routine imaging is not routinely recommended for MNE but US may be used for assessment.

MANAGEMENT

Nocturnal enuresis is a stressful condition for both child and parent, which can lead to social isolation, low self-esteem and anxiety.

Children < 5 years should not be actively treated.

Providing information to parents and demystifying the condition is paramount.

Behavioural

Conservative strategies may include emptying bladder before bedtime, reducing evening fluids, avoiding caffeinated drinks and parents waking the child up to void at their later bedtime.

Pharmacological

Desmopressin (ADH analogue) given 200–400mcg PO before bed (nasal spray no longer advised due to risk of overdose) produces an anti-diuretic response. [40]

Success rates of 70% can be achieved.

Relapse rates are high after stopping treatment (50%) unless structured discontinuation is applied. [41]

Can be used in conjunction with oxybutynin in case of small bladder capacity; however, the condition would no longer be considered to be solely MNE.

Alarm Treatment

Enuresis alarm activates when the child wets to wake them up; best form for arousal disorder.

Child and parents need to persevere for weeks/months to achieve results; however, success rates of ≤ 70% can be expected, with low relapse rates. [42]

URINARY TRACT INFECTIONS IN CHILDREN

EPIDEMIOLOGY

Under 12 months of age:

- UTI more common in boys vs. girls
- More common in uncircumcised vs. circumcised boys.

The most common bacterium found in community-acquired UTI is E.coli (75%).

Other species such as Klebsiella, Enterobacter, Pseudomonas are more frequent in nosocomial UTI.

40% children with UTI have underlying urinary tract abnormality (the most common pathology is VUR).

Increased risk of an underlying urinary tract abnormality if the UTI presented with fever.

CLASSIFICATION

There are 5 classification systems for UTI (site and severity most important in acute setting):

1. <u>According to site</u>
   - Lower urinary tract (cystitis) vs. upper urinary tract

2. <u>According to episode</u>
   - *Persistent*, implies re-emergence of same pathogen
   - *Recurrent*, implies infection with different pathogen (E.coli may re-occur as different serotype)
   - *Atypical*, which according to NICE 2022 applies to: [43]
     - Seriously ill/septic patient
     - Palpable abdominal mass
     - Infection with non-E.coli pathogen
     - Failure to respond to treatment with suitable antibiotics within 48 hours

3. <u>According to severity</u>
   - *Simple* UTI, child may have low-grade pyrexia and feel systemically well

- *Severe* UTI, child has fever > 39°, dehydration and systemic malaise
4. According to symptoms
   - Asymptomatic bacteriuria/UTI vs. symptomatic UTI
5. According to complicating factors
   - *Uncomplicated*, suggests UTI in a morphologically and functionally normal urinary tract, immuno-competent patient, usually eradicated with oral antibiotics
   - *Complicated*, refers to UTI in neonates, children with pyelonephritis and patients with morphologically and/or functionally abnormal urinary tract.

DIAGNOSTIC EVALUATION

The history should consider the following specific aspects:

- First vs. recurrent episodes (enquire regarding prior severity and treatment received)
- Screen for known or possible structural abnormalities of urinary tract
- Assess for any associated bowel dysfunction
- Family/sibling history of UTI or VUR
- Associated medical comorbidities e.g. diabetes, immunosuppression.

Physical examination should evaluate:

- Vital parameters and temperature (fever is most common symptom of UTI in infants > 3 months)
- Abdomen, flank, genitalia
- Back (stigmata of spina bifida).

Urine should be collected for analysis preferably prior to antibiotic administration.

Clean catch, involves parent catching mid-urine specimen in clean container; the glans or separated labia should be cleaned prior to procedure.

Suprapubic aspirate is the most sensitive method to obtain uncontaminated urine sample in children.

Urine dipstick is appealing as readily available providing rapid result; however:

- Bacterial conversion of nitrate to nitrite takes 4 hours in bladder (infants void often)
- Not all pathogens convert nitrate to nitrite.

Positive nitrite finding has high specificity for UTI.

If urine dipstick is positive, confirmation by urine culture is strongly recommended.

IMAGING

US urinary tract is generally first-line radiological investigation – in 15% of cases abnormalities are found.

Abnormal US and concerning clinical history warrant further imaging (usually DMSA).

NICE 2022 has specific recommendations for imaging schedules in paediatric UTI for different age groups (see Tables 2–4).

Table 2 – NICE 2022 imaging schedule for children < 6 months [43]

Test	Responds to treatment within 48 hours	Atypical UTI	Recurrent UTI
US during acute infection	NO	YES	YES
US within 6 weeks	YES	NO	NO
DMSA 4–6 months after UTI	NO	YES	YES
MCUG	NO	YES	YES

Table 3 – NICE 2022 imaging schedule for children > 6 months and < 3 years [43]

Test	Responds to treatment within 48 hours	Atypical UTI	Recurrent UTI
US during acute infection	NO	YES	NO
US within 6 weeks	NO	NO	YES
DMSA 4–6 months after UTI	NO	YES	YES
MCUG	NO	NO	NO

Table 4 – NICE 2022 imaging schedule for children > 3 years [43]

Test	Responds to treatment within 48 hours	Atypical UTI	Recurrent UTI
US during acute infection	NO	YES	NO
US within 6 weeks	NO	NO	YES
DMSA 4–6 months after UTI	NO	NO	YES
MCUG	NO	NO	NO

VIVA Referring to the NICE 2022 Guidelines paediatric UTI imaging schedule is an FRCS (Urol) favourite and so this is particularly worth memorising. I would also recommend generally reading through the entire NICE 2022 Guideline "Urinary tract infection in under 16s: diagnosis and management" as the document nicely takes you through the key principles anyway.

MANAGEMENT

The child should be resuscitated systematically according to Airway-to-Exposure protocol.

Follow the paediatric Sepsis-6 protocol where appropriate (be aware that paediatric baseline ranges of vital parameters differ between age groups).

Antibiotics administered based on local guidelines, allergy status, previous culture results, patient age and clinical severity of UTI.

Children should be admitted to the paediatric ward and joint care provided with paediatric team.

CAP is not routinely recommended following first-time UTI (NICE 2022).

DIFFERENCES IN SEX DEVELOPMENT

DSD are congenital conditions in which the development of chromosomal, gonadal and/or anatomical sex is atypical.

Estimated to affect 1 in 4,500 births.

DSD can present diagnostically:

- *Prenatal*, based on karyotype and US findings
- *Neonatal*, based on genital examination
- *Delayed*, based on early or late puberty.

The paediatric urologist plays a major role in the neonatal presentation.

DSD management requires a dedicated MDT which includes geneticists, neonatologists, paediatricians, endocrinologists, gynaecologists, psychologists.

Gender assignment should not be rushed until definitive diagnosis is made. Urgent child naming is not encouraged. Registry offices allow for delays in child registration in these circumstances.

DSD is divided into the following categories:

- Sex-chromosome DSD
- 46XY DSD
- 46XX DSD.

EVALUATION

Detailed history should be taken to enquire: [2]

- Parental consanguinity
- Sibling DSD/abnormal genitalia/deaths
- Failure to thrive of the neonate
- Maternal exposure to drugs (steroids, contraceptives).

Physical examination should include assessment of: [2]

- Phallus length and appearance
- Palpable gonads (which would almost certainly be testes, which excludes 46XX DSD)
- Number and location of openings in perineum (e.g. hypospadias)
- Fusion of labio-scrotal folds, hymenal ring.

Micropenis

Micropenis is a small but otherwise normally formed penis with a stretched length < 2cm. [44]

The penis is stretched and measured on dorsal aspect from the pubic symphysis to the glans tip. The scrotum may be underdeveloped and testes palpable but small.

Karyotyping is mandatory, endocrine assessment (LH, FSH, testosterone) and referral to paediatric endocrinologist advised.

Consider central causes (hypothalamic/pituitary) vs. testicular.

In proven androgen sensitivity, androgen therapy is recommended.

SEX CHROMOSOME DSD

These are disorders of gonadal differentiation and development, usually due to absent or disordered genetic material.

Typically occurs during meiosis (1 or 2) due to non-disjunction. Failure of separation leads to one gamete with 22 chromosomes and one with 24 (pure 45 X and 47 XXY karyotypes).

Mosaicism results from non-disjunction during mitosis at blastocyst stage (note that dysgenetic gonads are at significant higher risk of subsequent malignancy).

Klinefelter's Syndrome (47 XXY)

One of the most common chromosomal disorders (1:1,000 male births), diagnosed by karyotyping. [45]

Involves at least one extra X-chromosome in addition to Y-chromosome such that total chromosome number is 47+ (i.e. 47 XXY, rarely 48XXXY, 49XXXXY or 46XY/47XXY mosaicism).

Typical features include: [46]

- Gynaecomastia, female fat distribution, absent facial hair
- Small firm testes, azoospermia
- Elevated FSH/LH, testosterone is low in 50%
- Usually infertile (presence of sperm suggests mosaicism).

Phenotypical manifestations are more pronounced in proportion to number of extra X-chromosomes.

8x risk of breast cancer vs. normal males; also increased risk of Leydig and Sertoli cell tumours.

Klinefelter's cannot be cured; however, a number of treatments may help:

- Testosterone replacement
- Reduction mammoplasty for gynaecomastia (and risk of breast cancer)
- Surveillance for breast and testicular malignancy.

Turner's Syndrome

Incidence 1:2,500

Chromosomal abnormality in which all or part of one of the X-chromosomes is missing or altered.

45X female (occasionally 45X/46XX mosaicism; rarely 45X/46XY but important as high risk of virilisation and gonadoblastoma).

Phenotypic features: female sex, failure of secondary sexual differentiation, streak ovaries, primary amenorrhoea, short stature, webbed neck, widespread nipples, short fourth metacarpal. [47]

Associated congenital abnormalities include coarctation of aorta, bicuspid aortic valve, horseshoe kidney, renal agenesis (reduced life expectancy due to cardiovascular conditions).

Turner's syndrome cannot be cured; however, a number of treatments may help:

- Excision of streak gonad in those with Y-chromosome material
- Surveillance for cardiovascular and renal abnormalities.

Mixed Gonadal Dysgenesis

Typically 45X/46XY mosaicism – wide spectrum of clinical manifestations.

Streak gonad one side, testis (often undescended) on other with corresponding Mullerian and Wolffian ducts, phallic enlargement but with uterus and vagina.

Increased risk of gonadal tumours involving testis (gonadoblastoma) and Wilms' tumour.

Mixed gonadal dysgenesis and Wilms' tumour (WT) commonly associated with Denys–Drash syndrome (triad of ambiguous genitalia, WT and glomerulonephritis).

VIRILISATION OF 46XX FEMALE (46XX DSD)

Virilisation of 46XX female due to either foetal androgen (CAH) or excess maternal androgens (e.g. androgen-secreting tumours of ovary or adrenal).

The most common type is CAH.

Congenital Adrenal Hyperplasia

CAH accounts for 90% of all infants with ambiguous genitalia.

Autosomal recessive disorder due to 21-hydroxylase deficiency (95% of cases). [48]

Mutation of 21-hydroxylase gene on chromosome 6 (conversion to inactive CYP21A gene).

Diagnosis – elevated 17α-hydroxyprogesterone.

75% of patients present with salt-wasting and 25% with simple virilisation.

Impaired hydrocortisone production, resulting in compensatory increase ACTH and testosterone, presents with "salt-losing crisis" (dehydration, low sodium) due to aldosterone deficiency.

This is a neonatal emergency – requiring IV fluids to maintain blood pressure, UE check and potassium-lowering agents, mineralocorticoid and glucocorticoid supplementation.

INADEQUATE VIRILISATION OF 46XY MALE (46XY DSD)

46XY with defects of testosterone production/metabolism resulting in varying degrees of feminisation.

The most common type is CAIS.

Complete Androgen Insensitivity Syndrome

CAIS is caused by androgen resistance.

With relevant family history, karyotyping can be performed at birth, otherwise difficult to detect.

X-linked recessive: mutation of androgen receptor located on long arm of chromosome X.

Phenotype/external genitalia are female; however, internal genitalia are rudimentary/absent. Lower 2/3 blind-ending vagina. Testes may be palpable in inguinal canal. [49]

May be detected on investigation for primary amenorrhea (raised LH and testosterone).

Management includes:

- Inguinal orchidectomy due to future malignancy risk
- Oestrogen replacement therapy
- Vaginoplasty.

5α-Reductase Deficiency

Autosomal recessive condition (mutation of 5αR type 2 gene). [50]

Patients are born with male gonads which can be normal, ambiguous or include normal female genitalia; however, only affects those with a Y-chromosome.

Virilisation will become apparent at puberty and adults never get BPH.

MISCELLANEOUS PAEDIATRIC UROLOGY

EMBRYOLOGY OF KIDNEY

In order of appearance, the embryonic kidney transitions from pronephros, to mesonephros, to metanephros – these all develop from the intermediate mesoderm.

The first two regress in utero; however, the metanephros (forms at gestation day 28) becomes the permanent kidney.

Renal calyces and pelvis, ureter and collecting ducts arise from the ureteric bud.

Transitional zone of the prostate and bulbourethral glands arise from the urogenital sinus.

Vas, seminal vesicle, epididymis, ejaculatory ducts, bladder trigone and central zone of the prostate arise from the mesonephric (Wolffian) ducts.

By week 12, the urachus involutes to become the median umbilical ligament. [51]

PAEDIATRIC FLUIDS

Weight (kg)	Fluid Rate
Up to 10kg	4mL/kg/hour for the first 10kg
10–20kg	2mL/kg/hour for the next 10kg
> 20kg	1mL/kg/hour for every kg over 20kg

Estimated circulating blood volume in child is 80mL/kg.

Fluid bolus for children is 10–20mL/kg.

WILMS' TUMOUR

EPIDEMIOLOGY

Incidence 1:10,000 (commonest intra-abdominal tumour of childhood).

20% of all paediatric malignancies, 80% of genito-urinary malignancies.

Majority present < 5 years of age (75%).

Male and female equally affected, bilateral in 5%.

PATHOLOGY

Wilms' tumour contains metanephric blastema, primitive renal tubular epithelium and connective tissue components (appearing grey in colour like cerebral tissue). [52]

Histological sub-types include favourable (well-differentiated) and anaplastic (poorly differentiated).

Molecular relevance is WT1 tumour suppressor gene (11p13) mutation or deletion.

DIAGNOSTIC EVALUATION

Most common presentation is palpable abdominal mass (90%).

Other symptoms include visible haematuria (50%), hypertension (50%) and abdominal pain.

Associated syndromes include Denys–Drash (ambiguous genitalia), Beckwith–Wiedemann (macroglossia) and horseshoe kidney. [53]

US is first-line radiological investigation – upon finding a mass, patient would require standard CT thorax/abdomen/pelvis for completion staging.

Percutaneous biopsy confirmation is not mandatory in context of convincing radiological evidence.

MANAGEMENT

Most children with Wilms' tumour have neo-adjuvant chemotherapy prior to surgical resection, which may include vincristine, actinomycin D, doxorubicin, carboplatin.

Surgical excision may then be followed by adjuvant chemo- or radiotherapy.

Staging [54]

Stage 1 – tumour limited to kidney, no capsular invasion, completely excised

Stage 2 – tumour outside kidney but completely removed

Stage 3 – intra-abdominal/peritoneal/IVC involvement

Stage 4 – haematogenous/extra-abdominal lymph node involvement

Stage 5 – bilateral tumours

RHABDOMYOSARCOMA

Very rare tumour of mesenchyme, resembling skeletal muscle.

May involve genito-urinary tract, typically bladder base, prostate, para-testicular, uterus and vagina.

Increased risk in Li–Fraumeni syndrome (p53 mutation).

Embryonic forms have the better prognosis (most bladder tumours are embryonal).

NEUROBLASTOMA

Tumour arising from neuro-ectoderm – 50% occur in the adrenal gland and remainder along the sympathetic chain.

Patients with neuroblastoma tend to be more symptomatic compared to Wilms' tumour.

Median age at diagnosis is 2 years.

Poor prognostic sign is deletion of short arm of chromosome 1.

MIBG scan is highly sensitive.

PRUNE BELLY SYNDROME

Genetic condition almost always affecting boys.

Name arises for the wrinkled skin appearance present on the abdomen, typical triad involving:

- Abdominal wall defects
- Cryptorchidism (often intra-abdominal) which may be bilateral, patient typically infertile
- Genito-urinary defects (dilated ureter and bladder, VUR, detrusor failure).

REFERENCES

1. Hindryckx A, De Catte L (2011). Prenatal diagnosis of congenital renal and urinary tract malformations. *Facts, Views & Vision in ObGyn, 3*(3), 165.

2. Radmayr C, Bogaert G, Bujons A, et al. (2024). EAU Guidelines Paediatric Urology. Available at: https://d56bochluxqnz.cloudfront.net/documents/full-guideline/EAU-Guidelines-on-Paediatric-Urology-2024.pdf [last accessed 26 June 2024].

3. Skoog SJ, Peters CA, Arant BS (2010). Pediatric vesicoureteral reflux guidelines panel summary report: clinical practice guidelines for screening siblings of children with vesicoureteral reflux and neonates/infants with prenatal hydronephrosis. *Journal of Urology, 184*(3), 1,145–1,151.

4. Alsaywid BS, Saleh H, Deshpande A (2010). High grade primary vesicoureteral reflux in boys: long-term results of a prospective cohort study. *Journal of Urology, 184*(4), 1,598–1,603.

5. Mohanan N, Colhoun E, Puri P (2008). Renal parenchymal damage in intermediate and high grade infantile vesicoureteral reflux. *Journal of Urology, 180*(4S), 1,635–1,638.

6. Darge K, Riedmiller H (2004). Current status of vesicoureteral reflux diagnosis. *World Journal of Urology, 22*(2), 88–95.

7. RIVUR Trial Investigators (2014). Antimicrobial prophylaxis for children with vesicoureteral reflux. *New England Journal of Medicine, 370*(25), 2,367–2,376.

8. Brandström P, Jodal U, Sillén U (2011). The Swedish reflux trial: review of a randomized, controlled trial in children with dilating vesicoureteral reflux. *Journal of Pediatric Urology, 7*(6), 594–600.

9. Abhyankar A, Taghizadeh AK (2018). Paediatric Urology. In: *Viva Practice for the FRCS (Urol) and Postgraduate Urology Examinations*, second edition, CRS Press, London.

10. Hodges SJ, Patel B, McLorie G (2009). Posterior urethral valves. *Scientific World Journal, 9*, 1,119–1,126.

11. Hennus PML, de Koprt LMO, Bosch JLH, et al. (2014). A systematic review on the accuracy of diagnostic procedures for infravesical obstruction in boys. *PLoS One*, 9(2), e85474.

12. Nasir AA, Ameh EA, Abdur-Rahman, et al. (2011). Posterior urethral valve. *World Journal of Pediatrics, 7*(3), 205.

13. Rittenberg MH, Hulbert WC, Snyder HM, et al. (1988). Protective factors in posterior urethral valves. *Journal of Urology, 140*(5 Part 1), 993–996.

14. Scott JES (1985). Management of congenital posterior urethral valves. *British Journal of Urology, 57*(1), 71–77.

15. Sarhan O, El-Ghoneimi A, Hafez A (2010). Surgical complications of posterior urethral valve ablation: 20 years experience. *Journal of Pediatric Surgery*, *45*(11), 2,222–2,226.
16. Brown T, Mandell J, Lebowitz RL (1987). Neonatal hydronephrosis in the era of sonography. *American Journal of Roentgenology*, *148*(5), 959–963.
17. Sparks S, Viteri B, Sprague BM, et al. (2013). Evaluation of differential renal function and renographic patterns in patients with Dietl crisis. *Journal of Urology*, *189*(2), 684–689.
18. Weizer AZ, Silverstein AD, Auge BK, et al. (2003). Determining the incidence of horseshoe kidney from radiographic data at a single institution. *Journal of Urology*, *170*(5), 1,722–1,726.
19. Lippe B, Geffner ME, Dietrich RB, et al. (1988). Renal malformations in patients with Turner syndrome: imaging in 141 patients. *Pediatrics*, *82*(6), 852–856.
20. Gairdner D (1950). The fate of the foreskin: a study of circumcision. *Obstetrical & Gynecological Survey*, *5*(5), 699.
21. Larke NL, Thomas SL, dos Santos Silva, I, et al. (2011). Male circumcision and penile cancer: a systematic review and meta-analysis. *Cancer Causes & Control*, *22*(8), 1,097–1,110.
22. Summerton DJ, McNally J, Denny AJ, et al. (2000). Congenital megaprepuce: an emerging condition–how to recognize and treat it. *BJU International*, *86*(4), 519–522.
23. Stec AA, Thomas JC, DeMarco RT, et al. (2007). Incidence of testicular ascent in boys with retractile testes. *Journal of Urology*, *178*(4), 1,722–1,725.
24. Pirgon Ö, Dündar BN (2012). Vanishing testes: a literature review. *Journal of Clinical Research in Pediatric Endocrinology*, *4*(3), 116.
25. Esposito C, Vallone G, Savanelli A, et al. (2009). Long-term outcome of laparoscopic Fowler-Stephens orchiopexy in boys with intra-abdominal testis. *Journal of Urology*, *181*(4), 1,851–1,856.
26. Duckett JW (1989). Hypospadias. *Pediatr Rev*, *11*(2), 37–42.
27. Orkiszewski M (2012). A standardized classification of hypospadias. *Journal of Pediatric Urology*, *8*(4), 410–414.
28. Netto JMB, Ferrarez CEP, Leal AAS, et al. (2013). Hormone therapy in hypospadias surgery: a systematic review. *Journal of Pediatric Urology*, *9*(6), 971–979.
29. Shanberg AM, Sanderson K, Duel B (2001). Re-operative hypospadias repair using the Snodgrass incised plate urethroplasty. *BJU International*, *87*(6), 544–547.
30. Koski ME, Makari JH, Adams MC, et al. (2010). Infant communicating hydroceles – do they need immediate repair or might some clinically resolve? *Journal of Pediatric Surgery*, *45*(3), 590–593.

31. Stylianos S, Jacir NN, Harris BH (1993). Incarceration of inguinal hernia in infants prior to elective repair. *Journal of Pediatric Surgery, 28*(4), 582–583.
32. Austin PF, Bauer SB, Bower W, et al. (2014). The standardization of terminology of lower urinary tract function in children and adolescents: update report from the Standardization Committee of the International Children's Continence Society. *Journal of Urology, 191*(6), 1,863–1,865.
33. Yagci S, Kibar Y, Akay O, et al. (2005). The effect of biofeedback treatment on voiding and urodynamic parameters in children with voiding dysfunction. *Journal of Urology, 174*(5), 1,994–1,998.
34. Kilicoglu G, Aslan AR, Oztürk M, et al. (2010). Vesicovaginal reflux: recognition and diagnosis using ultrasound. *Pediatric Radiology, 40*(1), 114.
35. Berry AK, Zderic S, Carr M (2009). Methylphenidate for giggle incontinence. *Journal of Urology, 182*(4), 2,028–2,032.
36. Watemberg N, Shalev H (1994). Daytime urinary frequency in children. *Clinical Pediatrics, 33*(1), 50–53.
37. Hoebeke P, Bower W, Combs A, et al. (2010). Diagnostic evaluation of children with daytime incontinence. *Journal of Urology, 183*(2), 699–703.
38. Lottmann HB, Alova I (2007). Primary monosymptomatic nocturnal enuresis in children and adolescents. *International Journal of Clinical Practice, 61*, 8–16.
39. Läckgren G, Hjalmås K, Gool JV, et al. (1999). Committee Report: Nocturnal enuresis: a suggestion for a European treatment strategy. *Acta Paediatrica, 88*(6), 679–690.
40. Dehoorne JL, Raes AM, Van Laecke E, et al. (2006). Desmopressin toxicity due to prolonged half-life in 18 patients with nocturnal enuresis. *Journal of Urology, 176*(2), 754–758.
41. Gökçe MI, Hajıyev P, Süer E, et al. (2014). Does structured withdrawal of desmopressin improve relapse rates in patients with monosymptomatic enuresis? *Journal of Urology, 192*(2), 530–534.
42. Glazener CM, Evans JH, Peto RE (2005). Alarm interventions for nocturnal enuresis in children. Available at: https://www.cochranelibrary.com/cdsr/doi/10.1002/14651858.CD002911.pub2/abstract [last accessed 8 June 2020]
43. NICE – Urinary tract infection in under 16s: diagnosis and management. Available at: https://www.nice.org.uk/guidance/ng224/resources/urinary-tract-infection-in-under-16s-diagnosis-and-management-pdf-66143835667141 [last accessed 10 July 2024].
44. Wiygul, J, Palmer LS (2011). Micropenis. *Scientific World Journal, 11*, 1,462–1,469.
45. Nielsen J, Wohlert M (1991). Chromosome abnormalities found among 34910 newborn children: results from a 13-year incidence study in Århus, Denmark. *Human Genetics, 87*(1), 81–83.

46. Bojesen A, Gravholt CH (2007). Klinefelter syndrome in clinical practice. *Nature Clinical Practice Urology, 4*(4), 192–204.

47. Stochholm K, Juul S, Juel K, et al. (2006). Prevalence, incidence, diagnostic delay, and mortality in Turner syndrome. *Journal of Clinical Endocrinology & Metabolism, 91*(10), 3,897–3,902.

48. Speiser PW, White PC (2003). Congenital adrenal hyperplasia. *New England Journal of Medicine, 349*(8), 776–788.

49. Hines M, Ahmed SF, Hughes IA (2003). Psychological outcomes and gender-related development in complete androgen insensitivity syndrome. *Archives of Sexual Behavior, 32*(2), 93–101.

50. Okeigwe I, Kuohung W (2014). 5-Alpha reductase deficiency: a 40-year retrospective review. *Current Opinion in Endocrinology, Diabetes and Obesity, 21*(6), 483–487.

51. Das JP, Vargas HA, Lee A, et al. (2020). The urachus revisited: multimodal imaging of benign & malignant urachal pathology. *British Journal of Radiology, 93*, 20190118.

52. Kaste SC, Dome JS, Babyn PS, et al. (2008). Wilms tumour: prognostic factors, staging, therapy and late effects. *Pediatric Radiology, 38*(1), 2–17.

53. Rivera MN, Haber DA (2005). Wilms' tumour: connecting tumorigenesis and organ development in the kidney. *Nature Reviews Cancer, 5*(9), 699–712.

54. Kalapurakal JA, Dome JS, Perlman EJ, et al. (2004). Management of Wilms' tumour: current practice and future goals. *Lancet Oncology, 5*(1), 37–46.

PAEDIATRIC UROLOGY MCQS

1. What is the most common aetiological cause of antenatally detected hydronephrosis?
   A) VUR
   B) Ureterocoele
   C) PUJO
   D) PUV
   E) Renal cyst

2. In which of the following scenarios would you not be more inclined to consider continuous antibiotic prophylaxis in an infant with antenatal diagnosis of unilateral hydronephrosis?
   A) History of oligo-hydramnios
   B) Uncircumcised male
   C) Presence of high-grade hydronephrosis on US
   D) Presence of hydro-ureteronephrosis on US
   E) Strong sibling history of confirmed VUR

3. Which of the following factors is not known to suggest an increased chance of spontaneous resolution of VUR in children?
   A) Absence of concomitant LUTD
   B) Young age at presentation (< 3 years)
   C) Male gender
   D) Lower grade (1–3)
   E) Asymptomatic patient

4. Which of the following statements regarding VUR in children is true?
   A) The collecting system is not dilated in Grade III
   B) In screened populations the prevalence of VUR is less than 30%
   C) Renal DMSA uptake is increased in areas of acute inflammation
   D) UTIs are more common in boys with VUR as their grade of reflux tends to be higher
   E) In Grade II reflux the entire ureter is dilated but does not reach renal pelvis

5. Which of the following statements regarding VUR in children is incorrect?
    A) 80% of Grade I–II cases will self-resolve
    B) ≤ 50% of Grade III–IV cases will self-resolve
    C) Teflon used for endoscopic treatment of VUR contains PTFE
    D) Deflux® contains hyaluronic acid
    E) The intra-vesical Lich–Gregoir procedure can be used for reimplantation treatment of VUR

6. What is the most accurate figure for incidence of PUJO in newborns?
    A) 1:250
    B) 1:500
    C) 1:1,500
    D) 1:3,000
    E) 1:5,000

7. Which of the following statements is true?
    A) Ectopic ureter is more common in males than females
    B) Ureterocoele is more common in males than females
    C) PUJO is more common in males than females
    D) Bedwetting at any age is more common in females than males
    E) Urachal remnant is more common in females than males

8. What is the most accurate figure for incidence of horseshoe kidney?
    A) 1:200
    B) 1:400
    C) 1:600
    D) 1:800
    E) 1:1,000

9. Which of the following corticosteroid creams would you not use to treat phimosis in a 7-year-old boy?
    A) Betamethasone 0.025%
    B) Betamethasone 0.05%
    C) Mometasone furoate 0.1%
    D) Hydrocortisone 1%
    E) Clobetasone butyrate 1%

10. *Up to what percentage of pre-term male infants will have UDT?*
    A) 25%
    B) 35%
    C) 45%
    D) 55%
    E) 65%

11. *Regarding hypospadias, which of the following statements is false?*
    A) The TIP technique for repair should not be used in anterior hypospadias
    B) Incidence rate of hypospadias has increased over the last 25 years
    C) Distal hypospadias is the most common type
    D) The rates of associated cryptorchidism or inguinal hernia with hypospadias are similar
    E) Vast majority of complications after hypospadias repair surgery occur within the first 12 months of the operation

12. *Which of the following is not a recognised surgical technique for hypospadias repair?*
    A) Chiavari hypospadias repair
    B) Koyanagi hypospadias repair
    C) Byar's hypospadias repair
    D) Bracka hypospadias repair
    E) Onlay-tube-onlay hypospadias repair

13. *Which anatomical area of the brain is responsible for detrusor sphincter co-ordination?*
    A) Cerebellum
    B) Thalamus
    C) Medulla
    D) Pons
    E) Corpus callosum

14. *Which of the following statements regarding day-time lower urinary tract symptoms in children is false?*
    A) Interrupted voiding is in more severe terms than staccato voiding
    B) UTIs usually disappear after successful treatment of dysfunctional voiding
    C) Cerebral cortex is responsible for inhibition of micturition reflex
    D) Bladder overactivity in children is most commonly seen at ages 7–9 years
    E) Cerebral cortex is responsible for voluntary initiation of micturition

15. *What is the correct formula for calculating estimated bladder capacity (in mL) in children?*

    A) (Age +1) x 20
    B) (Age + 1) x 30
    C) (Age + 1) x 40
    D) (Age + 2) x 20
    E) (Age + 2) x 30

16. *Which of the following statements regarding the use of oral oxybutynin in children is false?*

    A) 5mg BD for 7-year-old child is a standard acceptable starting dose
    B) It is not licensed for use under the age of 5 years
    C) Pyloric stenosis is a contraindication
    D) Reduced sweating is a side-effect
    E) It is safe to use with methylphenidate

17. *Regarding monosymptomatic nocturnal enuresis, which of the following statements is false?*

    A) If both parents suffered with bedwetting, chance of child being affected is up to 77%
    B) Genetic associations have been identified with loci on chromosome 13
    C) Desmopressin should not be prescribed if the child has SIADH
    D) 200mcg OD is an acceptable starting dose of desmopressin for a 6-year-old boy
    E) Bedwetting affects up to 6% of adolescents

18. *According to NICE 2022 Guidelines, a 4-month-old male infant with UTI is recommended to:*

    A) Have an US during acute infection if responding well to treatment
    B) Have an MCUG performed if the UTI are recurrent
    C) Have an MCUG even if the US is normal, in a child that responded well to treatment
    D) Have a DMSA within 3 months after the acute infection
    E) Have an US within 6 weeks, if the UTI was atypical

19. *According to NICE 2022 Guidelines, a 5-year-old female with UTI is recommended to:*

    A) Have an US during the acute infection, if these are recurrent
    B) Have an MCUG if the UTI was atypical
    C) Have an US during the acute infection, if this is atypical
    D) Have a DMSA within 3 months after the UTI, if this was atypical
    E) Have an US within 6 weeks, if the UTI was atypical

20. *According to NICE 2022 Guidelines, which of the following is not a criterion to define atypical UTI in children?*

    A) Raised creatinine
    B) Poor urine flow
    C) Septicaemia
    D) Positive MSU culture of E.coli
    E) Bladder mass

21. *Which of the following is the correct enzyme abnormality most likely to be found in congenital adrenal hyperplasia?*

    A) 17-hydroxylase deficiency
    B) 19-hydroxylase deficiency
    C) 21-hydroxylase deficiency
    D) 11ß-hydroxylase excess
    E) 13ß-hydroxylase excess

22. *Which hormone is typically found to be elevated in classic congenital adrenal hyperplasia?*

    A) 15ß-hydroxyprogesterone
    B) 17α-hydroxyprogesterone
    C) 19-hydroxyprogesterone
    D) 21-hydroxyprogesterone
    E) 23-hydroxyprogesterone

23. *Which of the following are not abnormalities associated with Turner's syndrome?*

    A) Tricuspid aortic valve
    B) Shortening of fourth metacarpal
    C) Shortening of fifth metacarpal
    D) Cubitus valgus
    E) Scoliosis

24. *Where does the mesonephros originate from in renal embryology?*

    A) Lateral plate mesoderm
    B) Mesenchyme
    C) Prechordal plate
    D) Intermediate mesoderm
    E) Primitive streak

25. *Where does the ureteric bud arise from around the fifth week of gestation?*

    A) Pronephric duct
    B) Metanephric duct
    C) Intermediate mesoderm
    D) Mesenchyme
    E) Mesonephric duct

STATION 4
EMERGENCY UROLOGY

BLADDER TRAUMA

EPIDEMIOLOGY

Bladder is urological organ that most suffers iatrogenic injury – most common procedure causing perforation is TURBT (external injuries may arise from laparoscopic surgery, for example).

Risk factors – older age, female gender, large tumour, tumour location on dome, previous perforation

RTAs most common cause of blunt bladder injury, followed by industrial trauma and falls.

60–90% of blunt bladder trauma have associated pelvic fractures (i.e. polytrauma is very common).

Pelvic fractures are associated with bladder injury in 3% of cases.

CLASSIFICATION

Bladder traumas are primarily classified into (as it guides further management):

- *Intra-peritoneal* (IPR)
- *Extra-peritoneal* (EPR)
- Combined IPR/EPR.

Bladder trauma can also be categorised by aetiology:

- *Non-iatrogenic* (blunt or penetrating)
- *Iatrogenic* (internal and external).

Intra-Peritoneal

The peritoneum overlying the bladder is breached allowing urine to escape into peritoneal cavity.

Ruptures tend to occur due to sudden rise in intra-vesical pressure (e.g. direct blow to distended bladder). The dome is the weakest point, where rupture is most likely to occur.

Intra-operative signs include low return of irrigation fluid, abdominal distension and bladder not filling.

Extra-peritoneal

Pelvic fractures are almost always associated with extra-peritoneal fractures.

Injury usually caused by distortion of pelvic ring and shearing of anterolateral bladder wall near the bladder base at the fascial attachments.

DIAGNOSTIC EVALUATION

The principal sign of bladder injury is visible haematuria.

Classic triad for bladder perforation:

- Lower abdominal pain, inability to void and visible haematuria.

Bladder injury may be detected cystoscopically directly at the time of injury – dark hole seen with bowel on the other side – no further on-table imaging required.

Indications for further bladder imaging in trauma are:

- VH + pelvic fracture
- NVH + high-risk pelvic fracture (disruption of pelvic circle with displacement > 1cm)
- Blunt urethral trauma and high injury severity score.

If urinary ascites occurs, blood tests for UE will show pseudo-rise in creatinine due to urine reabsorption via peritoneal cavity membrane.

IMAGING

The preferred imaging modality to detect non-iatrogenic or suspected iatrogenic bladder injury (when not noted intra-operatively) is cystography.

Cystoscopy is the preferred method for detecting intra-operative bladder injuries.

(Stress) Cystography

Requires catheterisation (be aware of potential urethral trauma).

Must be performed with > 300mL of water-soluble contrast (e.g. 50:50 mix), in order to distend the bladder and adequately diagnose perforation.

(For children, 60mL + 30mL for every year of age up to 400mL total.)

Sub-filled bladder may result in clot/omentum/bowel loop plugging a perforation.

AP and post-drainage films are taken.

IPR reveals contrast in or throughout peritoneal cavity highlighting bowel loops (CT may even reveal contrast around the liver).

EPR will reveal flame-shaped areas of extravasation in peri-vesical soft tissues.

Plain and CT cystography have comparable sensitivity (95%) and specificity (100%).

CT cystography (300mL of contrast into bladder via catheter and CT of pelvis) is superior at identifying bony fragments and can detect other abdominal injuries.

CTU is not a reliable imaging modality for detecting bladder injury – as the bladder is compliant and the amount of contrast excreted from CTU may not fill it sufficiently to note perforation.

Cystoscopy

Allows accurate localisation of bladder injury in relation to trigone and ureteric orifices.

A bladder that does not fill despite irrigation suggests large perforation; the surgeon must also palpate the abdomen for distension due to irrigation fluid in peritoneal cavity.

AAST Bladder Injury Scale

Table 1 – The AAST's bladder trauma scale [1]

Grade	Description of Injury
I	*Haematoma* (contusion) and/or partial-thickness *laceration*
II	*Laceration* – EPR injury with laceration < 2cm
III	*Laceration* – EPR injury (laceration ≥ 2cm) or IPR injury (laceration < 2cm)
IV	*Laceration* – IPR injury (laceration ≥ 2cm)
V	*Laceration* – IPR or EPR bladder injury extending to bladder neck or trigone/ureteric orifices

PREVENTION

VIVA   You may be asked in your viva how you would try to reduce your intra-operative risk of causing iatrogenic bladder injury, and you could consider mentioning the following:

- Give general anaesthesia with muscle paralysis
- Reduce current on diathermy settings
- Small, short controlled swipes with the diathermy loop
- Keep the bladder under-filled during cystoscopy
- Obturator nerve block.

For abdominal procedures carrying a significant risk of bladder injury, insert catheter at start.

MANAGEMENT

For trauma cases, initial management adopts systematic Airway-to-Exposure assessment of the patient, adhering to ATLS principles with a multi-disciplinary approach.

Resuscitation should include administration of broad-spectrum antibiotics as per local guidelines.

Extra-peritoneal Injury

Most EPR bladder injuries do not require surgical repair and can be managed conservatively:

- Broad-spectrum antibiotics
- Close observation of vital parameters
- Urethral catheter on free drainage for > 10 days followed by repeat cystography.

EPR injuries may be repaired when there are other injuries that require abdomino-pelvic surgery anyway (e.g. pelvic bone fragments, recto-vaginal injuries) to reduce the risk of infective complications.

Repair using 2-layer closure with 2'0 vicryl (absorbable) sutures (water-tight single-layer closure is equally acceptable).

Persisting extravasation (i.e. failure to heal) may also warrant delayed surgical repair of EPR.

Intra-peritoneal Injury

IPRs should always be managed by formal surgical repair, as intra-peritoneal urine extravasation can lead to peritonitis, sepsis and death.

Repair by lower midline laparotomy and single/double layer closure with absorbable sutures.

Catheter should be inserted and cystography performed after > 10 days.

IPR can be managed conservatively if small and delayed recognition after surgery, when the patient is clinically well and no signs of fever or peritonitis, via close observation.

Penetrating Injury

Bladder rupture due to penetrating injury mandates emergency surgical exploration. Debridement of any devitalised bladder tissue is advised.

The entirety of bladder wall and ureteric orifices must be inspected and primary closure advised.

FOLLOW-UP

Continuous bladder catheter drainage required to keep the intra-vesical pressure low.

Repeat cystography is recommended > 10 days after injury. If this shows ongoing extravasation, catheter should again be left on free drainage and scan repeated in 7 days.

TESTICULAR TRAUMA

EPIDEMIOLOGY

Most civilian trauma is blunt injury, usually unilateral (only 1% are bilateral).

More common in younger men, due to increased risk of RTAs and participation in contact sports.

Penetrating injury is most commonly due to firearms, affects both testes in 30%, and is associated with concomitant injuries in 70%.

Rarer causes – self-mutilation (psychosis), animal bites

CLASSIFICATION

Haematocoele occurs when bleeding is confined within the tunica vaginalis.

Intra-parenchymal (intra-testicular) bleeding occurs within the testis itself.

Testicular dislocation implies repositioning of the testis within superficial inguinal ring, the inguinal canal or abdominal cavity.

Testicular rupture implies disruption of the tunica albuginea.

DIAGNOSTIC EVALUATION

Patient *history* should address specifically:

- Mechanism/time of injury
- Presence and evolvement of pain/swelling
- Infective risk factors for penetrating injuries.

Patient *examination* should assess specifically:

- Whether testes are palpable, tender, smooth and intact
- Degree of scrotal swelling (quantify size and compare to contra-lateral testis).

IMAGING

Scrotal US is the diagnostic imaging modality of choice for assessing scrotal trauma.

Primary aim of US is to detect integrity of tunica albuginea (specificity 75%, specificity 64%) and vascularity of testis.

Heterogenecity within testis on US suggests an intra-testicular bleed may have occurred.

MANAGEMENT

Trauma patients should be resuscitated systematically in an A-to-E sequence, adhering to ATLS principles and adopting a multi-disciplinary management strategy.

Penetrating testicular trauma patients should:

- Undergo urgent scrotal exploration, wash-out and debridement of non-viable tissue
- Be given prophylactic antibiotics + tetanus prophylaxis are recommended.

Haematocoeles due to trauma should:

- Be managed conservatively if small and uncomplicated (ice, elevation, rest)
- Be treated surgically if large (> 3x size of contra-lateral testis) due to concern of raised pressure within scrotum that can lead to testicular ischaemia
- Orchidectomy rates are higher in delayed (80%) vs. early (< 3 days) surgical intervention.

Testicular dislocation following trauma should:

- Be replaced manually and a delayed orchidopexy offered
- Be offered immediate orchidopexy if manual reposition cannot be performed.

Testicular rupture following trauma should:

- Be taken urgently to theatre for exploration and the tunica albuginea closed with 4'0 absorbable sutures if the testis is viable e.g. 4'0 vicryl
- Undergo orchidectomy if tissue is non-viable.

Consider sperm banking in cases of severe bilateral testicular injury.

RENAL TRAUMA

EPIDEMIOLOGY

Renal trauma occurs in < 5% of all cases of major trauma (protected as retro-peritoneal structures, therefore requires considerable force and likely collateral injuries present).

Incidence is 5 per 100,000 population – higher for young men.

Vast majority of injuries in Europe are *blunt* trauma (97%) rather than *penetrating*, and most can be managed without surgical intervention.

Renal pedicle injuries are rare in blunt trauma (< 5%) and can be due to rapid deceleration injuries.

Most common causes of blunt injuries include RTAs, falls from height and sporting injuries.

Penetrating injuries are more common in urban areas, mainly involving stab or gunshot wounds to the flank, and are usually more severe than blunt injuries.

DIAGNOSTIC EVALUATION

Patient *history* should focus on the relevant factors:

- Mechanism and time of injury
- Any <u>blood in the urine</u>
- Previous urological history
- Relevant medical history to include anti-coagulation status and pre-existing renal disease.

Patient *examination* should initially adhere to ATLS principles, adopting a multi-disciplinary approach along with A+E/orthopaedics/general surgery/anaesthetics.

Perform systematic A-to-E examination recording vital signs. VH is the key finding; however, if urine is clear then urinanalysis should be performed to look for NVH.

The lowest recorded blood pressure should be documented as it may determine need for CT scan.

VIVA You would be expected in your viva to be able to succinctly run through an A-to-E evaluation of a very sick or trauma patient. I would therefore strongly recommend you familiarise yourself with the ATLS and CCrISP algorithms, which you can find online. Broad concepts to mention:

- A*irway* (know your airway adjuncts) and C-spine control
- B*reathing* – high-flow oxygen via non-rebreathe mask, know saturations and respiratory rate
- *Circulation* – large-bore IV access + fluids, record blood pressure + heart rate, cross-match
- D*isability* – GCS score
- E*xposure* – assess temperature, remove clothing and full secondary survey.

IMAGING

CT scan with contrast is the investigation of choice.

CT allows accurate grading of injury, assessment of contra-lateral kidney and injuries to other organs.

Indications for CT in a stable patient following renal trauma (EAU 2023):

- Associated visible haematuria
- Associated NVH and one episode of hypotension
- History of rapid deceleration injury and/or significant associated injuries
- Penetrating trauma
- Clinical signs of renal trauma (flank pain/bruising, tender palpable mass).

Adults with no visible haematuria, normal BP and no significant mechanism of injury do not require routine initial CT imaging (chance of significant injury 0.2%).

Lower threshold for imaging in children due to paediatric kidneys being less protected during trauma.

Haemodynamically unstable patient may preclude CT imaging and need direct transfer to theatre.

CT should ideally be performed as a 3-phase study:

- *Arterial* phase to assess for vascular injury showing "blush"/ extravasation

- *Nephrographic* phase to assess parenchymal contusions and lacerations

- *Delayed urographic* phase (after 5–10 minutes) to identify collecting system/ureteric injuries.

GRADING

The AAST grading system is based primarily on CT findings, and is also used in UK practice.

Table 2 – The AAST's renal trauma scale [1]

Grade	Description of Injury
I	*Contusion* or non-expanding sub-capsular haematoma, without laceration
II	*Haematoma* – non-expanding perirenal haematoma *Laceration* – parenchymal laceration ≤ 1cm deep (without urinary extravasation)
III	*Laceration* – parenchymal laceration > 1cm deep (without urinary extravasation)
IV	*Laceration* – extending into collecting system with urinary extravasation *Vascular* – segmental renal artery/vein injury with contained haematoma, vessel thrombosis causing renal infarction
V	*Laceration* – shattered kidney *Vascular* – main renal artery/vein laceration, or avulsion of hilum, or devascularised kidney with active bleeding

Image 1 – AAST grading of renal trauma

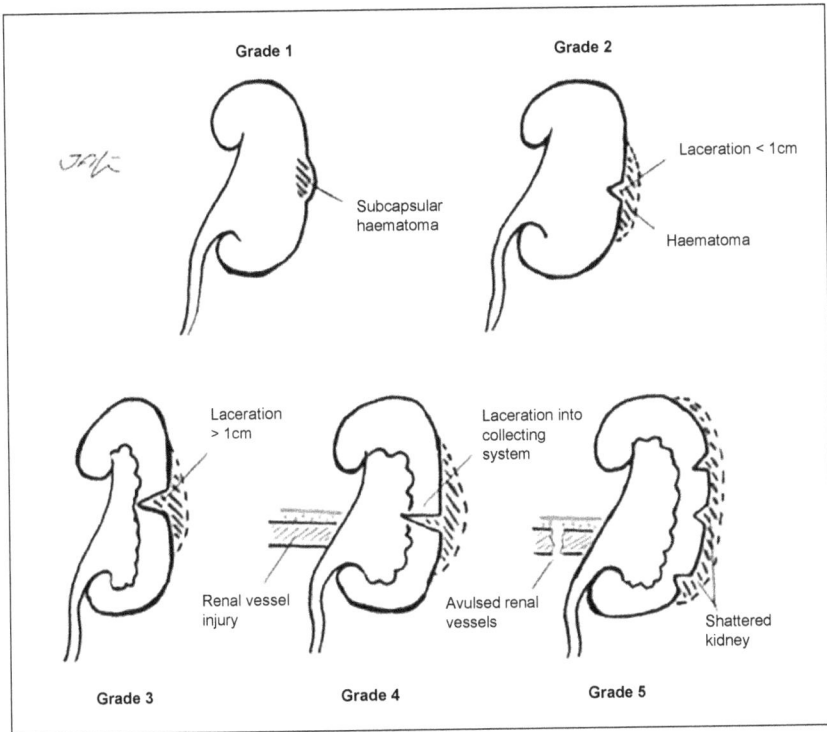

Grade 1

Grade 2

Subcapsular haematoma

Laceration < 1cm

Haematoma

Laceration > 1cm

Laceration into collecting system

Renal vessel injury

Avulsed renal vessels

Shattered kidney

Grade 3

Grade 4

Grade 5

MANAGEMENT

Haemodynamic stability is the primary criterion for the management of all renal injuries.

Non-operative management is treatment of choice for most blunt renal trauma injuries:

- Bed rest
- Serial blood tests and regular vital parameter observation
- Delayed re-imaging.

It is associated with lower nephrectomy rate and no increased long-term morbidity.

Grade 4 and 5 renal trauma patients can be managed conservatively if haemodynamically stable without any active bleeding. (However, requirement for subsequent intervention is higher.)

The potential complications of conservative management of renal trauma include:

- *Early*, such as secondary haemorrhage, urinoma formation requiring drainage/stenting, infection, abscess formation, AVF or pseudo-aneurysm formation
- *Late*, such as hypertension and fibrosis (Page kidney), renal insufficiency, chronic pyelonephritis, renal artery thrombosis.

Selective Angioembolisation

IR selective angioembolisation has a key role in non-operative management of blunt renal trauma.

Can be utilised for all grades of injury; likely to be most beneficial in high-grade injuries (IV and V), to treat active extravasation/bleeding, AVF and pseudoaneurysm formation.

Main renal artery can be embolised as life-saving measure, allowing a more controlled nephrectomy.

Any uncontrolled bleeding will require surgical exploration.

Urinary Extravasation

90% of these injuries will heal spontaneously and do not require surgical exploration.

Associated bowel injuries with urinary extravasation is an indication to explore.

Prescribe broad-spectrum antibiotic, monitor for fever or persisting pain (urinoma) and for significant extravasation, consider placing a ureteric stent +/- IR percutaneous drain.

SURGICAL EXPLORATION

There is a trend toward ongoing resuscitation and embolisation, as opposed to surgical exploration.

Emergency exploration for blunt and penetrating renal trauma may be indicated if:

- Haemodynamically unstable Grade 5 injury
- Other abdominal injuries need exploring (e.g. leaking bowel injury) and expanding/pulsatile haematoma is found at laparotomy (i.e. leave a stable detected haematoma alone).

The aim of surgical exploration after renal trauma is vascular control and renal salvage.

If pre-operative CT was not performed due to critical condition, arrange one-shot on-table IVU.

Surgical exploration is performed as follows:

- Generous midline laparotomy from sternum to pubis
- Small bowel gently retracted away to expose retro-peritoneum
- Incise peritoneum over aorta above the inferior mesenteric artery
- Superior dissection to locate the renal arteries and veins which can be ligated
- Reflect the colon to expose the kidney.

If haematoma is found to be non-expanding and non-pulsatile, most can be left alone, as exploration increases chance of subsequent nephrectomy.

Most kidneys will not function after arterial injury – arterial reconstruction may only be indicated if diagnosed very quickly in solitary kidneys or bilateral injuries.

PENETRATING INJURIES

The broad principles of management of penetrating renal injuries are similar.

Penetrating injury is an indication to undergo CT regardless of haematuria status, therefore even minor grades of injury may be detected.

High grades (IV and V) are likely to require urgent surgery and renal exploration.

EAU 2024 Guidelines for Penetrating Renal Trauma [2]

Figure 1 – EAU Guidelines for Penetrating Renal Trauma

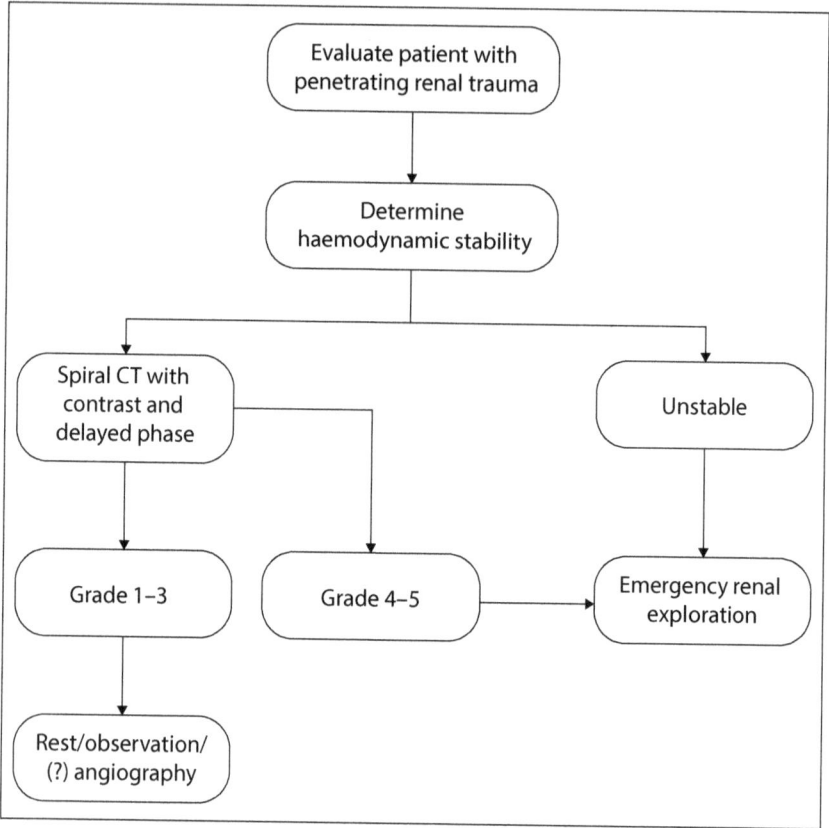

FOLLOW-UP

Risk of complications in conservatively treated patients increases with injury grade.

Repeat CT 2–4 days after Grade 3–5 injury should be considered, particularly if worsening flank pain, onset of fever or falling haematocrit.

Decline in long-term renal function correlates with increasing injury grade. DMSA can evaluate further.

Follow-up should include annual BP measurement and UEs.

URETERAL TRAUMA

EPIDEMIOLOGY

Ureteric trauma accounts for < 2.5% of all trauma to urinary tract.

Iatrogenic trauma during surgery is the commonest cause (80%) – often missed and delayed recognition, resulting in significant morbidity.

Iatrogenic injuries include suture ligation, clamp crushing, partial/complete transection, thermal injury or ischaemia from devascularisation.

Gynaecological operations are the commonest cause of iatrogenic injuries to the ureter.

Prophylactic stenting before complex pelvic surgery may help detect ureteric injuries during surgery, but does not reduce risk of injury occurring (however, it is more expensive and time consuming).

EAU 2024 recommends prophylactic ureteric stents prior to high-risk cases.

External causes include RTAs in 1/3 of cases (blunt deceleration avulsing ureter from renal pelvis) and gunshot (2% of all wounds) and should be suspected in any penetrating injury.

DIAGNOSTIC EVALUATION

The injury may be suspected intra-operatively, in which case it can be dealt with immediately; however, often the injury will not become apparent for days/weeks after surgery.

Patient history or history from colleague should enquire regarding:

- Details of surgical procedure/difficulties/indication (read operation note)
- Past medical history to include abdo-/gynae-/urological surgery, RTx
- Flank pain
- Haematuria (only present in 50% of injuries)
- Urinoma, fever/sepsis, persisting high drain output, abdominal swelling, ileus.

Drain fluid (where applicable) should be tested for urea and creatinine, and should have higher creatinine than serum (drain fluid creatinine > 300μmol/L suggests urine).

IMAGING

Post-operative Scenario/External Cause

CTU is ideal investigation; extravasation of contrast is the hallmark sign of ureteral injury.

Hydronephrosis, mild ureteral dilatation or urinoma may however be the only radiological signs.

US may show hydronephrosis; however, insufficient investigation as for example a complete transection leaks urine into peritoneal cavity with no obstruction or hydronephrosis.

For patients with a nephrostomy, antegrade nephrostogram will aid in confirming diagnosis.

Intra-operative Scenario

Direct, by full mobilisation of the ureter by packing bowel out the way and examining the full length (lower end is more difficult).

Retrograde ureterography is a very accurate method via cystoscope to look for contrast extravasation and should be undertaken bilaterally.

On-table IVU is technically difficult and unreliable in diagnosis.

GRADING

The AAST has defined a grading system for ureteral injuries (see Table 3).

Table 3 – The AAST's ureteric trauma scale [1]

Grade	Injury Description	Management Options
I	Contusion/haematoma only	Conservative +/- stent
II	Laceration < 50% transection	Stent +/- suture
III	Laceration ≥ 50% transection	Stent +/- suture Uretero-ureterostomy +/- stent
IV	Complete transection < 2cm of devascularisation	Ureteric reconstruction or temporary nephrostomy
V	Complete transection > 2cm of devascularisation	Ureteric reconstruction or temporary nephrostomy

MANAGEMENT

Management options for ureteral trauma depend on:

- Whether injury is recognised intra-operatively or delayed
- Grade and level of injury
- Other associated clinical factors (e.g. active infection, concomitant traumatic injuries)
- Skill-set of surgeon and centre, available resources (e.g. robotic surgery).

For iatrogenic injuries detected *intra-operatively*, the optimal time for repair is immediate, except:

- Evidence of active infection at the proposed repair site
- Patient unsafe/unstable for prolonged general anaesthesia (ligate and insert nephrostomy).

For iatrogenic injuries detected following a *delay*, consider urgent nephrostomy insertion +/- ureteric stent and delaying definitive repair in early elective planned setting (EAU 2024).

SURGICAL RECONSTRUCTION

Most minor intra-operative injuries can be managed with stent, antibiotics and observation, provided full ureter has been visually inspected/complete retrograde study and minor entity established.

Options for ureteric surgical reconstruction are summarised in Table 4. [3]

Ureteric Stenting

Endo-urological treatment of ureteral injuries by stenting is the first step in most cases.

Can be performed via retrograde or antegrade route.

Stent should remain in situ for minimum of 6 weeks. Patient can be listed for stent removal under GA and on-table retrograde study to ensure resolution of injury.

Proximal/Mid-ureteral Injury

For ureteral injuries < 3cm in length:

- Primary uretero-ureterostomy
- If primary anastomosis not possible, consider uretero-calycostomy.

For extensive ureteral loss, consider transuretero-ureterostomy (proximal stump of ureter is transposed across midline and anastomosed to contra-lateral ureter).

Distal Ureteral Injury

Distal injuries should undergo reimplantation as blood supply to distal ureter is jeopardised.

Psoas hitch is reconstructive operation for more distal injuries:

- Bladder is opened via surgical incision (held with two stay sutures)
- Bladder pulled up by inserting index finger and is secured to psoas muscle, to reduce distance between ipsilateral distal ureter and bladder
- Contra-lateral superior vesical pedicle is also divided to aid this manoeuvre
- Uretero-neocystostomy is then performed (Image 2).

Boari flap involves tubularisation of flap of bladder to extend from bladder to ureter, an option for ureteric reimplantation when diseased segment is long (e.g. > 5cm) (Image 3).

The base of the flap should be broader than the tip, to reduce the risk of flap ischaemia.

Long-segment Ureteral Injury

Long-segment ureteric injuries are complex, long-term outcomes are poorer, and specialist centre input may be required due to limited case numbers.

Options for surgical reconstruction include:

- *Ileal-interposition*, where a segment of the ileum is used for replacement
- *Downward nephropexy and long Boari flap*
- *Auto-transplantation*, kidney is relocated to pelvis and vessels anastomosed to iliac vessels
- *Buccal ureteroplasty*, if previous reconstruction attempts have failed.

Image 2 – Psoas hitch for ureteric injury

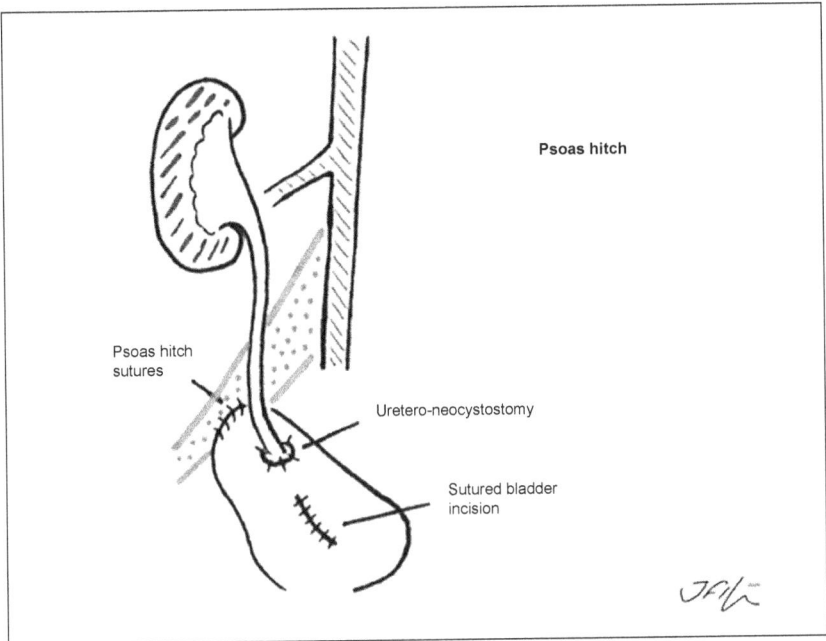

Psoas hitch

Psoas hitch sutures

Uretero-neocystostomy

Sutured bladder incision

Image 3 – Boari flap for ureteric injury

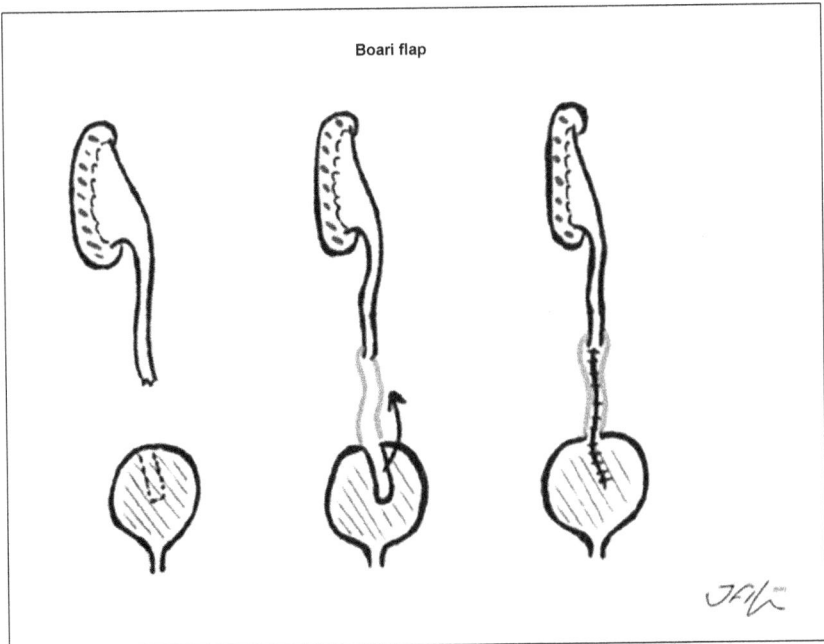

Boari flap

Table 4 – Options of surgical repair for ureteric injuries divided by location of injury

Injury Location	Surgical Option for Reconstruction
Distal ureter	Uretero-ureterostomy Primary reimplantation Psoas hitch or Boari flap
Mid-ureter	Uretero-ureterostomy Boari flap Transuretero-ureterostomy
Proximal ureter	Uretero-ureterostomy Uretero-calycostomy Transuretero-ureterostomy
Complete avulsion or injury	Ileal interposition Renal auto-transplantation

Principles underpinning ureteric reconstruction are tension-free, spatulated anastomosis with fine absorbable sutures (5'0/6'0), placement of stent and drain.

Consider further additional protective omental interposition.

URETHRAL TRAUMA

EPIDEMIOLOGY

Iatrogenic injury is the most common type of urethral trauma (particularly during male catheterisation).

Bulbar (anterior) urethra is the most common site affected by blunt trauma, as it is compressed against the pubic symphysis in straddle/kicking/RTA injuries.

Blunt posterior urethral injuries are almost always related to pelvic fractures.

Penetrating injuries are rare e.g. dog bite, gunshot, foreign-body insertion for auto-erotic stimulation.

AETIOLOGY

ANTERIOR (NON-IATROGENIC)

Most common cause is straddle/kick injury causing bulbar urethra to crush against pubic symphysis.

Other causes include penile fracture, foreign-body insertion into urethra and penetrating wounds.

POSTERIOR (NON-IATROGENIC)

Most injuries to the posterior urethra are related to pelvic fractures (RTAs, crush injury, falls).

Urethral injuries are not directly life-threatening; however, their association with concomitant pelvic fractures and/or thoraco-abdominal injuries can be (i.e. clinical prioritisation).

Surgically these injuries are described as either *partial* or *complete* ruptures.

Complete ruptures due to shearing effect of bone disruption, feature a gap between disrupted ends of the urethra. These ends will retract and eventually fibrous tissue fills the space in between.

The prostate (fixed to symphysis via pubo-prostatic ligaments) and the membranous urethra (fixed in the urogenital diaphragm) move in different directions.

These injuries are also called pelvic fracture urethral distraction defects (PFUDD).

Delayed morbidity associated with posterior urethral injuries includes strictures, ED, incontinence.

IATROGENIC

Urethral instrumentation is the most common cause of urethral trauma in the Western world and can affect all segments of the urethra, leading to stricture formation.

Catheterisation

Most strictures caused by catheterisation affect the bulbar urethra.

Size and type of catheter have an important bearing on urethral stricture formation. Smaller gauge and silicone catheters are associated with lower urethral morbidity.

Balloon inflation in the anterior urethra is also a potential cause of injury.

Local catheter training programmes are important and should be implemented (EAU 2024).

Trans-urethral Surgery

Strictures following trans-urethral surgery may arise from size mismatch between scope and urethra, such that urethra is sufficiently stretched to be effectively ischaemic whilst scope is in situ.

Strictures may arise from diathermy dispersion – insulation with ample lubrication may reduce risk.

Stricture rates associated with mono- and bipolar trans-urethral resections are comparable.

Cancer Treatment

Both RTx and BTx treatments for pelvic cancers are recognised causes of urethral strictures.

Anastomotic strictures are recognised complication of RP surgery (risk 1–5%).

DIAGNOSTIC EVALUATION

Patient *history* should enquire specifically regarding:

- Mechanism of injury
- Passage of blood per urethra (cardinal sign of urethral injury)
- Difficulty voiding (often associated with complete rupture)
- Lower abdominal pain.

Patient *examination* should assess specifically for:

- Palpable bladder (suggesting inability to void)
- Pattern of bruising to perineum, groin and abdomen (consider butterfly-wing pattern)
- DRE for pelvic haematoma (soft, boggy swelling), blood on the glove (rectal injury in 5% pelvic fractures) and high-riding prostate (pushed up by haematoma).

Note that it is safe and acceptable to attempt gentle passage of a urethral catheter in the context of pelvic fracture. Any resistance should result in abandoning and inserting SPC.

Failure to insert a catheter may suggest urethral injury.

IMAGING

Retrograde urethrography (RU) is diagnostic investigation of choice for suspected urethral injury.

> **VIVA** You may be asked in your viva how to perform RU. Familiarise yourself with this technique:

- 12F catheter placed in fossa navicularis
- Inflate balloon to 2mL to create a seal preventing contrast leakage
- Flush 20mL of water-soluble contrast whilst employing fluoroscopy
- Patient placed 30% oblique, with hip + knee flexed (may not be possible in trauma scenario)
- In trauma patient, C-arm is oblique rather than patient (bulbar urethra is superimposed on itself).

The distinction between complete and partial injury is not always clear.

Contrast extravasation on RU is pathognomic for urethral injury:

- Urethral extravasation with bladder filling suggests partial rupture
- Massive extravasation without bladder filling suggests complete rupture.

If an SPC is in situ, an antegrade urethrogram can be performed with contrast via SPC.

If a urethral catheter has been successfully inserted (which excludes complete rupture) you may pass a 6F NGT alongside it and perform RU to exclude extravasation.

There is a physiological urethral narrowing as it passes through pelvic floor; may mimic stricture on RU.

GRADING

The AAST has defined a grading system for urethral injuries (Table 5).

Table 5 – The AAST urethral trauma scale [1]

Grade	Description	Treatment Options
I	Contusion	No treatment required
II	Stretch injury	Conservatively (with SPC or urethral catheter)
III	Partial disruption	Conservatively (with SPC or urethral catheter)
IV	Complete disruption (> 2cm separation)	Immediate endoscopic realignment vs. delayed urethroplasty
V	Complete disruption (transection with ≥ 2cm separation)	Immediate endoscopic realignment vs. delayed urethroplasty

MANAGEMENT

Commence systematic A-to-E ATLS protocol assessment engaging a multi-disciplinary approach.

Broad-spectrum antibiotics as per local guidelines should be given if urological injury suspected.

One attempt at gentle urethral catheterisation is permissible even in context of pelvic fracture.

Failed urethral catheterisation mandates SPC insertion, which may be US-guided; however, may require open cystostomy if bladder is collapsed.

> **VIVA** A patient with traumatic urethral injury is a good example of a situation where non-urological injuries/factors likely take clinical priority – you should therefore approach a relevant viva scenario cognisant of this concept and make it clear in your viva answer. Ensure you state you will see patient urgently, approach/assess via A-to-E ATLS protocol, work with colleagues in other specialities etc.

ANTERIOR URETHRAL INJURIES (MALE)

Contusions without rupture can be managed by 12F catheter insertion and removal in 7 days.

Small lacerations can be managed by simple closure.

Partial ruptures can have temporary urinary diversion via SPC (urethral catheter may complete the rupture), repeat voiding cysto-urethrogram in 2 weeks, remove SPC if normal.

Complete ruptures without extensive tissue loss or apparent infection (e.g. bite wound) should be offered immediate anastomotic repair, for example in injuries associated with penile fractures.

If unsuitable local surgical skill-set or active infection, can delay, divert via SPC and give antibiotics.

Long-term outcomes are comparable between immediate vs. delayed urethroplasty; however, the main advantage to patient if done immediately is significantly reduced time to spontaneous voiding.

Penetrating injuries require urgent exploration:

- Small defects can be treated by spatulation of both ends and primary anastomosis
- Longer defects may require staged repair with temporary SPC.

POSTERIOR URETHRAL INJURIES (MALE)

Posterior urethral injuries occur most commonly in trauma and must be prioritised accordingly.

Single gentle attempt at catheterisation is permissible; excludes significant urethral injury if successful.

SPC via US guidance as means of urinary diversion is desirable as it allows:

- Urine output monitoring in critically ill patient
- Avoids development of urinary retention in obtunded patients
- Minimise urinary extravasation and its associated sequalae such as infection and/or fibrosis.

Partial Ruptures

Can be managed with urethral catheter or SPC in situ for > 4 weeks, as most will heal; follow-up RU confirming healing is, however, essential prior to removing catheter.

Early realignment is an option if patient is stable; beneficial as reduces stricture rates vs. temporary urinary diversion via SPC, with any ensuing stricture likely to be shorter and easier to treat.

Early realignment should be performed endoscopically (rather than open) via cystoscopy-guided wire insertion over which a catheter is passed and kept in situ > 4 weeks.

Subsequent strictures treated by urethrotomy if short, or anastomotic urethroplasty if long/complex.

Complete Rupture

A complete injury will not heal and formation of obliterated urethral segment is inevitable if patient was treated with SPC urinary diversion alone.

Permanent SPC may be suitable option if poor performance status and/or severe disability.

If surgical reconstruction is appropriate, the timing of intervention is classified as:

- *Immediate*, implying within 48 hours from injury (not recommended)
- *Delayed primary*, implying 2 days to 6 weeks after the injury
- *Deferred*, implying > 3 months after the injury.

Deferred repair following complete posterior urethral rupture is preferred (EAU 2024) as:

- Patient can recover from major trauma (likely to allow lithotomy position)
- Pelvic haematoma/urinary extravasation can reduce (urethral ends come closer together, reducing length of defect and need for mobilisation during primary anastomosis)
- Prostate descends to normal position allowing more accurate assessment of urethral defect
- Better outcomes (bleeding, stricture formation, incontinence, impotence) vs. immediate repair.

Most PFUDDs will be short and amenable to one-stage perineal anastomotic repair.

Scar tissue is excised, both healthy urethral ends are spatulated with the key objective of achieving successful <u>tension-free anastomosis</u>.

If significant loss of length occurred, urethral mobilisation required to achieve tension-free anastomosis.

This can be achieved by:

- Separating crura at base of penis (where they first come together and run parallel, potential gain for the first 5–7cm from the base where they then fuse)
- Spatulate dorsal ends and suture skin/buccal mucosa for anastomosis.

Early urethroplasty is only advisable in PFUDD cases associated with bladder neck involvement, as injury here compromises intrinsic sphincter mechanism leading to incontinence.

FEMALE URETHRAL INJURY

Urethral injuries in females are very rare, with pelvic fractures being the main aetiological cause.

Usually involve longitudinal tears of anterior wall associated with vaginal laceration.

Urethral injury in a female patient with pelvic fracture should be suspected if blood noted at vaginal introitus, associated VH, urinary retention and/or labial swelling.

Distal injuries can be left unrepaired as no disruption to continence mechanism.

Primary anastomosis performed retropubically (proximal injury) or transvaginally (mid-urethral injury).

EAU 2024 recommends *early* repair (within 7 days) as this is associated with lowest complication rates.

METASTATIC SPINAL CORD COMPRESSION

Defined as spinal cord compression (SCC) by direct pressure and/or vertebral collapse by metastases or direct extension of malignancy that threatens neurological disability.

EPIDEMIOLOGY

Majority of SCC cases with an underlying urological cause are due to metastatic prostate cancer.

Only 2/3 of patients with SCC presenting unable to walk/stand recover any function within 1 month.

95% of patients will complain of back and/or nerve root pain and have positive bone scan.

20% have multi-level spinal metastatic infiltration.

DIAGNOSTIC EVALUATION

Patient *history* should enquire specifically regarding:

- Onset, duration and progression of neurological symptoms
- Red-flag symptoms including night-time pain, pain lying flat, weight loss
- Known history of prostate cancer and patient's latest PSA
- Previous spinal pathology/surgery.

Patient *examination* should include:

- Full peripheral neurological examination of lower limbs
- Anal tone and sensation (S2–4).

Imaging modality of choice is emergency full MRI of the spine with contrast.

MANAGEMENT

The patient should be assessed/approached in a systematic A-to-E fashion, involving a multi-disciplinary approach with other specialities (e.g. orthopaedics, oncology, palliative care).

The local MSCC co-ordinator should be informed.

Patient should be nursed flat with neutral spine alignment.

Initial treatment involves high-dose corticosteroids (e.g. dexamethasone) +/- PPI cover.

Degarelix for castration can be prescribed if patient is known to have prostate cancer, or PSA is found to be very high and radiological imaging confirming metastatic disease.

Definitive treatment includes fractionated targeted RTx to spine, or urgent neurosurgical spinal decompression which may require transfer to tertiary care centre.

PENILE FRACTURE

EPIDEMIOLOGY

Most commonly caused by sexual intercourse by penis slipping out of vagina and striking pubic symphysis, other causes include masturbation and rolling over in bed.

Penile fracture is more likely to occur during sexual intercourse if patient is underneath.

5–10% of cases are associated with a urethral injury. [4]

AETIOLOGY

Penile fracture is due to the rupture of the tunica albuginea of the erect penis.

The tunica albuginea is 2mm thick in flaccid state, but thins to 0.25mm during erection and is therefore more vulnerable to rupture if penis is forcibly bent.

The tunica is thinnest in the ventral area of the penis, therefore the most common site for fractures to occur is at the region of the ventral penile base.

DIAGNOSTIC EVALUATION

The diagnosis of penile fracture should be clinical, based on history and examination findings; however, further investigations can aid location of the fracture site and thus planning of surgical repair.

Patient *history* should address in particular:

- Nature of precipitating event (vigorous sex, position during intercourse)
- Sudden onset penile pain associated with a popping sound
- Rapid penile detumescence following the moment of injury
- Any blood seen per urethra or history of VH.

Patient *examination* should assess for:

- Gross penile bruising and swelling, termed *"aubergine sign"*
- Bruising to perineum, scrotum and lower abdominal wall (ruptured Buck's fascia)
- Palpable defect of tunica albuginea over site of tear
- Stigmata of urethral injury, including blood per meatus, painful voiding, retention of urine.

IMAGING

US of penis can detect site of tunica albuginea tear, but is inferior to MRI.

MRI can detect small tunica tears (tape penis to the lower abdominal wall during scan) and is considered superior to all other imaging techniques.

RU or flexible cystoscopy may be used to evaluate urethral injury, either pre-operatively or on table.

MANAGEMENT

Early exploration and repair (within 24 hours) recommended as treatment of choice (BAUS).

Surgical repair should be performed even more urgently if there is associated urethral injury (BAUS).

Conservative treatment (ice, anti-inflammatories, abstinence from sex) is associated with higher incidence of penile fibrosis (35 vs. 5%), ED (62 vs. 5%) and penile curvature.

| VIVA | If you are asked about management of penile fracture in your viva, it is worth familiarising yourself with the relevant *BAUS consensus document on penile fracture* published in 2018 [5] and letting the examiner know that you are referring to this resource.

SURGICAL REPAIR

Traditional approach to penile fracture repair:

- Gently pass 12F catheter, if successful then cystoscopy not required to assess for urethral injury
- Circumferential de-gloving incision proximal to corona
- Identify tunica albuginea defect site, evacuate any overlying haematoma
- Repair defect with 2'0 PDS interrupted (absorbable)
- Repair any urethral injuries with 4'0 PDS over catheter (consider on-table RU)
- May complete with circumcision if patient agreeing/consented.

A local longitudinal incision centred over area of fracture can be used as alternative surgical approach.

The patient is advised to abstain from sexual intercourse for > 6 weeks after surgery.

Complications include penile curvature and erectile dysfunction.

PRIAPISM

EPIDEMIOLOGY

Priapism is a prolonged and unwanted erection, in absence of sexual stimulus, lasting > 4 hours.

> 95% of all priapism episodes are of the *"ischaemic"* type.

Sickle cell disease is the most common cause in childhood (> 60% of cases) and > 20% of adults (lifetime risk of priapism in sickle cell patients is 1/3, approx.).

PATHOPHYSIOLOGY

Ischaemic priapism for > 4 hours is considered akin to a compartment syndrome.

Histological changes that sequentially occur in ischaemic priapism include:

- Interstitial oedema
- Progressive destruction of sinusoidal epithelium
- Exposure of basement membrane after 24 hours
- Smooth muscle necrosis with fibrosis after 48 hours.

Emergency intervention required to prevent irreversible necrosis/fibrosis which causes permanent ED.

The duration of untreated priapism is the most significant predictor for subsequent development of ED.

CLASSIFICATION

The two common types of priapism are *ischaemic* (low flow) and *non-ischaemic* (high flow).

A rare sub-type is *stuttering* (recurrent) priapism.

Ischaemic (Low Flow)

Ischaemic priapism occurs due to veno-occlusion (intra-cavernosal pressures > 80mmHg) and is the most common form of priapism (> 95%) and requires emergency intervention.

Characterised by <u>painful</u> and <u>rigid</u> erection, with low or absent cavernosal blood flow.

Blood gas sampling from corpora cavernosa reveals hypoxia, acidosis and appears dark in colour.

Non-ischaemic (High Flow)

Non-ischaemic priapism occurs due to unregulated arterial flow.

Presents as <u>painless</u> and <u>semi-rigid</u> erection.

Usually arises from previous trauma and subsequent fistula formation; corporal blood gas readings will be similar to arterial blood; this condition is usually self-limiting.

Recurrent (Stuttering)

Usually seen in sickle cell disease.

Commonly high-flow type of priapism (can also be low-flow), featuring frequent prolonged and painful erections which are generally self-limiting.

Management relies on optimising the underlying haematological condition.

AETIOLOGY

Priapism can be primary (idiopathic) in nature.

Secondary causes of priapism include:

- Intra-cavernosal injections – papaverine, alprostadil
- PDE5i drugs – carefully counsel sickle cell patients when prescribing
- Haematological – leukaemia, sickle cell disease
- Trauma – resulting in AVF formation
- Infective – malaria, rabies, genito-urinary sepsis
- Oncological – infiltrating pelvic malignancy.

DIAGNOSTIC EVALUATION

Main aims of history and examination are to identify aetiological cause and sub-type of priapism.

Patient History

Key points in patient *history* of priapism include:

- Time of onset of erection and presence/absence of sexual stimulus
- Presence of pain
- Previous episodes of priapism and treatment received
- Drug history to include prescription and online medications for ED
- History of pelvic trauma, known pelvic malignancy, sickle cell disease.

Patient Examination

Assess/resuscitate patient in systematic A-to-E manner, provide analgesia, obtain chaperone.

The following should be carefully examined:

- Penis, rigid and tender shaft with soft glans (low flow)
- Abdomen, palpable mass/organomegaly which may suggest advanced malignancy
- DRE, to assess for locally advanced prostate cancer.

Baseline Investigations

Blood tests (FBC, UE, clotting profile) for haematological malignancies.

Aspirate blood from corpora using large (e.g. 19-gauge) butterfly/cannula for blood gas analysis:

- Ischaemic priapism yields acidotic blood gas parameters with high pCO_2
- Non-ischaemic priapism yields similar blood gas parameters to normal arterial blood.

IMAGING

Routine imaging not required to distinguish between low- vs. high-flow priapism (blood gas parameters).

Penile Doppler US can be used as adjunct/alternative to aid this diagnostic distinction:

- Ischaemic priapism reveals minimal/absent flow in cavernosal arteries and corpora
- Non-ischaemic shows high-peak systolic velocities (possible fistula).

MRI of penis may help evaluate viability of corpora in refractory/prolonged cases to aid decision for early penile prosthesis insertion.

MANAGEMENT (LOW FLOW)

VIVA   If you are asked about management of priapism in your viva, it is worth familiarising yourself with the relevant *BAUS consensus document on priapism* published in 2018 [6] and letting the examiner know that you are referring to this resource. You must specify this is a time-sensitive urological emergency and you would see the patient immediately without delay.

The aim of any treatment is to restore penile flaccidity, prevent damage to corpora, avert risk of ED.

BAUS categorises management strategies into:

- *Priapism < 48 hours* (shunting should be attempted if aspiration unsuccessful)
- *Priapism 48–72 hours* (offer MRI + US Doppler and consider prosthesis if no perfusion)
- *Priapism > 72 hours* (shunting likely to be futile and consider early prosthesis insertion).

Sickle cell patients require oxygenation, rehydration and liaising with haematologist. Stuttering cases can be offered daily dose etilefrine as preventive strategy in select cases (BAUS).

ASPIRATION OF CORPORA

Offer penile block with 10mL of 1% lidocaine (if pain is issue).

Insert large (19-gauge) butterfly/cannula into corpus cavernosum:

- Either through lateral penile shaft
- Or through the glans penis into tip of corpus cavernosum.

Aspirate stagnant blood from corpora (send for gas analysis) until draining fresh red, corpora can be flushed with saline to bust clots, aspirate ≤ 150mL as detumescence expected with this amount.

Attempt corpora aspiration for any priapism duration; however, the longer the history, the less likely aspiration will be to have a meaningful result.

INTRA-CAVERNOSAL PHENYLEPHRINE

Proceed to instillation of α-adrenergic agonist if aspiration unsuccessful for any priapism duration.

Phenylephrine is drug of choice due to high selectivity for α-1 adrenergic receptor; however, due to potential cardiovascular side-effects the patient should be in monitored bed.

Less preferable alternative is metaraminol; however, greater risk of adverse cardiovascular side-effects.

VIVA   You will be expected to know and confidently describe how you would draw up and administer phenylephrine to treat priapism refractory to aspiration. I recommend memorising the following:

- Obtain phenylephrine ampoule (available as 10mg in 1mL)
- Dilute 1mL ampoule in 19mL saline (thus preparing a 20mL syringe) – strength is 500µg/mL
- Inject 0.5mL (i.e. 250µg) as aliquot, directly into corpora
- Repeat every 10 minutes, to a maximum dosage of ≤ 1mg within one hour.

SURGICAL MANAGEMENT

Penile shunt surgery should only be considered when bedside treatments have failed and priapism duration implies there is a chance of meaningful successful outcome (i.e. < 72 hours).

Shunt surgery aims to provide exit for ischaemic blood from corpora to restore normal circulation.

Distal shunting procedures should be attempted before proximal techniques.

Distal Shunts

Winter shunt procedure:

- Insert Tru-cut biopsy needle through glans penis into tip of corpus cavernosum to create fistula
- Easy to perform

T-Shunt procedure:

- Point size-11 blade at glans and stab directly through it into the tip of the corpora
- Rotate the blade 90° away from urethra and then pull out; can perform bilaterally
- Manual penile compression to express out congealed blood
- Close glans incision wound with 3'0 vicyrl (absorbable)

Al-Ghorab shunt procedure:

- Bilateral excision of cone segments of distal tunica albuginea creating corporo-glandular shunt
- Subsequent glans closure with 3'0 vicyrl (absorbable)

Proximal Shunts

Quackle's technique and *Grayhack's* procedure are recognised proximal shunt operations.

Overall efficacy of proximal shunt procedures is questionable – likely high rates of ED.

No particular proximal shunting technique is proven superior than any other.

Consider taking an intra-operative smooth muscle biopsy to evaluate for necrosis, which can have medico-legal implications as well as manage patient expectations and need for prosthesis.

Penile Prosthesis Insertion

Prolonged ischaemic priapism (> 72 hours) leads to necrosis, fibrosis with penile shortening.

The resulting ED is likely to be permanent and refractory to medical therapy.

BAUS recommends early penile prosthesis insertion to avert the corporal fibrosis that will develop with longer delays, which make prosthesis insertion more challenging and less successful.

Offer early malleable prosthesis first, to maintain length/girth and prevent curvature from fibrosis, this can then be exchanged to inflatable device later on with option of cylinder upsize if needed.

There are no clear indications of when to insert prosthesis; however, relative indications include:

- Prolonged ischaemic priapism > 72 hours
- Biopsy of corporal smooth muscle proving necrosis
- Failure of aspiration, phenylephrine and shunting surgery
- MRI evidence of fibrosis and absent perfusion of US Doppler.

MANAGEMENT (HIGH FLOW)

Most common cause of high-flow priapism is blunt groin trauma leading to AVF formation.

Trauma leads to laceration of cavernosal artery leading to high-flow fistula between artery and sinusoidal tissue, which is unregulated and leads to erection.

Patient history may report local trauma, non-painful erections and sexual function possible; clinical examination reveals semi-rigid and non-tender erection.

Corporal aspiration of bright red blood reveals blood gas readings similar to arterial blood.

Confirm diagnosis with penile US Doppler study.

High-flow priapism is not an emergency as penis is not ischaemic – aspiration is not required.

Patient can be discharged after investigations and confirmation of diagnosis:

- Many can be managed conservatively
- Super-selective embolisation is an option for those wanting treatment (use autologous clot or fat).

Anti-androgens (e.g. bicalutamide) can be used, but only in adults.

Figure 2 – Treatment of ischaemic priapism scheme [6]

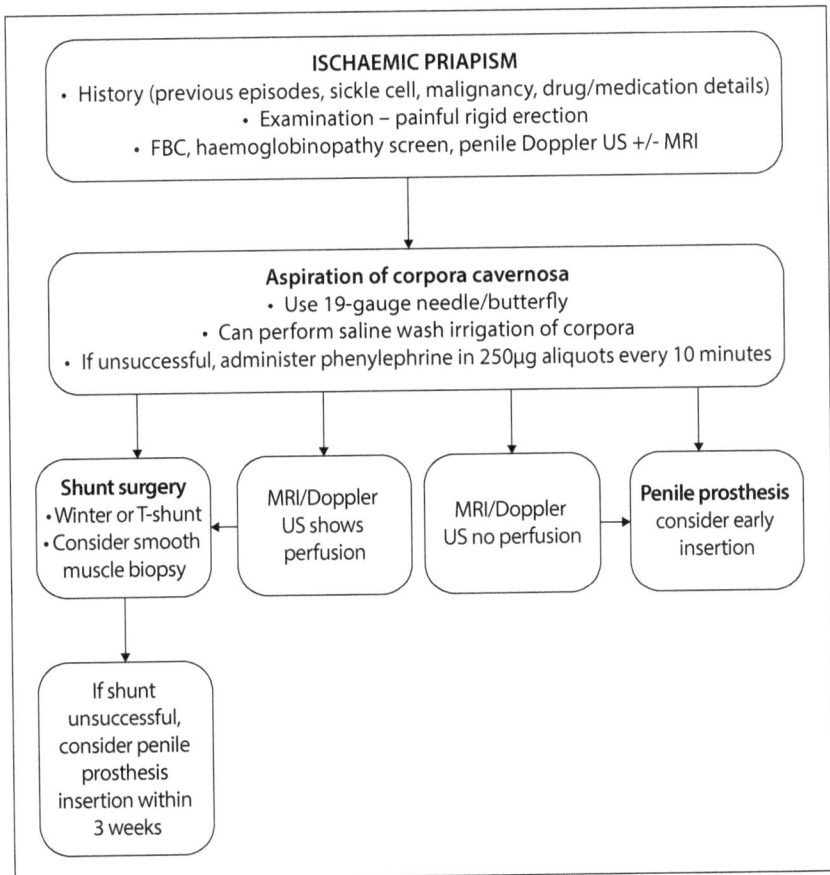

SEPSIS, ANAPHYLAXIS AND BIOCHEMICAL EMERGENCIES

DEFINITIONS OF SEPSIS

Sepsis – life-threatening condition that arises when the body's response to infection causes injury to its own tissues and organs (WHO 2024). [7]

Severe sepsis – sepsis associated with hypotension, organ hypoperfusion and dysfunction, leading to lactic acidosis, oliguria or alteration in mental state.

Septic shock – sepsis with hypotension despite fluid resuscitation along with end-organ hypoperfusion leading to lactic acidosis, oliguria or alteration in mental state.

Refractory septic shock – resistant to fluid resuscitation and pharmacological intervention.

SEPSIS-6 CARE BUNDLE PROTOCOL

Sick/trauma patients should be systematically assessed/resuscitated in an Airway-to-Exposure manner, and in particular with suspected sepsis, according to the *Sepsis-6 care bundle*.

Sepsis-6 has 6 components – 3 IN (oxygen, fluids, antibiotics) and 3 OUT (urine output, lactate, cultures).

Table 6 – The Sepsis-6 bundle [8]

Sepsis-6 Component	Notes
(IN) Oxygen	15L/minute via non-rebreathe mask
(IN) IV Fluids	Large-bore IV access, 1,000mL Hartmann's bolus
(IN) Antibiotics	Broad-spectrum according to local guidelines
(OUT) Monitor urine output	Insert urinary catheter and monitor urine output hourly
(OUT) Lactate	Take blood sample
(OUT) Blood cultures	Take blood cultures ideally before antibiotics

VIVA │ In your viva you will be asked to assess and treat sick patients.
I recommend you say: *"I will see the patient immediately and assess/resuscitate them in a systematic A-to-E manner as per CCrISP protocol. If fever is recorded or I suspect sepsis, I will ensure all components of the Sepsis-6 bundle are complete".* Needless to say, you therefore need to be broadly familiar with the CCrISP algorithm so I recommend you have a read about it online.

Identifying sepsis can be challenging and different screening tools have been proposed – however, there is no standardised international consensus on which tool should be used.

NICE 2024 recommends using NEWS2 to assess patients ≥ 16 years with suspected sepsis. [9]

NEWS2

Simple aggregate scoring system allocated to physiological measurements:

- Respiratory rate
- Oxygen saturations
- Systolic blood pressure
- Pulse rate
- Level of consciousness or new confusion
- Temperature.

VIVA │ You may be asked in your viva which physiological parameters make up the NEWS2 score. Make sure you know all of them confidently as this is a basic question and you use these scores in your daily clinical practice.

Systemic Inflammatory Response Syndrome (SIRS)

SIRS is the body's response to both infectious and non-infectious stimuli. Sepsis may lead to SIRS, as well as non-infectious stimuli such as burns, pancreatitis and trauma.

SIRS criteria were formerly used as tool to identify sepsis; however, has since fallen out of favour. [10]

Criteria for diagnosis of SIRS are listed in Table 7 – at least 2 of the criteria must be present.

Table 7 – The SIRS criteria [11]

Temperature	> 38°C or < 36°C
Heart Rate	> 90/minute
Respiratory Rate	> 20/minute or $PaCO_2$ < 32 mmHg (< 4.3 kPa) or need for mechanical ventilation
WCC	< 4 x 109/L or > 12 x 109/L or > 10% presence of immature neutrophils

qSOFA Score

qSOFA is a bedside test to aid identification of patients with suspected infection who are at greater risk of poorer outcome outside ITU.

qSOFA is not supported as a treatment prompt or diagnostic tool by the UK Sepsis Trust. [12]

The components of the qSOFA score are: [13]

- Low blood pressure (systolic ≤ 100mmHg)
- Raised respiratory rate (≥ 22/minute)
- Altered mental state (GCS < 15).

SOFA Score [14]

An alternative scoring system for sepsis is the sequential organ failure assessment score (SOFA):

- Respiratory (PaO_2)
- Cardiovascular (MAP)
- Renal (urine output or creatinine)
- Coagulation (platelet count)
- Neurology (GCS)
- Liver (bilirubin).

Used to monitor a patient's stay on ITU, assessing organ system function, to predict clinical outcomes.

ANAPHYLAXIS

Management of anaphylaxis for the urologist:

- Secure patient airway, give high-flow oxygen, obtain IV access and place cardiac monitoring
- Give 0.5mL of 1:1,000 adrenaline (IM) (i.e. 500mcg)
- Give 10mg of chlorphenamine (IV) + 200mg of hydrocortisone (IV)
- Request immediate help via EMRT call.

BIOCHEMICAL EMERGENCIES

HYPERKALAEMIA

Request ECG – possible changes include tall tented T-waves, wide QRS complex.

Management of hyperkalaemia for the urologist:

1. Protect myocardium – 10mL of 10% calcium gluconate
2. Drive K+ into cells – 10units of actrapid in 50mL of 50% glucose + 5mg salbutamol (neb)
3. Deplete total body K+ – calcium resonium 15mg (PO) TDS

Repeat ECG if hyperkalaemia-related changes were noted on initial trace, consider cardiac monitoring.

Regularly re-check K+ (and blood sugar) until this has come down into safe range.

If dangerous hyperkalaemia persists despite medical therapy, critical care and renal medicine must be urgently contacted to consider commencing emergency dialysis.

HYPERCALCAEMIA

Features – confusion/altered GCS/coma, thirst/dehydration, muscle weakness, arrhythmias

Obtain ECG – possible change includes shortened QT interval.

Urgent treatment is required if Ca2+ > 3.0mmol/L (check PTH, albumin and renal function).

Management of hypercalcaemia for the urologist:

1. Aggressive rehydration – 4–6L of 0.9% saline (IV) over 24 hours (consider loop diuretic if patient is overloaded)
2. Bisphosphonates (IV) e.g. zoledronic acid 4mg
3. Treat underlying cause e.g. thiazide diuretics, rhabdomyolysis.

If dangerous hypercalcaemia persists despite medical therapy, critical care and renal medicine must be urgently contacted to consider commencing emergency dialysis.

Equation for corrected calcium = (measured total Ca2+) + 0.02(40 – serum albumin)

TESTICULAR TORSION

EPIDEMIOLOGY

Testicular torsion is a twist of the spermatic cord, strangulating blood supply to testis and epididymis.

May occur at any age; however, there is a bi-modal distribution of incidence with the main peak around puberty (12–18 years) and a smaller peak within first year of life.

CLASSIFICATION

Extra-vaginal Torsion

Most commonly occurs in first year of life (can occur pre- or postnatally)

Incomplete fixation of gubernaculum to scrotal wall, resulting in entire testis and tunica vaginalis twisting in vertical axis on the spermatic cord, outside the tunica vaginalis.

Intra-vaginal Torsion

Most common form of testicular torsion found in adolescents.

Usually due to congenital *bell-clapper deformity*, whereby the testis not attached posteriorly to inner scrotum by the mesorchium, such that it is free-floating and can rotate more readily.

DIAGNOSTIC EVALUATION

Patient *history* should enquire in particular regarding:

- Time/nature/activity at the onset of pain (often waking from sleep)
- Any previous similar self-limiting episodes (to suggest intermittent torsion)
- Any previous scrotal surgery or exploration.

Patient *examination* should evaluate:

- Tender affected testicle (rather than just superior pole, suggesting torted hydatid)
- Absent cremasteric reflex (sensitivity close to 100%, specificity 66%)
- High-riding and horizontal lie testis

- Mild fever
- Elevation of testicle does not ameliorate symptoms (negative *Prehn's sign*).

Urine dipstick test is usually normal in testicular torsion.

Cremasteric reflex

Elicited by stroking the inner surface of the thigh in males – immediate contraction of the cremaster muscle which draws ipsilateral testis superiorly.

Sensory pathway – stimulation of ilio-inguinal nerve

Motor pathway – activation of genital branch of the genito-femoral nerve

IMAGING

Testicular torsion is a <u>clinical</u> diagnosis and the gold-standard management for suspected testicular torsion is urgent scrotal exploration in theatre.

The use of radiological investigations should <u>not</u> delay patient transfer to theatre.

Doppler colour US can have a role in patients where clinical features are equivocal and there is no clinical indication for urgent exploration (sensitivity < 90% and specificity < 95%).

US is operator dependent and the presence of arterial flow can be misleading in early cases of torsion; furthermore, persisting arterial flow does not exclude the diagnosis of torsion.

Radionuclide scrotal scan (^{99m}Tc) is most accurate imaging technique to detect reduced radioisotope uptake; however, it is time consuming and not readily available.

MANAGEMENT

Urgent exploration is gold standard – perform whenever there is clinical suspicion of testicular torsion.

The two most important determinants for testicular salvage rates are:

- Time between symptom onset and surgical de-torsion
- Degree of cord twisting (worse if > 360° rotation).

Salvage rates correlate with number of hours after onset of pain.

Testicular fixation should be performed on affected testicle (if viable) with 3'0 prolene using 3-point technique (medial, lateral, antero-inferior).

Contra-lateral fixation should be performed if testicular torsion found or thought to have been highly likely on initial patient history and examination.

Upfront insertion of prosthesis is not advised at time of orchidectomy – can be offered after delay.

Impact on Fertility

The impact of testicular torsion on fertility remains unclear and evidence is conflicting.

Early surgical intervention with successful de-torsion is likely to preserve fertility.

If the condition is not treated urgently and the testis becomes infarcted, there is a risk of abscess/sinus formation, breaking down the BTB with subsequent risk of infertility.

Blood–testis Barrier (BTB)

BTB is a barrier between blood vessels and Sertoli cells of seminiferous tubules, formed by tight/adherens/gap junctions by intracellular adhesion molecules.

BTB serves to control environment in which germ cells develop (e.g. blocks entry cytotoxic agents).

If BTB is breached, sperm may enter bloodstream and immune system mounts auto-immune response against the unique sperm antigens only expressed by these cells.

The anti-sperm antibodies may bind to sperm and reduce fertility.

TRANS-URETHRAL RESECTION OF PROSTATE SYNDROME

EPIDEMIOLOGY

TURP syndrome is an iatrogenic condition arising from absorption of large volumes of irrigation fluid (1.5% glycine) during endo-urological surgery (typically TURP – can occur in PCNL or TURBT).

Since the advent of bipolar TURP, TURP syndrome has become much less common.

AETIOLOGY

During TURP there is 20mL/minute fluid absorption (i.e. 1.2L/hour) directly into peri-prostatic venous plexus (delayed absorption in retro-peritoneal and peri-vesical spaces).

1.5% glycine is hypotonic with respect to plasma (plasma ~280mmol/L, glycine ~220mmol/L).

Glycine is dealt with in the body as follows: [15]

- [Liver]: (90%)   glycine -> ammonia + glycolic acid + H2O (lowers Na+ concentration)
- [Kidney]: (10%)   glycine -> atrial natriuretic peptide (ANP).

The 3 main factors underpinning the clinical signs and symptoms of TUR syndrome include:

1. Dilutional hyponatraemia
2. Fluid overload
3. Effects of glycine toxicity.

Dilutional Hyponatraemia

Hypotonic glycine in bloodstream leads to osmotic shift of water from plasma into the brain causing confusion, nausea, reduced GCS, coma, cerebral herniation and death.

Glycine also induces osmotic diuresis and loss of sodium, further exacerbated by ANP natriuresis.

Table 8 – Symptoms noted with lowering concentrations of serum sodium

Sodium Concentration (mmol/L)	Symptoms
130–135	Asymptomatic
120–130	Restlessness, confusion
115–120	Nausea
< 115	Seizures, coma

Fluid Overload

Pulmonary oedema by fluid overload results in shortness of breath, cyanosis and hypertension. Patient may need critical care transfer for respiratory support and careful diuretic titration.

Later features include bradycardia and marked systolic hypotension.

Glycine Toxicity

Glycine is an inhibitory neurotransmitter in the retina – excess glycine slows down impulses from the retina to the cerebral cortex, which may manifest as patient reporting seeing flashing lights.

Glycine results in bradycardia due to cardio-toxic side-effects.

MANAGEMENT

TURP syndrome management can be divided into prevention, recognition and treatment.

Prior to listing a patient for TURP, they should be deemed anaesthetically fit and their pre-operative serum sodium must be checked and treated if low, before the surgery takes place.

PREVENTION

The following strategies can be employed to reduce the risk of TURP syndrome:

- *Operative time*, limited to < 60 minutes (consider staged procedures)
- *Gland size selection*, avoiding TURP for extremely large prostates (refer for HoLEP)
- *Bipolar resection*, which uses normal saline as the irrigation fluid

- *Reduce height* of irrigation bag
- *Spinal anaesthesia*, allows earlier syndrome recognition as patient can report symptoms.

If procedure is inevitably prolonged, the anaesthetist may consider administering IV furosemide.

RECOGNITION

Offer TURP under spinal anaesthesia, provided medically safe and patient's wishes respected.

Spinal anaesthesia allows assessment of altered mental state and patient-reported flashing lights.

TURP syndrome signs noted under GA may include hypertension due to fluid overload (early) or arrhythmias and bradycardia (late).

Addition of 1% ethanol in irrigant allows alcohol breath level monitoring to estimate volume of excess absorbed fluid.

TREATMENT

Intra-operative recognition mandates termination of procedure as soon as safely possible.

Mild cases: – Give 40mg IV furosemide (causes loss of more water than sodium)

         – Close observation

         – Repeat UEs

         – Inform critical care outreach

Severe cases: – Give 40mg IV furosemide

         – Immediate critical care outreach review and transfer to high-dependency

         – Invasive BP monitoring, central line insertion, intubation, consider mannitol

Hyponatraemia correction aimed at < 1mmol/L/hour to avoid central pontine myelinolysis.

Components of Common IV Fluids

Normal saline – 154mmol/L Na+ + 154mmol/L Cl-

1.5% glycine – 15g of glycine per litre

Hartmann's – 131mmol/L Na+ + 111mmol/L Cl- + 29mmol/L HCO3- + 5mmol/L K+ + 2mmol/L CA2+

5% glucose – 278mmol/L glucose (50g)

URETHRAL STRICTURES

A urethral stricture refers to scarring in sub-epithelial tissues of corpus spongiosum which results in narrowing of the urethral lumen.

True strictures can only affect the *anterior* male urethra, as the *posterior* urethra has no spongiosus tissue (hence posterior urethral narrowing is termed stenosis instead).

A short distal narrowing of the meatus without involving the navicular fossa is called *meatal stenosis*.

AETIOLOGY

The anterior urethra is most frequently affected (> 90%).

Causes of stricture disease vary according to geographical location in the world:

- *Inflammatory*, e.g. gonococcal urethritis, BXO
- *Trauma*, particularly straddle injuries
- *Iatrogenic*, such as urethral catheterisation, TUR surgery, prostate cancer surgery
- *Idiopathic* (often contain high levels of smooth muscle on biopsy).

CLASSIFICATION

Male urethral strictures can be classified based on their location, which affects their management: [16]

- *Anterior* (from meatus to urogenital diaphragm), subdivided into meatal, penile and bulbar
- *Posterior*, which has 3 segments (membranous, prostatic, bladder neck).

There is no universal definition for what constitutes a female urethral stricture.

Female stricture can be considered a fixed anatomical narrowing causing reduced urethral calibre, generally defined as < 14F size.

There is an EAU classification of stricture according to the degree of urethral narrowing. [16]

DIAGNOSTIC EVALUATION

Patient *history* should specifically address the following:

- Duration and onset of urinary symptoms (likely voiding LUTS predominant)
- Causative factors (e.g. urological history/trauma/STI)
- Previous treatment for urethral stricture disease.

Patient *examination* is often externally unremarkable; assess for BXO and/ or meatal pathology, bladder scan for chronic retention, stigmata of chronic renal disease.

Further investigations involve flexible urethroscopy, RU or uroflowmetry.

Flexible urethroscopy allows direct visualisation of the stricture.

RU in specialist centres is preferred as it more accurately details the length, location and number of urethral strictures – urethroscopy may not be able to pass the initial narrowed segment.

EAU 2024 recommends that RU be performed for men being considered for reconstructive surgery.

Uroflowmetry pattern seen in urethral stricture is plateau-shaped, with little change in Qmax (see Figure 3).

Figure 3 – Typical uroflowmetry trace of urethral stricture

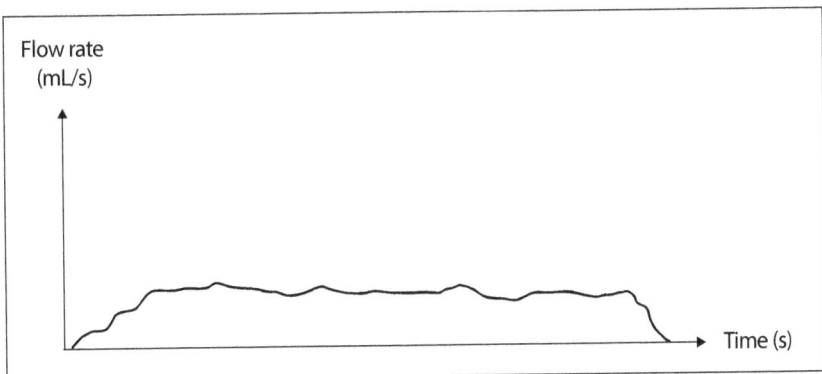

MANAGEMENT

Short Strictures (< 2cm)

Options include optical urethrotomy vs. urethral dilatation (neither treatment proven superior).

Urethral dilatation is preferable for strictures close to urinary sphincter mechanism.

Discharge with catheter in situ for 3–5 days and organise nurse-led TWOC.

Practice of post-treatment referral for ISD varies – potential benefit of ISD stabilising the stricture must be balanced vs. drawbacks (bleeding, UTI, increased complexity of subsequent strictures).

Intra-urethral corticosteroids (as catheter lubricant) can improve ISD outcomes and time to recurrence.

If patient is suitable future candidate for urethroplasty if required, preferable to avoid ISD training.

Stricture-free rates after first treatment are highly variable ($\leq$ 70%), reflecting the heterogenous nature of the condition; however, if recurrences occur they tend to happen within 12 months.

Stricture-free rates are much lower after treatment of recurrent disease – EAU 2024 does not recommend performing > 2 dilatations/urethrotomy if urethroplasty is a viable option. [16]

De-novo Short Strictures

Patients with recurrent strictures should be considered for ABU.

The prerequisites for ABU include:

- Recurrent short bulbar stricture < 2cm in length
- Pelvic-fracture related injury (distraction rather than stricture)
- Not appropriate for penile strictures due to risk of chordee.

Any anastomotic repair must be spatulated, tension-free and catheterised.

Curative in 90% at 10 years follow-up.

Complications include post-micturition dribble (division of bulbospongiosus) and recurrence.

Meatal Strictures

Open repair of distal urethral strictures can be in the form of Malone meatoplasty, skin flap meatoplasty or graft (skin/buccal mucosa) urethroplasty.

Long Strictures

Long bulbar strictures not amenable to ABU, alternative option is *substitution/free graft* urethroplasty.

Dorsal stricturotomy performed, placing dorsal patch (Barbagli procedure) using a buccal mucosa graft.

Success rates are inferior – 85% patency rates at 3 years deteriorating at 5% yearly such that by 10 years approximately half the patients develop recurrence.

This is not appropriate for RTx-related strictures as grafts will not take (i.e. genital skin flap).

Buccal Mucosa

This is the graft of choice in substitution urethroplasty because:
- Readily available in sufficient quantity
- Minimal morbidity to donor site
- Accustomed to wet environment
- Resistant to skin diseases
- Antimicrobial properties
- Behaves like full-thickness graft and thus takes well.

Graft-take will take approximately 96 hours.

Initial process undergoes two phases:
- *Imbibition* – graft obtains nutrients from host bed (graft temperature below core body)
- *Inosculation* – phase in which true micro-circulation is re-established in graft.

A successful graft will re-establish its blood supply by revascularisation.

Buccal mucosa has pan-laminar plexus, allowing it to be thinned during harvesting.

Dorsal placement of patch preferred as well-supported by cavernous bodies, preventing outpouching.

Full-thickness grafts include both dermis and epidermis; however, they are less likely to take as they are thicker than partial-thickness grafts and rely on less-robust sub-dermal plexus.

Partial-thickness skin grafts are deficient in collagen, therefore will contract and inferior cosmetically.

Female Strictures

Stricture and meatal stenosis is much rarer in women; management likely to be in specialist centre.

Offer urethral dilatation (which can be repeated) + 16F ISD.

Urethroplasty can be considered in women with recurrent disease and/ or unwilling to perform ISD; grafts reportedly have been harvested from vagina, buccal or lingual.

URINARY RETENTION

VIVA | All candidates approaching FRCS (Urol) will be proficient at
dealing with urinary retention and difficult catheterisation
scenarios, as this forms the bread and butter of our clinical
practice. However, logical thinking, prioritisation and
communication skills all form part of the marks awarded for any
viva station, so I have included systematic points below.

DEFINITIONS

Urinary retention is the inability to voluntarily pass urine (NICE): [17]

- *Acute* – medical emergency characterised by abrupt painful
  development of inability to pass urine (hours) requiring urgent
  catheterisation for symptomatic relief
- *Chronic* – gradual onset inability to empty bladder completely (over
  months/years), painless, characterised by PVR > 1L (no consensus as to
  PVR volume considered as significant)
- *Acute on chronic* – abrupt development of AUR in patient who
  previously had chronic retention.

For further details please refer to the "Treatment of BPH" section of Chapter
8, "Andrology & BPH".

From an emergency perspective, this section will focus on addressing sick
patients with urinary retention and the difficult catheter scenario.

DIAGNOSTIC EVALUATION

Approach/resuscitate patient in systematic A-to-E manner first if
haemodynamically unstable; if patient is acutely distressed due to pain,
appropriate to catheterise first and then take history.

Chronic retention is not a medical emergency unless there is upper-tract
compromise or sepsis.

Key factors in *history* from the patient:

- Time since last passed urine and increasing pain
- Precipitating factors such as constipation, new medication, UTI, spinal
  pathology

- Urological history (e.g. outflow surgery, stricture disease, urological cancer, previous AUR)
- Anti-coagulation status and previous abdominal surgery, if SPC is required.

Key factors in *examination* of patient:

- Abdominal examination for palpable tender bladder (corroborate with bedside bladder scan)
- Groin examination for foreskin, meatal or penile pathology
- DRE for size and contour of prostate
- Document details of catheter insertion and residual volume.

Collect blood tests (UEs, FBC) prior or soon after catheterisation, record NEWS2 score and assess need for in-patient admission (e.g. frailty, sepsis, diuresis, renal impairment, haematuria).

Complete Sepsis-6 bundle with broad-spectrum IV antibiotics if sepsis is suspected.

DIFFICULT CATHETERISATION

Challenging catheterisation can arise at various points along the way, thought of sequentially as:

- *Buried penis* – either due to morbid obesity or severe oedema
- *Phimosis* – may require dilatation with clip or emergency circumcision/ dorsal slit
- *Meatal pathology* – may require emergency dilatation
- *Urethral stricture* – may require cystoscopy-guided catheter over wire +/- urethral dilatation
- *Prostatic obstruction* – may require curve-tip or cystoscopy-guided catheter over wire.

Always utilise smallest size of catheter that is, however, sufficiently large to ensure effective drainage of urine and avoid recurrent blockages (e.g. 14F).

Bedside portable flexible cystoscopy kits can be of assistance if available.

Percutaneous needle aspiration of urine from the bladder can relieve pain and buy time.

SPC insertion has associated morbidity and small but not insignificant mortality rate (1–2%) and in an emergency, measures should be taken to try to avoid this option if possible.

VIVA | If you are discussing SPC insertion in your viva, I recommend you quote the BAUS SPC practice guidelines [19] to the examiner, and familiarise yourself with this document.

Contraindications to SPC insertion:

- Known bladder or undiagnosed visible haematuria
- Uncorrected coagulopathy or active prescription of anti-coagulant
- Pregnancy
- Presence of subcutaneous vascular graft in suprapubic region.

Complications include infection, bleeding, discomfort, bowel injury requiring laparotomy, mortality.

BAUS 2020 recommends that US guidance should be used if bladder is not readily palpable.

SPC insertion using trocar kit is acceptable if bladder is fully distended and palpable.

Cystoscopic guidance aids bladder distension and allows clinician to confirm catheter entry into bladder; however, it does not reduce the risk of bowel injury.

Open cystostomy can be considered for complex cases unsuitable for trocar insertion and likely reduces the risk of bowel injury, at cost of increased morbidity due to surgical wound size.

REFERENCES

1. The American Association for the Surgery of Trauma. Injury Scoring Scale. Available at: https://www.aast.org/resources-detail/injury-scoring-scale#blatter [last accessed 29 May 2024].

2. Kitrey ND, Campos-Juanatey F, Hallscheidt P, et al. (2024). EAU Guidelines on Urological Trauma. Available at: https://d56bochluxqnz.cloudfront.net/documents/full-guideline/EAU-Guidelines-on-Urological-Trauma-2024_2024-04-11-083052_vlwe.pdf [last accessed 29 May 2024].

3. Sharma DM, Shergill IS, Arya M (2018). Urological emergencies, Part 2. In: Arya M, Shergill IS, Fernando HS, et al., *Viva Practice for the FRCS (Urol) and Postgraduate Urology Examinations*, second edition, CRC Press, London.

4. Amer T, Wilson R, Chlosta P, et al. (2016). Penile fracture: a meta-analysis. *Urologia Internationalis*, *96*(3), 315–329.

5. Rees RW, Brown G, Dorkin T, et al. (2018). British Association of Urological Surgeons (BAUS) consensus document for the management of male genital emergencies – penile fracture. *BJU International*, *122*(1), 26–28.

6. Dorkin T, Lucky M, Pearcy R, et al. (2018). BAUS consensus document for the management of male genital emergencies – priapism. *BJU International*, *121*(6), 835–839.

7. World Health Organization, Sepsis. Available at: https://www.who.int/news-room/fact-sheets/detail/sepsis [last accessed 9 April 2024].

8. The College of Emergency Medicine, Sepsis. Available at: https://www.rcem.ac.uk/docs/Sepsis/Sepsis%20Toolkit.pdf [last accessed 9 April 2024].

9. NICE (2024). Suspected sepsis: recognition, diagnosis and early management. Available at: https://www.nice.org.uk/guidance/ng51 [last accessed 26 May 2024].

10. Mignot-Evans L, Raaijmakers V, Buunk G, et al. (2021). Comparison of SIRS criteria and qSOFA score for identifying culture-positive sepsis in the emergency department: a prospective cross-sectional multicentre study. *BMJ Open*, *11*(6), e041024.

11. Comstedt P, Storgaard M, Lassen AT (2009). The Systemic Inflammatory Response Syndrome (SIRS) in acutely hospitalised medical patients: a cohort study. *Scandinavian Journal of Trauma, Resuscitation and Emergency Medicine*, *17*(1), 67.

12. The UK Sepsis Trust (2022). The Sepsis Manual, 6th edition. Available at: https://sepsistrust.org/wp-content/uploads/2022/06/Sepsis-Manual-Sixth-Edition.pdf [last accessed 9 April 2024].

13. Marik PE, Taeb AM (2017). SIRS, qSOFA and new sepsis definition. *Journal of Thoracic Disease*, *9*(4), 943.

14. Jones AE, Trzeciak S, Kline JA (2009). The Sequential Organ Failure Assessment score for predicting outcome in patients with severe sepsis and evidence of hypoperfusion at the time of emergency department presentation. *Critical Care Medicine*, *37*(5), 1,649.
15. Shergill IS, Jameel B (2018). Urological Emergencies, Part 1. In: Arya M, Shergill IS, Fernando HS, et al., *Viva Practice for the FRCS (Urol) and Postgraduate Urology Examinations*, second edition, CRC Press, London.
16. Lumen N, Campos-Juanatey F, Dimitropoulos K, et al. (2024). EAU Guidelines on Urethral Strictures. Available at: https://d56bochluxqnz.cloudfront.net/documents/full-guideline/EAU-Guidelines-on-Urethral-Strictures-2024.pdf [last accessed 5 June 2024].
17. NICE (2024). LUTS in men. Available at: https://cks.nice.org.uk/topics/luts-in-men/ [last accessed 31 May 2024].
18. Ahluwalia RS, Johal N, Kouriefs C, et al. (2006). The Surgical Risk of Suprapubic Catheter Insertion and Long-term Sequelae. *Annals of Royal College of Surgeons of England*, *88*(2), 210–213.
19. Hall SJ, Harrison S, Harding C, et al. (2020). British Association of Urological Surgeons suprapubic catheter practice guidelines – revised. *BJU International*, *126*(4), 416–422.

EMERGENCY UROLOGY MCQS

1. Which of the following statements regarding bladder trauma is true?
    A) AAST definition of Grade IV bladder injury is IPR injury with laceration $\geq$ 3cm
    B) AAST definition of Grade II bladder injury is EPR injury with laceration $\leq$ 3cm
    C) Concomitant urethral injuries are common in bladder trauma due to pelvic fracture
    D) 2'0 ethilon can be used for bladder injury repair
    E) Risk of bladder perforation during mid-urethral sling surgery for SUI is lower in obturator route compared to retropubic route

2. Which of the following regarding renal trauma is false?
    A) Hypertension in Page kidney is believed to arise from activation of the renin-angiotensin-aldosterone system
    B) Page kidney does not tend to cause hypertension if contra-lateral kidney is healthy
    C) AVF usually present with delayed VH
    D) Overall rate of patients who undergo nephrectomy during exploration is 30%
    E) AAST Grade 3 injury is renal parenchymal laceration > 1cm depth without urine extravasation

3. Which of the following sutures would you choose to use for primary uretero-ureterostomy to treat an iatrogenic ureteric transection?
    A) 5'0 prolene
    B) 5'0 ethilon
    C) 5'0 polyglactin
    D) 5'0 polypropylene
    E) 5'0 silk

4. *Which of the following statements regarding ureteric injuries is true?*

   A) Knife wounds are the most common cause of penetrating ureteric injury
   B) Prophylactic pre-operative stenting reduces the risk of iatrogenic ureteric injury
   C) If auto-transplantation is required, the renal vessels are anastomosed to the iliac vessels
   D) Culp de Weerd pelvic spiral flap should not be used in proximal injuries if there is a stricture
   E) Buccal ureteroplasties should not be used for management of long-segment ureteric injuries

5. *Which of the following statements regarding urethral trauma is true?*

   A) Urethral injuries due to pelvic fractures in women are best repaired early (within 7 days)
   B) Incidence of urethral injury during male catheterisation is approximately 45 per 1,000
   C) Early realignment of partial posterior urethral injury increases risk of ED
   D) For men with PFUDD causing complete rupture, suprapubic diversion with delayed urethroplasty has stricture-free success rates of up to 60%
   E) Immediate urethroplasty is preferable in small complete ruptures following bite injury

6. *What is the most appropriate short-term steroid prescription for a patient presenting with suspected metastatic spinal cord compression?*

   A) Dexamethasone 4mg (PO) stat loading dose, followed by 2mg (PO) BD until oncology review
   B) Dexamethasone 16mg (PO) stat loading dose, followed by 8mg (PO) BD until oncology review
   C) Dexamethasone 8mg (PO) stat loading dose, followed by 1mg (PO) BD until oncology review
   D) Hydrocortisone 4mg (PO) stat loading dose, followed by 2mg (PO) BD until oncology review
   E) Hydrocortisone 8mg (PO) stat loading dose, followed by 1mg (PO) BD until oncology review

7. Which of the following medications is not associated with a known risk of priapism as uncommon undesired side-effect?

    A) Warfarin
    B) Fluoxetine
    C) Phentolamine
    D) Trimix
    E) Imatinib

8. Which oral medication can be offered to sickle cell patients as means to prevent recurrent episodes of ischaemic priapism?

    A) Eflornithine
    B) Dinoprostone
    C) Levocarnitine
    D) Etilefrine
    E) Phenelzine

9. Which of the following is not a component of the NEWS2 score?

    A) Oxygen saturations
    B) New confusion
    C) Heart rate
    D) Urine output
    E) Blood pressure

10. If a patient develops TURP syndrome after monopolar TURP using glycine as irrigant, which of the following serum abnormalities would you not expect to see?

    A) Hypoammonaemia
    B) Hyperglicenaemia
    C) Hyponatraemia
    D) Hypocalcaemia
    E) Hyperserinaemia

11. Which of the following locations or descriptions would not be classified as a stricture in male anterior urethra?

    A) Meatal
    B) Penile
    C) Bulbar
    D) Membranous
    E) Peno-bulbar

12. Which of the following best describes the reason why optical urethrotomy of penile urethral strictures may risk causing ED and should be avoided?

   A) Formation of iatrogenic AVF
   B) Provocation of venous leakage from corpora cavernosa
   C) Local fibrosis of corpora cavernosa due to inflammatory reaction
   D) Risk of chordee formation
   E) Sub-clinical iatrogenic injury to deep dorsal penile artery

BONUS CHAPTER
RENAL TRANSPLANTATION

Miss Fiona McCaig
(Consultant Urological and Renal Transplant Surgeon)

RENAL FAILURE

GFR describes the flow rate of fluid through the nephrons; it is the standard measure of kidney function.

GFR can be measured using clearance of a substance from plasma e.g. 51Cr EDTA.

This type of measurement is clinically impractical, therefore standardised formulae have been developed to calculate estimated GFR using creatinine.

Creatinine clearance is a surrogate for GFR and can be calculated using the Cockcroft–Gault, MDRD or CKD-Epi formulae.

Cockcroft–Gault estimates clearance of creatinine whereas the MDRD estimates GFR.

ACUTE KIDNEY INJURY

AKI describes a spectrum of injury to the kidney.

It is characterised by a sudden decline in renal excretory function over hours or days that can result in failure to maintain fluid, electrolyte and acid–base balance.

The most common cause of AKI is pre-renal failure. ATN occurs when there is persistent hypotension/hypovolaemia +/- nephrotoxins/sepsis.

AKI diagnosis is based on changes in serum creatinine and/or reduction in urine output. Causes include:

- Pre-renal (reduced perfusion of kidneys +/- hypotension)
- Intra-renal (structural damage to the kidney)
- Post-renal (due to urinary tract obstruction).

CLASSIFICATION OF CKD

CKD occurs in patients who have abnormalities of their kidney function/structure present for > 3 months.

The overall prevalence is 9.1%; men are more likely to progress to renal failure.

eGFR uses creatinine, age and gender to calculate a number.

CKD can be classified into levels of GFR divided into 5 main groups.

Note a normal eGFR is 90mL/min/1.73m2 or more. CKD staging is useful for planning and follow-up.

Alongside blood tests, urine is required to measure ACR.

There are 3 categories of albuminuria or proteinuria – A1, A2 and A3. Together these parameters are used to calculate risk (Table 1).

ESRF is the irreversible, long-term condition resulting from CKD for which regular dialysis treatment or transplantation is required.

Table 1 – GFR, ACR categories and risk of adverse outcomes

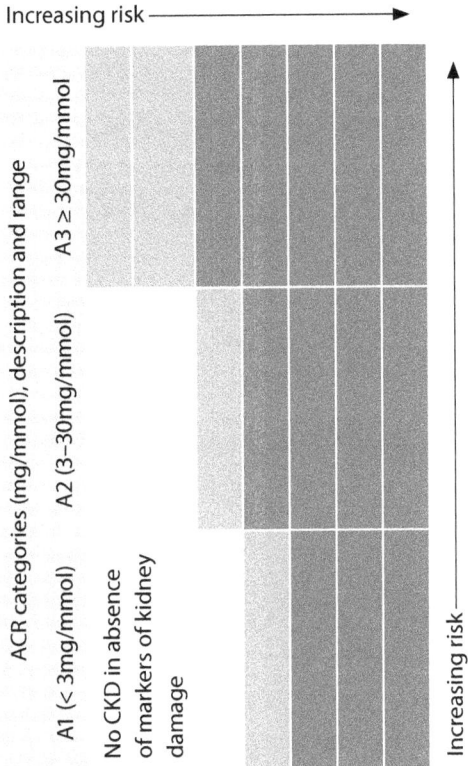

Increasing risk →

ACR categories (mg/mmol), description and range

GFR categories (mL/min/1.73m2) description and range		A1 (< 3mg/mmol)	A2 (3–30mg/mmol)	A3 ≥ 30mg/mmol
CKD I	GFR > 90	No CKD in absence of markers of kidney damage		
CKD II	GFR 60–89			
CKD IIIa	GFR 45–59			
CKD IIIb	GFR 30–44			
CKD IV	GFR 15–29			
CKD V	GFR < 15			
CKD Vd	on dialysis			

Increasing risk →

Key – shades represent risk of progression, morbidity and mortality from best to worse (light to dark)

The decision to start RRT should be made jointly with the patient, carers and attending medical team.

RRT includes haemodialysis, peritoneal dialysis and transplantation.

Indications for acute dialysis:

- Symptoms of uraemia (urea > 30mmol/L)
- Fluid overload, unresponsive to diuretics
- Biochemical abnormalities: severe hyperkalaemia (K > 6.5mmol/L or lower with ECG changes); severe metabolic acidosis (pH < 7.1)
- eGFR 5–7mL/min/1.73m2 if there are no symptoms
- Drug overdose with dialysable toxin.

DIALYSIS MODALITIES

1. Continuous haemofiltration (CVVH, CVVHD, CVVHDF, SCUF, CAVHD)

   - The most common modality in critical care, better suited for unstable patients.

2. Haemodialysis

   - Administered via an AVF, Vascath or central venous tunnelled line.
   - Each session of in-hospital dialysis lasts typically 4 hours.
   - Patients are often exhausted after dialysis.
   - Home dialysis is better tolerated but requires patients or their carers to cannulate their fistulae, unless there is a tunnelled line in situ.

3. Peritoneal dialysis

   - Patients taught to introduce fluid into their peritoneal cavity via a flexible peritoneal dialysis catheter tube, also known as a Tenckoff catheter.
   - Commonly inserted laparoscopically, can be placed via open incision (GA or local anaesthetic).
   - Typically have 2 cuffs which keep them in place.
   - Dialysate fluid absorbs toxins and is then drained and discarded.
   - Peritoneal dialysis is best for patients who still pass urine. It is the preferred modality for dialysis, resulting in less blood pressure shifts and reduced cardiovascular risk.

Peritoneal dialysis catheters are usually sited on the left, or the opposite side from any future transplant, as most first transplants are implanted on the right side due to the superficiality of the vessels.

Risks associated with peritoneal dialysis:

- Complications during Tenckoff catheter insertion – bleeding, blood transfusion, injury of adjacent structures, haemodynamic instability, infections
- Bowel dysfunction/constipation
- Catheter complications – catheter blockage, leakage of dialysis fluid around catheter
- Exit-site infection
- Peritoneal dialysis peritonitis

- Herniae
- Poor compliance
- Poor clearance
- Encapsulating peritoneal sclerosis.

Encapsulating peritoneal sclerosis is a rare but potentially life-threatening complication of long-term peritoneal dialysis.

Dialysis fluid is hyperosmotic, hyperglycaemic and acidic, causing chronic injury and inflammation to the peritoneum. Extensive thickening and fibrosis of the peritoneum occurs, resulting in the formation of a fibrous cocoon encapsulating the bowel, leading to intestinal obstruction.

Cases should be referred to specialist centres (in UK these include Manchester and Cambridge); treatment includes corticosteroids, peritonectomy and enterolysis alongside essential nutritional support.

The different modalities of dialysis are summarised in Table 2.

Table 2 – Summary of different modalities of dialysis

Critical Care CVVH	In-centre Haemodialysis	Home Haemodialysis	Peritoneal Dialysis - ADP	Peritoneal Dialysis - CAPD
Continuous temporary type of RRT/24hrs per day if required	2–3x per week	Shorter daily dialysis or nocturnal	Automated peritoneal dialysis	Continuous peritoneal dialysis
Via Vascath line, either femoral or jugular vein; the catheter has 2 separate lines (inflow and outflow)	Via AVF or tunnelled line	Via AVF or tunnelled line	Via peritoneal dialysis catheter; needs appropriate home setting	Via peritoneal dialysis catheter; needs appropriate home setting
Slower rate of fluid removal; indicated in low-blood-pressure, patients unable to tolerate HD or unstable	HD causes large swings in blood pressure, increasing cardiovascular risk	Lower cost and improved QOL in home therapies	Associated with improved survival	Associated with improved survival

CONTINUOUS HAEMOFILTRATION

- Continuous veno-venous haemofiltration (CVVH)
- Continuous veno-venous haemodialysis (CVVHD)
- Continuous veno-venous haemodiafiltration (CVVHDF), haemodiafiltration combines both diffusive and high-dose convective therapy
- Slow continuous ultrafiltration (SCUF)
- Continuous arterio-venous haemofiltration (CAVHD)

Differences between CVVH and Haemodialysis

CVVH involves filtration and fluid replacement, which run continuously. CVVH takes much longer than haemodialysis but is better tolerated from a cardiovascular point of view. It is useful in the critical care setting, for patients with cardiovascular instability.

Haemodialysis is a diffusive process using a semi-permeable membrane and a counter-current flow (contraflow) system to maintain a waste solute concentration which is always lower on the dialysate side of the membrane. The gradient persists along the entire length of the membrane.

Image 1 – Haemodialysis and haemofiltration

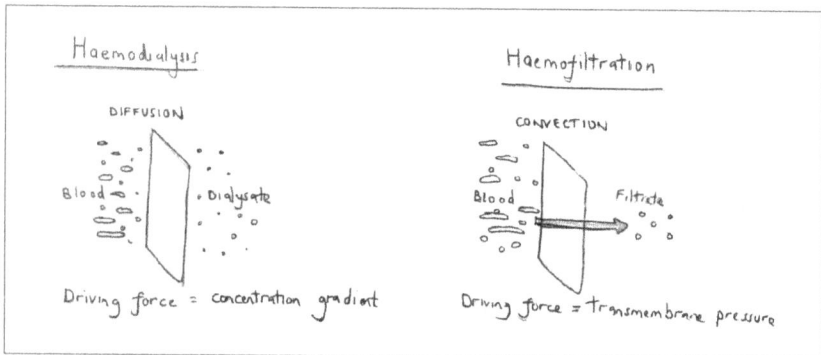

A dialyser works in the following way (Image 2):

- Blood enters the dialyser from the body
- Dialysate fluid is made to flow in counter-current direction to blood, taking away waste from it

- A membrane keeps blood and dialysate from mixing, but allows water to pass through
- Waste moves through the membrane from the blood into the dialysate
- Cleansed blood is then returned to the body.

Image 2 – Dialyser

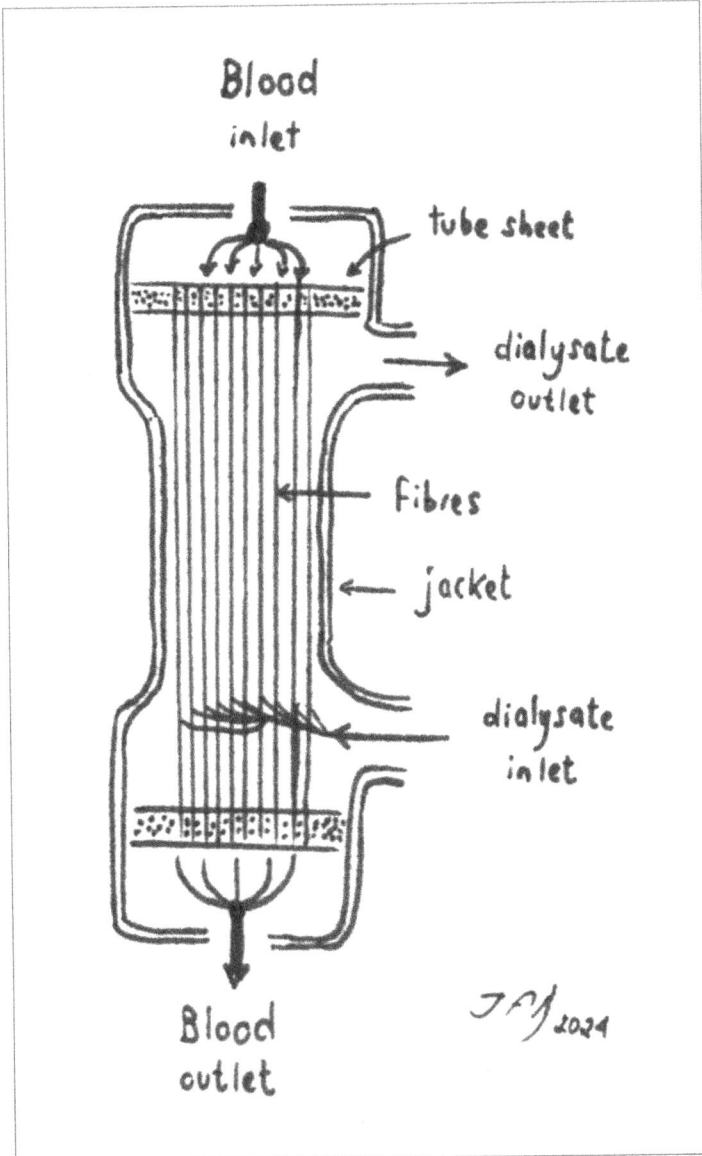

Blood inlet

tube sheet

dialysate outlet

Fibres

jacket

dialysate inlet

Blood outlet

JM 2024

Image 3 – Haemodialysis

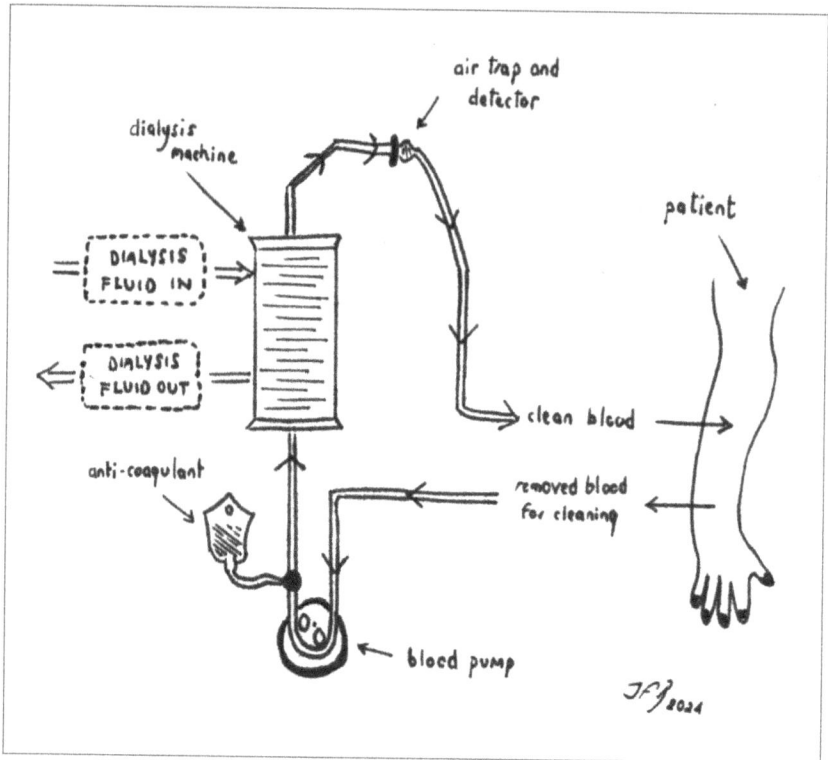

OPTIONS FOR HAEMODIALYSIS ACCESS – TYPES OF FISTULAE/CATHETERS/GRAFTS

The types of access include:

1. AVF

2. Central venous tunnelled line (Permcath)

3. Non-tunnelled central venous catheter (Vascath, used for temporary haemodialysis only, typically inserted into jugular or femoral vein)

4. Synthetic graft.

An AVF provides the best form of vascular access for successful dialysis. Ideally it should be fashioned within 6 months of a patient requiring dialysis.

Tunnelled central lines are an infection risk and are associated with superior vena cava stenosis and obstruction – they should be avoided whenever possible.

A Vascath can be inserted in an emergency setting to deliver haemodialysis or CVVH; however, it should be removed within 1–4 weeks.

Synthetic grafts are usually formed when access is running out. They typically include femoral loop grafts and have the advantage that they can be needled immediately after formation.

AVF options: start with the non-dominant hand

- Radio-cephalic
- Brachio-cephalic
- Brachio-basilic
- Synthetic grafts including femoral

Consider the most distal available site e.g. radio-cephalic. Gradually move proximally.

Image 4 – AVF

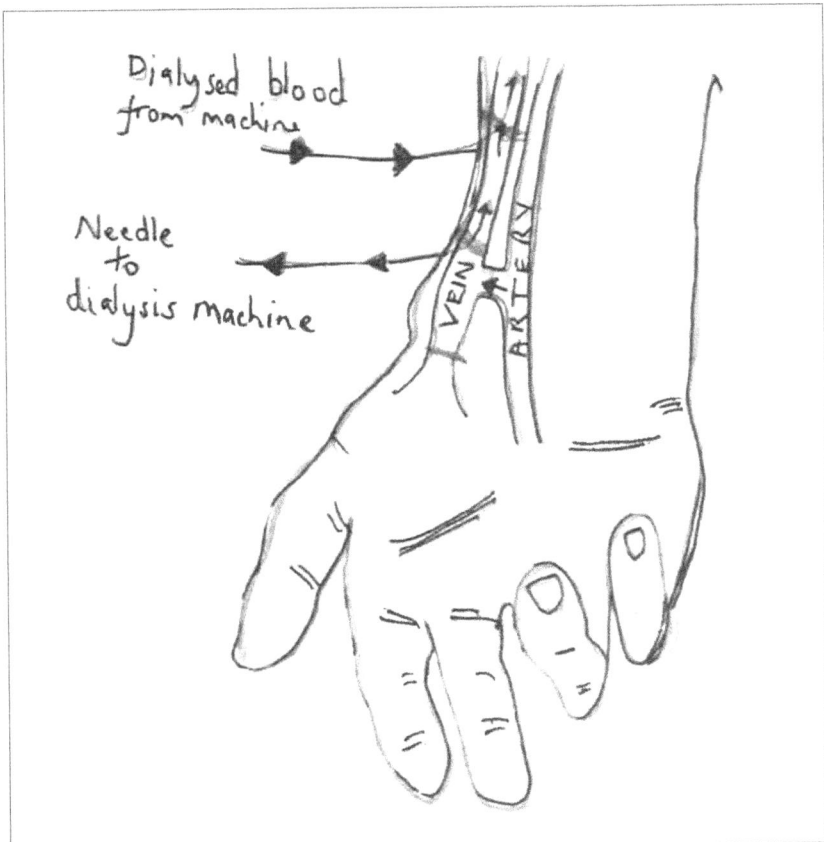

The complications of AVF include:

- Failure of procedure, failure of fistula to mature (therefore cannot be used)
- Infection, risk of bacteraemia and subsequent haemorrhage
- Thrombosis (lack of thrill)
- Nerve injury, numbness and coldness to the hand
- Bleeding (can be catastrophic)
- Steal syndrome (reduced blood flow to hand/peripheries, causing distal hypoxia/ischaemia/pain)
- Aneurysm formation
- Poor cosmesis.

An adult starting haemodialysis has a 50% 5-year mortality rate, therefore transplantation is the preferred option for RRT.

TYPES OF KIDNEY DONORS

Kidney donors can be broadly classified as living and deceased donors.

Live donors include *live related*, *live unrelated* and *directed* and *altruistic*.

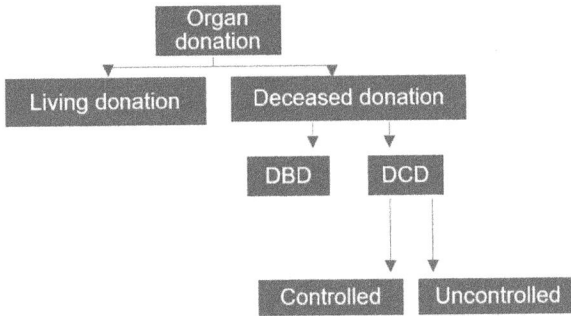

Deceased donors include DBD (donation after brain-stem death i.e. heart beating) and DCD (donation after circulatory death i.e. non heart beating).

There are two types of DCD, *controlled* and *uncontrolled*.

Controlled DCD death follows the planned withdrawal of life-sustaining treatments.

Uncontrolled DCD death refers to organ retrieval after an unexpected cardiac arrest. DCD donors can be further classified via the Maastricht classification, which describes mode of cardiac arrest (Table 3).

Table 3 – Maastricht categories of DCD donors

Maastricht Donor Type	Type of Death	Type of Organ Donation
Type I	Patient brought in dead	Uncontrolled donation
Type II	Unsuccessful resuscitation	Uncontrolled donation
Type III	Awaiting cardiac arrest	Controlled donation
Type IV	Cardiac death after brain-stem death	Uncontrolled donation
Type V	Cardiac arrest in a hospital in-patient	Uncontrolled donation

Extended criteria donors relate to deceased donors:

- \> 60 years
- 50–59 years with 2 of the following:
  - Hypertension
  - Terminal Cr > 133
  - Cerebrovascular cause of death.

All other donors are referred to as standard criteria donors.

CONTRAINDICATIONS TO BEING A LIVING KIDNEY DONOR

There are absolute and relative contraindications to living kidney donation.

The level of risk that a clinician and donor are prepared to accept when assessing relative contraindications is case-specific and requires very careful counselling.

The most common living donor transplants are parents to children and siblings to siblings.

Absolute contraindications include:

- Under 18 years
- Unable to give informed consent
- Psychiatric disorders or inadequate cognition
- Active drug or alcohol abuse
- Single kidney
- Morbid obesity (BMI > 40)
- Reduced GFR, age related
- Active untreated malignancy
- Active infections
- Uncontrolled diseases that may impact renal function e.g. hypertension/diabetes/renal calculi
- Pregnancy.

Table 4 – Advisory threshold GFR levels – considered acceptable for living kidney donation

Age (years)	Threshold GFR (mL/min/1.73m2	
	Male	Female
20–29	90	90
30–34	80	80
35	80	80
40	80	80
45	80	80
50	80	80
55	80	75
60	76	70
65	71	64
70	67	59
75	63	54
80	58	49

RENAL TRANSPLANTATION SURGERY

Renal transplantation improves both QOL and survival and is therefore the preferred modality of RRT.

HOW ARE ORGANS PRESERVED?

- **_Static cold storage, continuous cold perfusion, normothermic perfusion_**

Donor kidneys are cooled as quickly as possible after extraction – reducing the temperature to 4°C reduces its metabolism significantly.

Organ preservation solutions aim to minimise cellular changes and reduce ischaemia/hypoxia injury, which in turn improves graft survival.

Immediately after the kidney is removed, blood is flushed out using cold 4°C preservation fluid and then placed indirectly on ice (static cold storage).

This reduces the metabolic rate of the kidney to approximately 5%.

Prolonged cold ischaemic injury leads to delayed graft function and therefore the kidney should be transplanted as quickly as possible.

The kidney is often kept in static cold storage e.g. an ice box, until the time for implantation.

Alternatively, kidneys may be placed on a 'Lifeport' machine which continuously perfuses the organ with cold perfusate.

Normothermic machine perfusion is an emerging technique to perfuse the kidneys with warm, oxygenated red-cell-based plasma-free solution.

Preservation fluids include electrolytes, impermeants and buffers. Previously Marshall's (Soltran) was commonly used for kidneys; however, this is not currently available.

Most centres now use either HTK (Custodiol®) or Belzer University of Wisconsin (UW®) solutions.

Comparison of different preservation solutions:

1. Marshall's (Soltran) solution contains potassium citrate, sodium citrate, mannitol and magnesium sulphate.

2. HTK (Custodiol®) solution – contains histidine–tryptophan–ketoglutarate. Extracellular preservation solution with high sodium and low potassium concentration. Viscosity is similar to water, which reduces the time taken to cool the kidney.

3. Belzer University of Wisconsin (UW®) – intracellular preservation solution with low sodium and high potassium concentration. Contains lactobionate, raffinose, allopurinol, glutathione and adenosine. High viscosity which challenges tissue wash-out.

4. Collins solution – high potassium, high magnesium, low sodium concentrations which mimic composition of intracellular fluid. It is a phosphate-based solution with high glucose concentration which balances osmolarity.

5. Celsior® solution – extracellular preservation fluid which is high in sodium, low in potassium. Lactobionate and mannitol limit cellular oedema. Reduced glutathione was added as a free-radical scavenger.

Table 5 – Preservation fluids

	Solution				
	Marshall's (Soltran)	HTK (Custodiol®)	UW® Solution (Belzer)	Collins	Celsior®
Na+	Low	Low	Low	Low	High
K+	High	Low	High	High	Low
Buffer	Citrate	Histidine	Phosphate	Phosphate	Histidine
Impermeant	Mannitol citrate	Mannitol	Raffinose Lactobionate Hydroeyethyl starch	Glucose	Lactobionate Mannitol
Others	Magnesium sulphate	Histidine–tryptophan–ketoglutarate	Glutathione Allopurinol Adenosine Dexamethasone Insulin	Magnesium	Glutathione Glutamate

ISCHAEMIC TIMES

Every effort is made to limit both warm and cold ischaemic times (warm ischaemia is the most harmful).

Warm ischaemic time – time from cross clamp of renal artery or aorta, to perfusion with cold perfusate. A second warm ischaemic time occurs when the kidney is taken out of ice, up to the point where it is re-perfused with warm blood i.e. anastomotic time.

Cold ischaemic time – length of time organ is out of the body and cooled using cold perfusate fluid. This should ideally be < 18 hours, although kidneys have been implanted with > 24 hours cold time.

Recipient work-up should address the following points:

1. Is the recipient suitable for major surgery? (i.e. do they have any medical problems which may exclude them from transplantation e.g. unstable IHD or malignancy?)
2. Are there any anatomical problems that may preclude transplantation (e.g. severe calcification of iliac arteries)? Is there space for the kidney?
3. Is the patient's immune system sensitised and therefore difficult to match/at risk from rejection?
4. Will the patient develop recurrent renal disease in the kidney transplant e.g. FSGS?

BASIC ASPECTS TO RENAL TRANSPLANTATION

- Bench work: the kidney is thoroughly inspected for any areas of hypoperfusion, tumours or injuries before implantation. The surrounding fat is removed and the vessels/ureter are dissected out in preparation for implantation. The kidney continues to be stored in a cool environment until the recipient vasculature is ready for implantation.
- Right iliac fossa – the kidney is preferably implanted into the right iliac fossa, as the vascular structures are more superficial compared to the left. Subsequent transplants will be implanted on the opposite side.
- A Rutherford Morrison or Gibson incision is commonly used.
- Extra-peritoneal approach is standard.
- Most kidneys have single vessels, ~10–20% have multiple arteries or veins.

- The renal vein is commonly anastomosed to the external iliac vein in an end-to-side fashion; alternative strategies include the common iliac vein or IVC.

- The renal artery is commonly anastomosed to the external iliac artery, also end-to-side. Alternatives include the common iliac or internal iliac artery. The latter can be anastomosed end-to-end. The anastomoses can be performed onto the aorta if required. Another option is to perform an orthotopic transplant, although in practice this is rarely performed.

- Venous anastomosis first and then arterial is the standard order, but following this sequence is not mandatory.

- The uretero-vesical anastomosis is often performed using the Lich–Gregoir onlay technique. Alternatives include the tunnelled Politano–Leadbetter or U-stitch. The Lich–Gregoir technique is associated with fewer urological complications i.e. leaks, strictures and reflux. If access to the pelvis is difficult, a pelvi-ureteric (native ureter anastomosed onto donor renal pelvis) or uretero-uretero anastomosis can be performed.

- A urinary catheter and retro-peritoneal drain is left in situ at end of procedure.

Image 5 – The anastomoses in renal transplantation

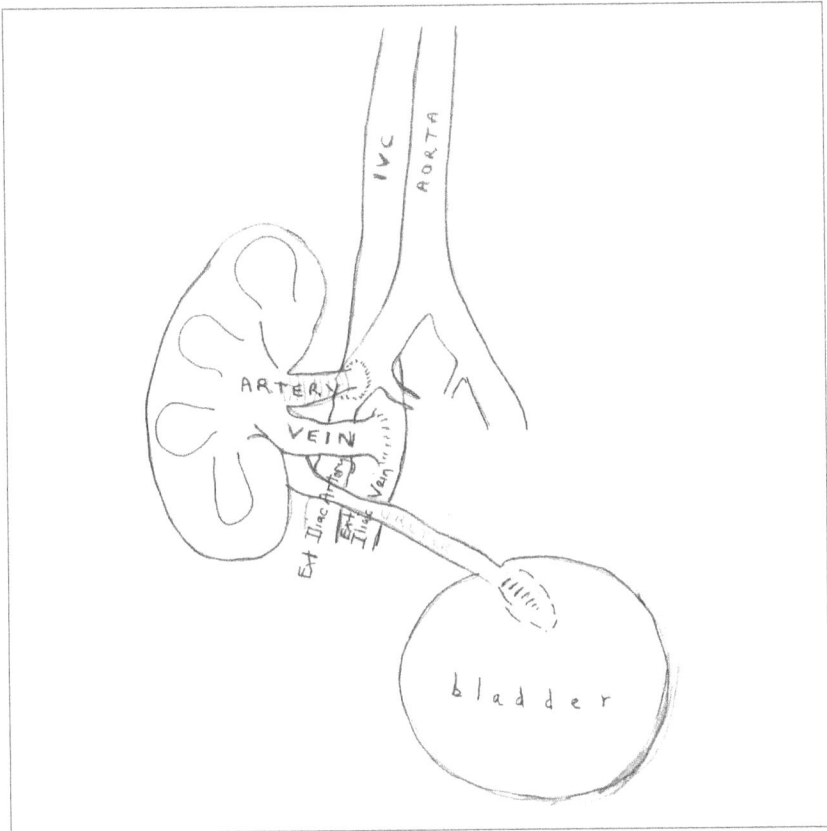

SURGICAL COMPLICATIONS

Vascular complications (1–2%):

- Bleeding
- Renal vein or artery thrombosis
- Renal artery stenosis
- Infarction/thrombosis of the kidney transplant
- Dissection of iliac artery leading to leg ischaemia
- Arterio-venous fistulas
- Pseudo-aneurysm

Urological complications (4–8%):

- Ureteral obstruction, kinking or stricture (2–4%)
- Urine leak/urinoma – manage aggressively due to risk of sepsis (PCN or take back to theatre)
- Stent migration/blockage

Infective complications:

- Wound infections, dehiscence, haematomas, lymphocoeles (0.5–20%; 4–8 weeks), deep infected collections
- Incisional hernia

Primary non function

Delayed graft function (patient will require dialysis within 2 weeks of transplant)

Gastro-intestinal complications:

- Bowel injury
- Internal hernia
- Peptic ulcer

Other complications:

- Infections e.g. UTI, chest infections, CMV, Epstein–Barr virus, herpes simplex virus, BK virus
- Hypertension
- Rejection, acute and chronic
- NODAT (new onset diabetes mellitus after transplantation)
- Persistent secondary hyperparathyroidism (38–77%)
- Increased risk of renal stones
- Malignancy – skin, Kaposi sarcoma, PTLD/lymphoma, urological cancers
- Long-term immunosuppression drug side-effects
- Transmission of infections or cancers to recipient from donor

Ureteric Stricture Management

Ureteric strictures usually occur distally due to ischaemia.

Another cause of strictures is BK virus.

Strictures can be managed by nephrostomy + antegrade ureteric stents.

Retrograde stent exchanges are technically challenging to perform and long-term stents often result in poor QOL.

Transplant recipients suffer less stent irritation/pain: the stent enters the bladder at the dome and therefore does not cause irritation of the trigone.

Stents are, however, associated with a high risk of obstruction and infection; the latter is particularly troublesome in the immunosuppressed recipient.

Ideally patients with strictures should be offered reconstruction.

It is important to know the bladder function/capacity and whether the native ureter can be used to perform a uretero-ureterostomy or even a uretero-pyelostomy if required.

For distal strictures, excision of the stenotic segment and reimplantation is performed i.e. ureteroneocystostomy. The bladder can be anastomosed directly onto the transplant renal pelvis or a psoas hitch/Boari flap may be required.

Alternatively, the recipient ipsilateral ureter can be used; an advantage is that VUR does not occur. This can be performed in an end-to-end or end-to-side fashion. Although the dissection required for reconstruction is often challenging, the success rate is ~80%.

Balloon dilatation is an alternative treatment of strictures; however, the long-term results are suboptimal compared with reconstruction.

TISSUE TYPING AND HLA MATCHING

Tissue typing of both recipient and donor are required. Both the ABO blood group and HLA are matched.

Blood groups were first discovered in the early 1900s.

The most common blood group is O – the universal donor and can be received by all blood types.

Blood groups A, B and AB can only receive blood or organs from the same blood group.

Blood-group O individuals lack A and B antigens, and develop antibodies to these antigens.

Humans generate antibodies against non-self blood-group antigens during their early years. ABO antigens are carbohydrate molecules present on the surface of RBCs and endothelial cells.

Hyperacute rejection occurs if organs are transplanted between ABO incompatible patients. It is an antibody-mediated type of rejection and is seen within minutes of implantation. Pre-existing antibodies against allograft donor blood-group antigens damage the graft.

Fortunately, hyperacute rejection is rare nowadays.

HLA are also known as the major histocompatibility complex (MHC) molecules; they are glycoproteins found on cell surfaces.

They are divided into class I and class II molecules.

Class I are found on the surface of all nucleated cells.

Class II molecules are found only on the surface of antigen-presenting cells (APCs).

HLA are encoded by genes located on chromosome 6 and present molecules to CD8 and CD4 T cells respectively.

There are 3 HLA class I genes (A, B and C), with extensive genetic variability. There are also 3 HLA class II genes (DP, DQ and DR).

In renal transplantation only A, B and DR mismatches are considered important and DR mismatches are more significant than A or B mismatches.

Each individual has two copies of each HLA gene and therefore the maximum number of mismatches that can occur between donor and recipient is 6. This worst mismatch would be described as a MM 2-2-2. The best mismatch would be a MM 0-0-0.

IMMUNOSUPPRESSION

Organs transplanted between genetically indistinguishable individuals (e.g. identical twins) will not be rejected. This knowledge paved the way for the first successful living-donor kidney transplant, performed at the Brigham Hospital in Boston in 1954.

The slightest difference between the donor's and the recipient's genetic material will cause graft rejection.

The development of anti-rejection drugs has allowed transplantation between genetically different patients.

The kidney transplant is often referred to as an allograft, "allo" being derived from the Greek for "other".

Patients are at high risk of rejection in the early transplant period. Rejection occurs due to T lymphocytes; depletion prior to allograft implantation therefore prevents rejection.

Immunosuppression drugs are therefore required – these can be divided into induction and maintenance immunosuppression.

In the UK the most common induction agent is IV Basiliximab, an anti-CD25 monoclonal antibody. Other centres may use IV lymphocyte depleting antibodies e.g. ATG (anti-thymocyte globulin) or Campath (monoclonal antibody alemtuzumab).

The induction regimen is often combined with IV methylprednisolone steroids.

Thereafter, the recipient will require maintenance immunosuppression; these are administered orally and usually consist of triple therapy e.g. a calcineurin inhibitor, anti-metabolite and steroid (a reducing dose of prednisolone).

Calcineurin inhibitors (CNIs) include ciclosporin and tacrolimus.

Anti-metabolites include azathioprine and mycophenylate mofetil (MMF). Both target T lymphocyte activation and proliferation.

The most common combination is tacrolimus, MMF and prednisolone.

Additional immunosuppressant drugs include mTOR inhibitors e.g. sirolimus and everolimus.

Immunosuppressant drugs have multiple undesirable side-effects including a susceptibility to cancers (PTLD and skin cancers in particular) and infections.

Side-effects of prolonged steroid use include cushingoid features: central obesity, moon face, hypertension, striae, osteoporosis, thin skin, bruising, reduced wound healing, avascular necrosis, peptic ulceration, glucose intolerance, predisposition to diabetes and proximal myopathy.

Some centres avoid the use of long-term steroids due to these side-effects.

CNIs are nephrotoxic and cause a tremor; the latter is dose dependent.

Ciclosporin specifically causes hirsutism and gingival hypertrophy.

Tacrolimus predisposes to new onset diabetes after transplant (NODAT) and is associated with 3x higher risk compared with ciclosporin.

Anti-metabolites inhibit purine production and DNA synthesis; their side-effects therefore include bone marrow suppression.

Gastro-intestinal upset including diarrhoea is commonly associated with MMF.

mTOR inhibitors are associated with poor wound healing, mouth ulceration, skin rashes, dyslipidaemia and interstitial pneumonitis. They also have anti-tumour properties and can be used if recipients develop cancers.

Other agents including lymphocyte-depleting ATG (anti-thymocyte globulin) is associated with an increased risk of CMV infection and PTLD. Most PTLD is driven by EBV infections (Epstein–Barr).

Delayed Graft Function

This is one of the commonest complications following kidney transplantation and is particularly common after DCD transplants.

It is defined by the need for dialysis within the first 14 days of transplantation.

Clinically the patient is often anuric with a climbing creatinine. More serious pathologies must be excluded e.g. renal vein thrombosis, rejection.

REJECTION

Transplant rejection can be classified into hyperacute, acute T-cell mediated, acute antibody-mediated and chronic types.

1. *Hyperacute rejection* occurs within minutes to hours following transplantation. Rapid arterial and venous thrombosis occurs, resulting in graft thrombosis and loss. It is caused by pre-formed donor-specific antibodies.

2. *Acute T-cell mediated rejection* (TMR) is also known as cellular rejection and occurs within the first 6 months. It is the commonest type, occurring in ~25% and most commonly within the first 6 months. T cells, phagocytes and B cells infiltrate the graft. The treatment is high-dose steroids +/- ATG (anti-thymocyte globulin).

3. *Acute antibody-mediated rejection* (AMR) occurs in ~4% and occurs within the first 6 months. It is treated by plasma exchange or immunoadsorption. Corticosteroids, ATG (anti-thymocyte globulin) and the CD20 antibody rituximab can be used.

4. *Chronic rejection* occurs after 1 month and occurs as a result of both immune and non-immune mechanisms. Treatment includes blood pressure control and minimising CNI exposure

Patients who present with deteriorating graft function should have an urgent US to exclude obstruction, urinalysis and urine culture, and should have their CNI levels checked e.g. tacrolimus level.

If no obvious cause is found, then an urgent biopsy should be undertaken to exclude rejection.

Acknowledgement to Mr Alistair Rogers, Newcastle upon Tyne Hospitals NHS Trust, for his help creating this chapter.

ANSWERS TO MCQS

Station 1: Urological Oncology 1

1. **D**
2. **B**
3. **B**
4. **E**
5. **D**
6. **C**
7. **A**
8. **A**
9. **C**
10. **B**
11. **B**
12. **E**
13. **D**
14. **D**
15. **C**
16. **A**
17. **E** – note it is cerebellar haemangioblastoma
18. **B**
19. **C**
20. **E** – phakomatoses are a group of multisystemic diseases which include tuberous sclerosis
21. **C**
22. **B** – ipsilateral adrenal gland involvement is T4, contra-lateral adrenal gland involvement is M1
23. **D**
24. **B**
25. **A** – correct Karnovsky performance status is < 80%
26. **E**
27. **A**

Station 2: Urological Oncology 2

1. **B** – UV in a study was shown to be protective vs. PCa (please refer to EAU 2023 – Prostate Cancer)

2. **D**

3. **D** – prognosis is unfavourable, basal cells are preserved, BRCA positive patients have a higher incidence of intraductal carcinoma of the prostate

4. **E**

5. **B**

6. **C** – FLAIR is used in almost all protocols for imaging the brain

7. **A**

8. **A** – majority of continence maintained by external urethral sphincter; however, internal lissosphincter at bladder neck has minor role and preserving has benefits for continence

9. **B** – please refer to EAU 2023 section 6.1.4.1.1.1.1

10. **A**

11. **D**

12. **C**

13. **E**

14. **E** – the correct figure for > 10-year survival is 95+% – Cancer Research UK is useful website for further information about UK incidence of testicular cancer

15. **E** – remember that testicular cancer staging has separate sections for regional lymph nodes as "clinical" or "pathological" – in this case the patient's nodes have only been staged clinically

16. **C**

17. **D**

18. **B**

19. **C** – if the patient consents accordingly at the time of banking, sperm can be used by their partner for insemination even after their death

20. **A**

21. **A**

22. **B**

23. **E**

24. **B**

25. **D** – BTx can be offered for lesions < 4cm in size, minimum RTx dose is 60Gy

Station 3: Paediatric Urology

1. **C**

2. **A**

3. **B** – increased change of spontaneous resolution of VUR if male gender, detected prior to first year of life, absence of renal scarring or LUTD, lower-grade disease

4. **B**

5. **E** – Lich–Gregoir can be used, but it is an extra-vesical technique

6. **C**

7. **C**

8. **B**

9. **E** – this preparation is too potent, the others are acceptable – make sure you chose one for your daily clinical practice that you state to the examiner

10. **C**

11. **A** – TIP can be used for anterior hypospadias repair, but only in absence of chordee

12. **A**

13. **D**

14. **D** – most common age is 5–7 years, also please make sure you learn the micturition cycle in good level of detail for the FRCS (Urol) exam

15. **B**

16. **A** – correct starting dose is 2.5mg BD (alternatively 5mg OD)

17. **E** – the correct figure is 1–2%

18. **B** – please note the DMSA is recommended 4–6 months after the UTI

19. **C**

20. **D**

21. **C**

22. **B**

23. **A**

24. **D**

25. **E**

Station 4: Emergency Urology

1. **E** – ethilon is non-absorbable, concomitant urethral injuries in context of pelvic fracture causing bladder injury are not that common (5–20%)

2. **B** – Page kidney is a unilateral process and will cause hypertension without affecting renal function (unless it is arising a single functional kidney)

3. **C** – sutures for ureteric repair must be absorbable (polyglactin is vicryl)

4. **C** – gunshot wounds most common penetrating

5. **A** – correct incidence 13 per 1,000 (approx.), no change to ED risk, stricture-free rate is > 80%

6. **B**

7. **E**

8. **D**

9. **D**

10. **A** – serum ammonia may be elevated

11. **D** – membranous is posterior urethra, peno-bulbar implies long stricture extending from penile urethra to bulbar region

12. **B**

ADDITIONAL MCQS

STATION 1:
UROLOGICAL ONCOLOGY 1 MCQS

1. *Which of the following tests has not been explored as a potential marker for detecting urothelial cancer in urine?*

   A) UroVysion
   B) BSP
   C) BTA stat
   D) ImmunoCyt
   E) UBC test

2. *Which of the following statements regarding PDD cystoscopy is false?*

   A) Under blue light, healthy bladder may appear red
   B) 5-ALA is converted to haem in cytoplasm of urothelial cells
   C) The trigone often fluoresces without malignant pathology
   D) Blue light has wavelength of 375–440nm
   E) Resection of a blue light abnormal area should be undertaken under white light

3. *Which of the following measurements is not routinely taken during CPEX testing?*

   A) Tidal volume (TV)
   B) Residual volume (RV)
   C) 12-lead ECG
   D) Respiratory exchange ratio (RER)
   E) Non-invasive arterial pressure (NIAP)

4. *On which chromosome is the VHL gene found?*

   A) 3
   B) 5
   C) 7
   D) 9
   E) 11

5. A newly diagnosed patient with RCC has a 7.5cm right-sided kidney tumour, with staging CT TAP revealing extension into the surrounding perirenal fat and contiguous adrenal gland, hilar lymph nodes are normal. What is the correct TNM staging for this patient?

A) T3aN0M1
B) T3bN0M0
C) T3cN0M1
D) T4N0M0
E) T4N0M1

6. Which of the following statements regarding the CARMENA trial is true?

A) Axitinib group was compared to axitinib + CN group in 1:1 randomisation
B) The primary end-point of the study was disease-free survival
C) Patients on anti-coagulants were excluded
D) The dose of axitinib was 50mg once daily
E) Axinitib alone was non-inferior to axitinib + CN in the primary end-point of the study

7. The histology from a radical nephrectomy report reads as: eosinophilic cells packed with mitochondria, acidophilic cytoplasm, microscopic nested architecture, myxoid stroma and areas of degenerative cytologic atypia. Which is the most likely underlying renal tumour that has been excised?

A) Leiomyosarcoma
B) Chromophobe RCC
C) Oncocytoma
D) Papillary type 1 tumour
E) Papillary type 2 tumour

8. A newly diagnosed patient with UTUC has undergone RNU and full staging CT. The primary tumour invades the renal parenchyma, a single positive lymph node of 3cm has been excised and there is no distant metastasis. What is the correct TNM staging for this patient?

A) T3aN1M0
B) T3aN2M0
C) T3N1M0
D) T3N2M0
E) T4N1M0

9. Which of the following is not a parameter as part of the International Metastatic RCC Database Consortium risk-stratification tool?

   A) Neutrophil count
   B) Serum calcium
   C) Haemoglobin
   D) Platelet count
   E) Time from diagnosis to treatment < 6 months

10. A newly diagnosed patient with 9cm renal tumour has thrombus extending into the IVC 3cm above the level of the renal vein orifice. Which of the following statements is true?

    A) This is T3b disease
    B) This is level 3 IVC involvement
    C) This is level 4 IVC involvement
    D) Cardiopulmonary bypass may be required for operative intervention
    E) Histology will most likely be papillary carcinoma

11. Which of the following is not a parameter on the Leibovich scoring system for risk stratification in RCC?

    A) Tumour necrosis
    B) Tumour size
    C) Tumour grade
    D) T-stage
    E) Sarcomatoid differentiation

12. Which of the following is not a recognised paraneoplastic symptom or syndrome associated with RCC?

    A) Polycythaemia
    B) Waldenstrom's macroglobulinemia
    C) Cushing's syndrome
    D) Galactorrhea
    E) Amyloidosis

13. On which chromosome does the gene mutation responsible for BHD occur?

    A) 13
    B) 15
    C) 17
    D) 19
    E) 21

14. *Which of the following statements regarding ileal conduit urinary diversion in radical cystectomy is false?*

   A) 15cm of ileum should be used
   B) Post-operative metabolic acidosis is less common than in neobladder formation
   C) Bricker technique involves spatulating and anastomosing each ureter to the serosa of the bowel separately
   D) Wallace 1 technique involves suturing the lateral walls of the spatulated ureters and anastomosing these to the anti-mesenteric part of the open bowel segment
   E) Entero-ureteric stricture rates between Wallace 1 and Bricker techniques are comparable

15. *Which of the following statements regarding lymph-node dissection in radical cystectomy is false?*

   A) Extended LND involves taking lymph nodes up to the inferior mesenteric artery
   B) 5-year CSS with positive nodal involvement is 40%
   C) 3 positive nodes in presacral group equates to N-stage 2 in TNM staging classification
   D) Post-operative pain and paraesthesia down the medial thigh suggest obturator nerve injury
   E) Anti-coagulation with LMWH can cause prolonged lymphorrhea

16. *Conventional total dose of fractionated radiation in EBRT for MIBC is:*

   A) 25–35Gy
   B) 35–45Gy
   C) 45–60Gy
   D) 60–70Gy
   E) 70–80Gy

17. *Which of the following statements regarding the POUT trial is true?*

   A) There is an agreed international consensus on benefit of adjuvant chemotherapy for UTUC
   B) Node-positive patients were excluded from the trial
   C) Patients with oligo metastasis were included in the trial
   D) Chemotherapy had to be given within < 90 days of RNU
   E) Patients with performance status ≤ 2 were included in the trial

18. *Which of the following statements regarding AML is false?*

    A) AML are the most common benign mesenchymal tumour
    B) 30% are due to tuberous sclerosis
    C) Familial AML grow faster than sporadic AML
    D) Everolimus is used to reduce AML volume in tuberous sclerosis
    E) Vascular component is in the form of thick-walled hyalinized
       vessels

19. *A full course of BCG (e.g. Lamm's regime) consists of how many doses of intra-vesical BCG?*

    A) 17
    B) 19
    C) 21
    D) 24
    E) 27

20. *What is the ARR of recurrence of bladder cancer by giving single instillation dose of MMC after first TURBT?*

    A) 6%
    B) 8%
    C) 12%
    D) 14%
    E) 16%

21. *Which of the following is not a factor used to predict bladder-cancer progression and recurrence in NMIBC, in the EORTC scoring system?*

    A) Tumour necrosis
    B) Presence of CIS
    C) Prior recurrence rate
    D) Tumour grade
    E) Tumour multi-focality

22. *Which of the following regarding urachal tumours is false?*

    A) The majority of cases are adenocarcinomas
    B) It is more common in men
    C) 5-year survival with RC ≤ 70%
    D) Tumours with polypoid configuration are more likely to seed
    E) The urachus is a fibrous remnant of the allantois and lies in the
       space of Retzius

23. *Which statement is correct regarding nephrological causes of visible haematuria?*

   A) Goodpasture's disease is an auto-immune condition where antibodies attack Bowman's capsule in the kidney
   B) Alport's syndrome involves a Y-linked collagen mutation
   C) Henoch–Schonlein purpura is a systemic vasculitis characterised by deposition of immunoglobulin-A complexes
   D) Nephrotic syndrome is associated with raised serum albumin
   E) Berger's disease involves deposition of IgG after a viral upper respiratory tract infection

24. *Which statement regarding intra-vesical BCG therapy is false?*

   A) Is used intra-venously for gastro-intestinal cancer
   B) Attaches to urothelium via laminin receptor
   C) Upregulates all of IL-2, IL-6 and IL-8
   D) Hepatic disorder is a common side-effect
   E) It is contraindicated in HIV

25. *Which of the following is not a recognised sequalae noted in patients who have previously undergone RC and urinary diversion?*

   A) Low cobalamin
   B) Hyperkalaemia
   C) Megaloblastic anaemia
   D) Hypomagnesemia
   E) Steatorrhea

STATION 2: UROLOGICAL ONCOLOGY 2 MCQS

1. Which of the following regarding abiraterone is false?

    A) It is an oestrogen receptor agonist
    B) It acts as a CYP17 inhibitor
    C) Strong history of cardiovascular disease is a contraindication
    D) Haematuria is a common side-effect
    E) Angina is a common side-effect

2. A newly diagnosed patient with prostate cancer has bilateral extra-capsular extension, with involvement of obturator lymph nodes and liver metastasis. What is his correct staging?

    A) T3aN1M1c
    B) T3aN2M1c
    C) T3bN1M1b
    D) T3bN1M1c
    E) T3bN1M1a

3. On which chromosome is PSA encoded?

    A) 13
    B) 15
    C) 17
    D) 19
    E) 21

4. Which of the following is not a criterion as part of the Wilson and Jungner criteria for screening?

    A) Facilities for diagnosis and treatment should be available
    B) The cost of case-finding should be balanced in relation to care cost as a whole
    C) There should be an agreed policy on whom to treat as patients
    D) There should be a recognised mortality rate for the condition
    E) The test should be acceptable to the population

5. Which of the following statements regarding the pathology of prostate cancer is true?

    A) 80–90% are adenocarcinomas
    B) A key feature is absence of staining for basal cell marker p53
    C) Peripheral zone cancers are less commonly associated with seminal vesicle extension
    D) 30–35% of cancers arise in the transitional zone
    E) 5% of cancers arise in the central zone

6. Which of the following statements regarding mpMRI of the prostate is false?

    A) PROMIS study excluded patients with PSA > 15
    B) 1.5T magnet is appropriate for use in this context
    C) Diffusion-weighted imaging appears dark in prostate cancer
    D) Water appears dark on T1 imaging
    E) DCE imaging is taken after gadolinium contrast

7. What is the most appropriate type of US probe required to perform TRUS biopsy?

    A) 4.5MHz
    B) 7.5MHz
    C) 9MHz
    D) 11MHz
    E) 13.5MHz

8. Regarding radical radiotherapy for prostate cancer, which of the following is not a component of the response to radiation?

    A) Repair
    B) Regeneration
    C) Repopulation
    D) Reassortment
    E) Reoxygenation

9. A patient with prostate cancer has had radical prostatectomy and full staging imaging. Histology shows tumour invading less than half of both lobes, positive lymph nodes were found in both external iliac groups and CT scan did not show any distant metastasis. What is the correct staging for this patient?

    A) T2cN1M0
    B) T2cN2M0
    C) T2bN1M0
    D) T2cN2M1a
    E) T2cN1M1a

10. Which of the following statements regarding brachytherapy for prostate cancer is true?

    A) Large prostate > 30cc is a contraindication
    B) It is a treatment option in T2c disease
    C) Low-dose brachytherapy uses Ir-192 seeds
    D) High bladder neck is a relative contraindication
    E) HIFU cannot be used as treatment option if brachytherapy fails

11. The following are all recognised side-effects of goserelin except:

    A) Azotaemia
    B) Alopecia
    C) Arthralgia
    D) Paraesthesia
    E) Prolongation of QT-interval

12. Which of the following is not a parameter of the Briganti nomogram 2018 for predicting lymph-node involvement of prostate cancer?

    A) Pre-operative PSA
    B) Maximum diameter of lesion on mpMRI
    C) Percentage of cores with prostate cancer on targeted biopsy
    D) Clinical stage on mpMRI
    E) Gleason grade group at systematic biopsy

13. Below what level of testosterone concentration should be achieved in castration therapy?

    A) < 75mg/mL
    B) < 50mg/mL
    C) < 25ng/dL
    D) < 75ng/dL
    E) < 50ng/dL

14. Regarding the physiology of androgen secretion, which of the following statements is false?

    A) Over-expression of Bcl-2 is associated with hormone refractory prostate cancer
    B) 5-AR type 1 converts testosterone to DHT
    C) The α and β sub-units of LH are encoded on different chromosomes
    D) Pasqualini syndrome is associated with high LH levels
    E) Leydig cells have a single nucleus

15. *Which of the following is not a sex cord stromal tumour?*
    A) Leydig cell tumour
    B) Sertoli cell tumour
    C) Adult granulosa cell tumour
    D) Sustentacular cell tumour
    E) Gonadoblastoma

16. *Which of the following regarding Leydig cell tumours is false?*
    A) There is no association with undescended testis
    B) 10% are bilateral at presentation
    C) Radiotherapy is ineffective in their treatment
    D) They cause gynaecomastia in adults
    E) Radical orchidectomy is the standard treatment

17. *Which of the following regarding half-life of tumour markers for testicular cancer is correct?*
    A) 36 hours for β-HCG and 5 days for α-FP
    B) 5 days for β-HCG and 36 hours for α-FP
    C) 12 hours for β-HCG and 3 days for α-FP
    D) 3 days for β-HCG and 12 hours for α-FP
    E) 24 hours for β-HCG and 12 hours for α-FP

18. *Elevation of LDH is recognised in all of the following conditions except:*
    A) Pancreatitis
    B) Haemolytic anaemia
    C) Haemangioblastoma
    D) Acute infectious mononucleosis
    E) Bone fracture

19. *What type of US probe transducer is best suited for performing testicular US?*
    A) 2–3kHz
    B) 3–4.5kHz
    C) 2–3MHz
    D) 3–4.5MHz
    E) 7–10MHz

20. A newly diagnosed patient with testicular cancer has tumour confined to the testis on radical orchidectomy specimen but with evidence of lympho-vascular invasion, CT showing single lymph-node metastasis of 3cm in greatest dimension and no distant metastasis. What is the correct staging for this patient?

   A) pT1N1M0
   B) pT2N2M0
   C) pT1N1M0
   D) pT2N2M0
   E) None of the above

21. Which of the following is not an indication to perform a contra-lateral testicular biopsy in a newly diagnosed patient with testicular cancer?

   A) Age < 40 years
   B) Testicular volume < 15mL
   C) History of undescended testis
   D) Johnsen score 1–3
   E) History of sub-fertility

22. Which of the following viruses are not screened prior to referring a patient for sperm banking?

   A) Hepatitis-B antibody
   B) CMV
   C) HIV-1
   D) HIV-2
   E) Hepatitis-C antibody

23. Which of the following statements regarding stage 1 NSGCT is correct?

   A) Induction chemotherapy is x1 cycle BEP
   B) Outside the retroperitoneum, the majority of micro-metastasis at presentation are in the liver
   C) Presence of vascular invasion on histology is associated with relapse risk of ≤ 28%
   D) 20% of recurrences occur after 12 months of treatment
   E) Embryonal component on histology is not an adverse factor

24. A 32-year-old male with seminoma in intermediate prognosis group has completed course of BEP chemotherapy. Post-treatment CT scan reveals residual 2cm residual volume retro-peritoneal disease. The most appropriate next step is:

    A) Continue surveillance
    B) Refer for PET scan
    C) Refer for RPLND
    D) Refer for biopsy of residual mass
    E) Give further chemotherapy

25. Regarding stage 1 seminoma, which of the following is false?

    A) Tumour size > 5cm is a risk factor
    B) Rete testis involvement is a risk factor
    C) Rete testis involvement alone has 16% risk of relapse
    D) No risk factors present has 12% risk of relapse
    E) None of the above

26. Regarding stage 1 seminoma, which of the following is true?

    A) For tumours confined to the testis, relapses after 5 years are very rare
    B) Adjuvant radiotherapy causes long-term bowel irritation in 20%
    C) Adjuvant radiotherapy is prescribed as 20Gy over 10 fractions
    D) Single-dose cisplatin is advised if risk factors present
    E) None of the above

27. Which of the following is false regarding ITGCN?

    A) Histology most commonly shows germ cells with enlarged hyperchromatic nuclei
    B) It is present up to 15% of the contra-lateral testes if all risk factors are present
    C) Cells are typically arranged along the basement membrane of the tubule
    D) Yolk-sac tumours do not arise from ITGCN
    E) Spermatocytic seminoma do not arise from ITGCN

28. Which of the following is not a risk factor for SCCa of the penis?

    A) HPV 18
    B) HIV
    C) UVA light
    D) UVB light
    E) Lymphoma

29. A 72-year-old male with type-2 diabetes and HIV presents to you with a painful blue papule on the penis. The most likely diagnosis is:

   A) Kaposi's sarcoma
   B) Primary syphilis
   C) Buschke–Lowenstein tumour
   D) Bowenoid papulosis
   E) Verrucous carcinoma

30. A newly diagnosed patient with penile cancer has histology showing sub-epithelial connective tissue invasion and Grade 2 SCCa, with CT showing metastasis in 5 unilateral inguinal nodes and lung metastasis. What is the correct staging?

   A) T1aN1M1a
   B) T1aN2M1a
   C) T1bN1M1a
   D) T1bN2M1a
   E) None of the above

31. A newly diagnosed patient with penile cancer has histology showing tumour invading both corpus spongiosum, 3 positive bilateral inguinal lymph nodes on radical lymphadenectomy specimen and no distant metastasis on CT. What is the correct staging?

   A) T1bN2M0
   B) T2pN3M0
   C) T2pN2M0
   D) T3pN2M0
   E) T3pN3M0

32. Which of the following imiquimod is false?

   A) A standard course is 4–6 weeks
   B) Asthenia is a common side-effect
   C) Patient should avoid having sexual intercourse during treatment
   D) Circumcision should be performed prior to offering treatment
   E) None of the above

33. Which of the following statements regarding the boundaries of the pelvic lymphadenectomy operation is false?

   A) Inferior margin is Cloquet's node
   B) Lateral margin is genito-femoral nerve
   C) Medial margin is bladder wall
   D) Superior margin is obturator nerve
   E) Proximal margin is iliac bifurcation

34. A newly diagnosed patient with penile cancer has histology showing invasion of sub-epithelial connective tissue with lympho-vascular invasion and Grade 1 SCC, there are no palpable lymph nodes and no enlarged nodes or distant metastasis on staging CT. What is the most appropriate next step?

   A) Offer surveillance
   B) Refer for US and FNA
   C) Refer for DSNB
   D) Refer for modified inguinal lymphadenectomy
   E) Refer for radical inguinal lymphadenectomy

35. Which factor in penile cancer histology does not increase the risk of lymph-node involvement?

   A) Sarcomatoid variant
   B) Helical growth pattern
   C) Urethral invasion
   D) Lympho-vascular invasion
   E) ≥ Grade 3 disease

STATION 3:
PAEDIATRIC UROLOGY MCQS

1. Which of the following statements regarding VUR is false?

    A) It is more common in Caucasian children compared to Afro-Caribbean
    B) It is more common in girls vs. boys
    C) The most common cause in females is duplication
    D) It tends to be diagnosed at a younger age in boys
    E) Grade 3 VUR is more common than Grade 1

2. At what gestational age does the urachus involute?

    A) 8 weeks
    B) 12 weeks
    C) 16 weeks
    D) 20 weeks
    E) 24 weeks

3. Regarding Wilms' tumour, on which chromosome is the WT1 gene found?

    A) 11
    B) 13
    C) 15
    D) 17
    E) 19

4. What is the most common enzyme abnormality in CAH?

    A) 21-hydroxylase deficiency
    B) 11β-hydroxylase deficiency
    C) 17α-hydroxylase deficiency
    D) 3 β-hydroysteroid deficiency
    E) 17β-hydroxylase deficiency

5. What is the most accurate incidence of horseshoe kidney?

    A) 1/200
    B) 1/400
    C) 1/600
    D) 1/800
    E) 1/1,000

6. A 2-year-old boy is successfully treated with oral antibiotics only for a klebsiella UTI and discharged. Which statement regarding his follow-up imaging is correct?

    A) He should have a US urinary tract within 4–6 weeks
    B) He should have an MCUG
    C) An US urinary tract at diagnosis is not required
    D) He should have a DMSA within 4–6 weeks
    E) None of the above

7. Which of the following is not a risk factor for developing hypospadias?

    A) Maternal use of iron supplements
    B) Paternal exposure to pesticides
    C) Increasing maternal age
    D) Oral contraceptive pill prior to pregnancy
    E) Excess intake of phytoestrogens

8. Orchidopexy to treat UDT delayed > 12 months has been associated with all of the following histological changes except?

    A) Delayed disappearance of gonocytes
    B) Reduced total numbers of germ cells per testicular tubule
    C) Reduced lipid quantity of Leydig cells
    D) Leydig cell hypoplasia
    E) Reduced number of adult dark (Ad) spermatogonia

9. Which of the following statements regarding ectopic ureter is false?

    A) In boys the ectopic orifice is rarely below the external sphincter
    B) Most common site of ectopic ureter drainage in boys is posterior urethra
    C) The upper moiety in a complete duplication tends to obstruct
    D) It is more common in girls
    E) It is less common than ureterocoele

10. A 6-year-old boy is referred to you as he passes urine every 15 minutes throughout the day, but generally sleeps through the night. He does not suffer with incontinence or any other LUTS. Which of the following is the most likely diagnosis?

    A) Ochoa syndrome
    B) Overactive bladder syndrome
    C) Hinman's syndrome
    D) Dysfunctional voiding
    E) Pollakiuria

11. *Which of the following statements regarding CAIS is false?*

    A) The Quigley scale uses 7 distinct classes to describe phenotypic grading
    B) The intra-abdominal gonads are testes
    C) Bone mineral density is typically higher than unaffected females
    D) Leydig cell testosterone is aromatised to oestrogen
    E) Mullerian ducts automatically develop in the absence of gonadal hormones

12. *Which of the following statements regarding horseshoe kidney is true?*

    A) The isthmus is typically anterior to L1–L2
    B) Horseshoe kidneys are more likely to develop upper-tract TCC
    C) The renal pelvis typically lies posteriorly
    D) The ascent of the kidney is typically inhibited by the superior mesenteric artery
    E) It is associated with Denys–Drash syndrome

13. *An MIBG scan is used to aid in the diagnosis of which paediatric tumour?*

    A) Rhabdomyosarcoma
    B) Neuroblastoma
    C) Nephroblastoma
    D) Germ cell tumour
    E) Hepatoblastoma

14. *A 6-week-old boy born at term is referred to you as the right testis was impalpable at the 6-week baby check by the GP. Indeed, your examination confirms these findings. What is the next most appropriate step?*

    A) EUA – if testis found in inguinal canal, proceed to laparoscopic right-sided orchidopexy
    B) EUA – if testis is found in scrotal sac, no further operating is required
    C) EUA – if no testis is palpable, proceed to laparoscopy and 2-stage Fowler–Stephens if viable testis found in the abdomen
    D) Refer for MRI
    E) No action is required at present

15. Which one of the following is not a criterion which defines an atypical UTI in children as per the NICE guidelines?

   A) Poor urine flow
   B) Raised creatinine
   C) Abdominal mass
   D) Raised white-cell count
   E) Klebsiella culture

16. Which of the following statements regarding ureterocoele is false?

   A) It may be associated with either moiety of a duplex kidney
   B) It is more common in girls
   C) Ectopic is more common than orthotopic ureterocoele
   D) Infected obstructed ureterocoele should be managed with urgent invasive surgical decompression
   E) Most ureterocoeles are associated with duplex kidneys rather than single system kidneys

17. Regarding the pharmacological therapy for MNE, which of the following statements is true?

   A) Desmopressin should not be prescribed via the sublingual route
   B) Fluid restriction along with desmopressin risks causing hyponatraemia
   C) Immediate release is more effective than modified release oxybutynin for MNE
   D) Oxybutynin is not licensed for children < 5 years of age
   E) Parents should be counselled that their child may lose weight with desmopressin

18. Which of the following statements regarding PUV in males is false?

   A) Vesicostomy is not known to decrease future bladder compliance and capacity
   B) Type 1 category of PUV is the most common
   C) 30% of paediatric ESRF can be attributed to PUV
   D) UDT is 10x more common in patients with PUV
   E) Thick-walled bladder on US is a better predictor of PUV compared to keyhole sign

19. *What is the correct estimated bladder capacity for a 6-year-old boy?*

    A) 120mL
    B) 160mL
    C) 180mL
    D) 210mL
    E) 230mL

20. *Which of the following statements regarding antibiotic prophylaxis in patients with VUR is false?*

    A) The RIVUR trial did not demonstrate any protective effect of antibiotic prophylaxis against paediatric hypertension
    B) The Swedish Reflux Study showed that antibiotic prophylaxis reduced rUTI in boys but did not protect against renal scarring
    C) Nitrofurantoin should not be used in children for prophylaxis if GFR < 45mL/minute
    D) Cefalexin is not licensed for the prophylaxis of rUTI in children
    E) The Swedish Reflux Study subjected its paediatric to invasive MCUG at start and end of trial

21. *Which of the following statements regarding UDT is true?*

    A) ≤ 90% of all UDT are palpable
    B) The Prentiss manoeuvre involves dividing the inferior epigastric vessels
    C) 1 in 2 retractile testes can later ascend and become effectively undescended
    D) 1 in 2 non-palpable testes are absent
    E) Success of hormonal therapy for UDT is not correlated to location of UDT

22. *Which of the following statements regarding the classification of VUR is false?*

    A) The ureters are not dilated in grade 1
    B) Refluxed urine reaches the renal pelvis in grade 2
    C) Grade 2 VUR is more common than grade 3
    D) The grading system does not apply to direct retrograde study via cystoscopy
    E) Grade 3 ureter is tortuous and deformed

23. *Which is the most common type of composition of stones found in children?*
    A) Calcium oxalate
    B) Uric acid
    C) Cystine
    D) Struvite
    E) Calcium phosphate

24. *Which of the following statements regarding paediatric hydrocoele is false?*
    A) Sclerosing agents use is limited due to risk of peritonitis
    B) Standard repairs (e.g. Lord's) should be used for secondary paediatric hydrocoeles
    C) Corrective surgery for a hydrocoele of the cord should excise the mass
    D) Patient ambulation does not affect non-communicating hydrocoeles
    E) The processus vaginalis persists in ≤ 30% of newborns

25. *Which of the following statements regarding prune belly syndrome is true?*
    A) Its eponymous name equivalent is Canavan's syndrome
    B) Pulmonary hypoplasia and oligohydramnios feature in category 3 of Woodard classification
    C) Single stage orchidopexy is rarely possible
    D) 1 in 3 will progress to ESRF requiring renal transplantation
    E) Malrotation is the most common gastro-intestinal associated abnormality

STATION 4:
EMERGENCY UROLOGY MCQS

1. *Which is the most appropriate choice of suture to repair the tunica albuginea of a ruptured testis due to traumatic injury?*

    A) 2'0 vicryl
    B) 4'0 vicryl
    C) 2'0 prolene
    D) 4'0 prolene
    E) 3'0 ethilon

2. *Which of the following is not a parameter that is part of the calculation of the SOFA score?*

    A) GCS
    B) Systolic blood pressure
    C) Platelet count
    D) Serum bilirubin concentration
    E) Serum creatinine concentration

3. *Which of the following histological changes occurs in untreated priapism?*

    A) Basement membrane exposure
    B) Green-stained collagen with picrosirius red
    C) Decrease in smooth muscle cells
    D) Increase in elastic system fibres
    E) All of the above

4. *By what process does a graft obtain nutrients from its host bed?*

    A) Diapedesis
    B) Active transport
    C) Inosculation
    D) Infiltration
    E) Imbibition

5. *What is the correct dose of adrenaline to be given as emergency treatment for anaphylaxis?*

    A) 0.5mL of 1:1,000 adrenaline (IM)
    B) 0.5mL of 1:10,000 adrenaline (IM)
    C) 1mL of 1:100 adrenaline (IM)
    D) 1mL of 1:1,000 adrenaline (IM)
    E) 1mL of 1:10,000 adrenaline (IM)

6. Which of the following is not an accepted indication to perform an emergency CT scan in the context of renal trauma?

    A) Concomitant fracture of the lower ribs
    B) History of rapid deceleration
    C) Non-visible haematuria with haemodynamic instability
    D) Visible haematuria with haemodynamic stability
    E) Systolic BP < 100mmHg

7. What is the most likely profile of biochemical abnormalities seen in TUR syndrome?

    A) Hyperkalaemia, hyponatraemia, hyperammonaemia
    B) Hypokalaemia, hyponatraemia, hyperammonaemia
    C) Hyperkalaemia, hyponatraemia, hypoammonaemia
    D) Hypokalaemia, hyponatraemia, hypoammonaemia
    E) None of the above

8. Which of the following is not a set parameter in the SIRS criteria scoring?

    A) Temperature < 36°C
    B) PaCO2 < 4.3KPa
    C) WCC > 14 x 109/L
    D) Heart rate > 90 beats/minute
    E) Presence > 10% immature neutrophils

9. Which of the following is false regarding the blood–testis barrier?

    A) Formed by punctate tight junctions between Sertoli cells
    B) Located on the luminal side of the basally positioned spermatogonia
    C) The formation of the barrier does not coincide with increasing numbers of spermatocytes
    D) The barrier is stabilised by espin proteins
    E) DHT induces the formation of the barrier; however, FSH alone does not

10. The correct equation for calculating the corrected calcium value is:

    A) (Measured total Ca2+) – 0.02(40 – serum albumin)
    B) (Measured total Ca2+) – 0.02(serum albumin – 40)
    C) (Measured total Ca2+) + 0.02(40 – serum albumin)
    D) (Measured total Ca2+) + 0.02(serum albumin – 40)
    E) (Measured total Ca2+) x 0.02(serum albumin – 40)

11. *Which of the following statements regarding penile fracture in male patient is true?*

    A) Right-sided corporal injuries are more common than left
    B) The most common site of injury to tunica albuginea is on the dorsal aspect of penis
    C) The sexual position with highest risk of penile fracture is male patient missionary on top
    D) USS may show hyper-echoic discontinuity in the normally echogenic tunica albuginea
    E) Bilateral corporal injuries do not increase the risk of urethral injury

12. *The correct dosage of intra-cavernosal phenylephrine to treat priapism is:*

    A) 100µg every 5–10 minutes, to a maximum of 0.5mg in 1 hour
    B) 250µg every 5–10 minutes, to a maximum of 2mg in 1 hour
    C) 100mg every 5–10 minutes, to a maximum of 0.5g in 1 hour
    D) 250mg every 5–10 minutes, to a maximum of 2g in 1 hour
    E) None of the above

13. *All of the following are recognised causes of priapism, except:*

    A) Buproprion
    B) Olanzapine
    C) Total parenteral nutrition
    D) Peritoneal dialysis
    E) Use of unfractionated heparin

14. *An 8-year-old boy has a clear history of acute testicular torsion for 5 hours, and you wish to proceed to scrotal exploration. Only his father is present. He has never been married to the boy's mother and is not on the birth certificate of his son. The mother is abroad for work and cannot be contacted anytime soon. His father refuses consent. What is the most appropriate course of action?*

    A) Proceed to operate – the father has no parental rights for consent
    B) Proceed to operate – evaluate whether boy is Gillick competent to consent
    C) Proceed to operate – via double signature consent from consultant colleague
    D) You cannot operate – respect the father's wishes
    E) You cannot operate – apply for emergency decision by the courts

15. *Regarding surgical intervention for ureteric injuries, which of the following is true?*

   A) In the unstable trauma patient with on-table incidental finding of ureteric transection, the affected ureter should not be ligated
   B) Psoas hitch procedure may injure the genito-femoral nerve, as this lies on the psoas muscle
   C) Psoas hitch procedure can be aided by division of the inferior vesical pedicle
   D) Prophylactic ureteric stenting prior to complex pelvic surgery reduces rates of ureteric injury
   E) AAST Grade 3 ureteric injuries cannot be managed by stenting alone

16. *Which of the following statements regarding testicular torsion is true?*

   A) Intra-vaginal torsion is most commonly seen in the first year of life
   B) Relief of pain by elevating the testis suggests the cause is epididymitis (negative Prehn's sign)
   C) The bell-clapper abnormality is a malformation of the processus vaginalis
   D) The absent cremasteric reflex is determined by the ilioinguinal nerve as afferent supply, and pudendal nerve as efferent
   E) Doppler US is the most accurate imaging technique, when clinically indicated

17. *Which of the following statements regarding shunt treatments for priapism is false?*

   A) Quackels procedure involves creating a shunt between corpora cavernosa and spongiosum at the level of the bulbar urethra
   B) Sacher approach involves a penoscrotal incision
   C) Greyhack procedure uses the saphenous vein anastomosed to the tunica albuginea
   D) Barry procedure uses the superficial vein of the penis anastomosed to the tunica albuginea
   E) Al-Ghorab procedure uses a dorsal sub-coronal incision

18. *The most appropriate initial hormone therapy for a patient newly presenting with lower-limb weakness, lower-back pain and a PSA of 3,500, is:*

   A) Goserelin 3.6mg stat then 3.6mg every 28 days
   B) Goserelin 10.8mg stat then 10.8mg every 12 weeks
   C) Degarelix 60mg stat then 20mg every 28 days
   D) Degarelix 120mg stat then 40mg every 28 days
   E) Degarelix 240mg stat then 80mg every 28 days

19. *Which of the following statements regarding Page phenomenon is false?*

   A) Results from external compression of the kidney
   B) Hypertension is caused by activation of the renin-angiotensinaldosterone system
   C) Decapsulation of fibro-collagenous shell can treat refractory hypertension
   D) There is a clear association between renal biopsies and Page kidney
   E) They do not occur in transplanted kidneys

20. *Which of the following statements regarding pharmacological treatment of priapism is false?*

   A) Phenylephrine is an option as an α-1 adrenergic receptor agonist
   B) Bicalutamide is an option as a competitive androgen inhibitor
   C) Terbutaline is an option as a β2-antagonist
   D) Metaraminol is an option as an α-1 adrenergic receptor agonist
   E) None of the above

ANSWERS TO ADDITIONAL MCQS

STATION 1: UROLOGICAL ONCOLOGY 1

1. B – BSP (bone sialoprotein) has not been used for urothelial cancer detection

2. A – healthy bladder is blue/purple, note also the trigone may appear abnormal as it is a common site of low-grade inflammation

3. B

4. A

5. D – ipsilateral adrenal gland is T4, contra-lateral adrenal gland is M1

6. C – the CARMENA trial evaluated sunitinib (A, D and E would all be correct if sunitinib were in the option), and note the primary end-point was OS

7. C

8. D

9. E – time from diagnosis to treatment < 12 months

10. A – tumour thrombus below hepatic veins but > 2cm above renal vein orifice is level 2, most likely histology is RCC

11. E

12. B

13. C

14. D – Wallace 1 involves suturing the medial walls of spatulated ureters together, and anastomosing this conjoined segment to the proximal end of the open bowel segment

15. A

16. D – typical dose is 60–66Gy in 30–32 fractions over 6 weeks

17. D – patients with any metastasis were excluded, performance status included 0–1 only

18. B – only 20% are due to tuberous sclerosis

19. E

20. C – essential fact for the viva station (not many study percentages of trial studies need memorising but it's fair to say this is one that does)

21. A

22. C – prognosis is poor and 5-year survival is < 50%

23. C

24. B – attaches to the fibronectin receptor

25. B – severe hypokalaemia may occur (also remember that cobalamin = vitamin B12)

STATION 2: UROLOGICAL ONCOLOGY 2

1. C – cardiovascular disease is a caution, not contraindication

2. A – you must know TNM staging inside out for all the cancers, it is a guarantee that you will be asked a question on this in the MCQ and/or viva

3. D

4. D

5. E – > 95% of prostate cancers are adenocarcinomas and the absent staining is for p63 (p53 is a tumour-suppressing gene)

6. C

7. B

8. B – recall the 4 "R"s of radiobiology

9. A

10. B

11. A

12. C – note that it is percentage of cores with "clinically significant" prostate cancer

13. E

14. D

15. D

16. B – 3% are bilateral at presentation

17. A

18. C

19. E

20. E – note that TNM for testicular cancer has an N-stage for both clinical lymph nodes and lymph nodes on pathology (i.e. after RPLND), in this case the nodes were evaluated on CT alone

21. B

22. B

23. D – induction chemotherapy is x3 BEP (upfront is x1), majority of micrometastasis outside the retroperitoneum are in the lung, relapse risk with vascular invasion is much higher at 48%

24. A – PET is advised if residual volume > 2cm

25. A – note it is tumour size > 4cm

26. C

27. B – if risk factors are all present, ITGCN is present in 1/3 contra-lateral testis

28. E – lymphoma can present on the penis as primary penile lymphoma; however, it is not otherwise a known risk factor for SCC of the penis

29. A

30. E – careful as TNM classification for penile cancer only has M0/1 as M-stage

31. C

32. C – sexual intercourse is permitted provided patient uses condom

33. D

34. A – the patient falls within the low-risk category

35. B

STATION 3: PAEDIATRIC UROLOGY

1. C – most common cause in females is ureterocoele

2. B

3. A

4. A

5. B

6. E – note that follow up DMSA is after 4–6 months

7. D – the contraceptive pill taken after conception has been shown to increase risk of hypospadias

8. C

9. A – in boys the ectopic orifice is never below the external sphincter

10. E – note that dysfunctional voiding is also known as Hinman's syndrome

11. C

12. B – horseshoe kidney has higher risk of Wilms' tumour and upper-tract TCC; however, not of RCC or other renal tumours

13. B

14. E – you should allow at least 3 months for the testis to drop into the scrotal sac spontaneously

15. D

16. A – if in a duplex system, a ureterocoele is always associated with the upper moiety

17. D – note that hyponatraemia is a common side-effect if the child is not fluid restricted along with the medication, counselling should also include weight gain

18. C – PUV is relatively rare, and so although 20–50% of PUV patients may progress to ESRF, actually the overall proportion of paediatric ESRF caused by PUV alone is much lower at 17%

19. D

20. B – the Swedish Reflux Study showed that antibiotic prophylaxis made no difference to boys in UTI rates and renal scarring; note that cefalexin can be used for prophylaxis – however, as per the BNF it is not licensed for this use

21. B – 80% of UDT are palpable, only 1 in 3 retractile testes will become undescended, only 1 in 5 impalpable testes are absent

22. A

23. A

24. E – the processus vaginalis persists in ≤ 90% of newborns

25. E

STATION 4: EMERGENCY UROLOGY

1. D – requires a fine absorbable suture

2. B – cardiovascular element is mean arterial pressure (MAP) = (2(diastolic BP) + (systolic BP)) / 3

3. E

4. E

5. A

6. E – a systolic blood pressure of < 90mmHg at any time after injury warrants emergency CT scan

7. A

8. C

9. C

10. C

11. A

12. E – the maximum dose in 1 hour is 1mg

13. D

14. A – if a father has never been married to the mother, and is not on the birth certificate, he has no automatic legal rights to the child; therefore, proceed on best interests due to time-sensitive nature of underlying pathology

15. B – note that it is the division of the superior vesical pedicle which is performed in psoas hitch

16. C

17. D

18. E

19. E – lymphocoele around a transplanted kidney can cause Page phenomenon

20. C – terbutaline is a β2-agonist

www.ingramcontent.com/pod-product-compliance
Lightning Source LLC
Chambersburg PA
CBHW040752220326
41597CB00029BA/4727